Congenital Anomalies: A Growing Concern

Congenital Anomalies: A Growing Concern

Edited by Marlon Whittaker

hayle medical
New York

Hayle Medical,
750 Third Avenue, 9th Floor,
New York, NY 10017, USA

Visit us on the World Wide Web at:
www.haylemedical.com

ISBN: 978-1-63241-885-2

Cataloging-in-Publication Data

Congenital anomalies : a growing concern / edited by Marlon Whittaker.
p. cm.
Includes bibliographical references and index.
ISBN 978-1-63241-885-2
1. Abnormalities, Human. 2. Growth disorders. 3. Newborn infants--Diseases. I. Whittaker, Marlon.
RG626 .C66 2020
618.32--dc23

Table of Contents

Preface

Congenital anomalies are birth defects that hamper the physical, intellectual and developmental health of individuals. These are divided into two chief types- structural disorders and functional disorders. In structural disorders, there are problems with the shape of a body part. In functional disorders, problems occur with the functioning of a body part. Functional disorders can be metabolic and degenerative. Some of the risk factors contributing to congenital anomalies include alcohol consumption, smoking, folate deficiency, poorly controlled diabetes, etc. Birth defects can be diagnosed by screening tests or may be visible at birth. The treatment of each anomaly is unique and depends on the defect. It may involve medication, surgery, therapy or assistive technology. This book presents researches and studies performed by experts across the globe on congenital anomalies. It strives to provide a fair idea about this condition and to help develop a better understanding of the latest advances in its assessment and treatment. For all readers who are interested in congenital anomalies, the case studies included in this book will serve as an excellent guide to develop a comprehensive understanding.

This book is a result of research of several months to collate the most relevant data in the field.

When I was approached with the idea of this book and the proposal to edit it, I was overwhelmed. It gave me an opportunity to reach out to all those who share a common interest with me in this field. I had 3 main parameters for editing this text:

1. Accuracy – The data and information provided in this book should be up-to-date and valuable to the readers.

2. Structure – The data must be presented in a structured format for easy understanding and better grasping of the readers.

3. Universal Approach – This book not only targets students but also experts and innovators in the field, thus my aim was to present topics which are of use to all.

Thus, it took me a couple of months to finish the editing of this book.

I would like to make a special mention of my publisher who considered me worthy of this opportunity and also supported me throughout the editing process. I would also like to thank the editing team at the back-end who extended their help whenever required.

Editor

1

Congenital Heart Disease: Genetic Aspect and Prenatal and Postnatal Counseling

Amal Zubani, Irfan Asra and Amjad Kouatli

Abstract

Cardiac malformation present at birth is an important component of pediatric cardiovascular disease. The etiology of congenital heart disease is multifaceted including environmental, genetic and stochastic factors. With the advancement of cardiac diagnostic and therapeutic techniques in the past decade, with relatively low morbidity and mortality, has led to more and more children with congenital heart disease living to adulthood. Therefore the role of prenatal and postnatal genetic counseling becomes even more paramount as there is a higher likelihood of these patients living to adulthood and having families of their own. Prenatal counseling allows for the expectant parents to understand the full ramifications of continuing the pregnancy and possible events after birth. It is a multidisciplinary approach to help parents reach an informed decision on how to best to proceed with the pregnancy. After the birth of the child with congenital heart defects, the course is significantly dependent on the type of cardiac lesion. Postnatally, if the lesion is amenable to surgery, therapeutics intervention is offered. The postnatal counseling session includes the possibility of performing advanced genetic testing to help determine the hereditary potential of the cardiac defect in future offspring.

Keywords: congenital heart disease, genetic syndromes, recurrence, counseling, genetic testing

1. Introduction

Congenital heart diseases (CHD) are the most common major fetal structural defects and leading cause of neonatal morbidity and mortality among birth defects. The medical and surgical management of these children has continued to progress rapidly such that, most of these patients now survive to adulthood. The estimated incidence of moderate and severe forms of CHD is 6 per 1000 live births [1]. However, fetuses with heart disease show unique diagnostic, therapeutic and sometimes ethical challenges. Treatment of the fetuses with CHD may expose the mother to significant risks, which may compete with the welfare of the mother [2, 3].

Advances in the field of prenatal imaging, and increasing experience in fetal cardiology and echocardiography over the last two decades has allowed for most heart defects to be well defined as early as the second trimester [4]. Pediatric cardiologists specializing in fetal medicine, play a critical role in help making an accurate diagnosis. In addition, these specialized physicians will be critical in providing prenatal counseling to help guide parents to understand the diagnosis and in the decision-making process. This counseling will give parents information about the fetus' heart defect and its expected outcomes. Fetal echocardiography has evolved since its inception, which now can provide precise details of cardiac structural and hemodynamic aberration in fetuses with CHD. During pregnancy, the sequential use of this modality can predict the evolution of disease in utero and transition to postnatal life. Such an approach allows for detailed prenatal counseling and detection of fetuses at high risk for morbidity and mortality. This allows for appropriate planning and postnatal management [5, 6]. Most CHD is well tolerated in utero, and does not present hemodynamic risks immediately. After birth, many of these babies, with simple cardiac lesion do not require specialized delivery care. However, some high-risk fetuses may develop hemodynamic instability soon after birth and may require immediate intervention [5]. With such infants it is highly recommended that these children be born at centers where a pediatric cardiac team and intensive care personnel are available to make appropriate therapeutics decisions and intervention, without delay.

Is the availability of a perinatal diagnosis of CHD is associated with improved surgical outcomes and less neonatal mortality? Some studies report a positive impact on outcomes while others showing no difference in outcomes compared to babies diagnosed with CHD after birth [7–19]. A recent meta-analysis evaluating the differences in pre-operative mortality rates between newborns with and without a prenatal diagnosis found that prenatal diagnosis of critical CHD improves neonatal pre-operative survival, and newborns with a postnatal diagnosis were more likely to die of cardiovascular compromise prior to planned cardiac surgery [20].

The etiology of CHD is multifaceted including environmental, genetic, and stochastic factors [21, 22]. Knowing the basis of the CHD will aid in the counseling of parents and help them to attain a complete understanding of the fetuses cardiac defect [23]. Although it will not change the course or management option, but it will allow for familial planning and future pregnancies.

2. Genetic syndromes

Genetic syndromes are defined as a consistent pattern of malformation caused by a genetic alteration. A malformation syndrome consists of multiple structural defects that are thought to be due to a single cause, even if the suspected cause has not yet been identified [24].

2.1. Noonan's syndrome

The Noonan phenotype includes characteristic facies (ptosis, hypertelorism, low set ears, and low posterior hairline), short stature, webbed neck and cardiac anomalies. Noonan syndrome occurs in I per 1000 to 1 per 2500 live births diagnosed clinically [25–27]. Cardiac anomalies are present in 80% of individuals [28]. In 70–80% of cases, the lesion is pulmonary stenosis, usually due to dysplastic pulmonary valve leaflets [25]. In 20–30% of affected individuals, the cardiac anomaly is in the form of a cardiomyopathy, which may be present at birth or develop later [25, 29].

Most of the cases of Noonan syndrome are sporadic, although families with a pattern of autosomal dominant inheritance are well known. Mutation in the gene PTPN11 on the chromosome locus 12q24.1 was noted in 45% of cases. Gelb et al. demonstrated a positive association between those with PTPN11 mutations and pulmonary stenosis [30]. Maternal transmission of the gene is three times more common than paternal transmission [28]. Prenatal testing can be established by chorionic villus sampling or amniocentesis, fetal ultrasound can show increased nuchal translucency, increased nuchal thickening, pleural effusions and generalized hydrops [31]. Developmental delays are always present, and intellectual disability is typically in the range of moderate mental retardation [28, 29]. Diagnosis in newborn baby may be difficult unless the cardiac lesion is severe, with either significant pulmonary stenosis or severe cardiomyopathy. The diagnosis can only be confirmed genetically if there is an affected parent with a recognized mutation [25, 27, 30].

2.2. Turner's syndrome

The classical Turner's syndrome phenotype includes short stature, webbed neck, renal anomalies, congenital lymphedema, ovarian dysgenesis and cardiac anomalies. In many, the features are sufficiently subtle to be overlooked until the teenage years. The prevalence of Turner's syndrome is 1 in 2500 female births [32]. The phenotype depends on whether the X chromosome is absent (45, X in almost 50% of patient) or structurally abnormal [33].

The most common presentation is spontaneous abortion with hydrops or lymphatic malformation in the neck or mediastinum. Cardiac anomalies are present in 30% of patients with Tuner Syndrome, bicuspid aortic valve (30%), coarctation of the aorta (10%) and hypoplastic left heart syndrome (HLHS); partial anomalous pulmonary venous connection is also associated with this syndrome. Aortic root dilatation is present in 5–10% of cases, associated with aortic root dissection in later life, this finding is mostly related to decreased numbers of smooth muscle and elastic fibers in the vascular walls [32]. Gotzsche et al. demonstrated a correlation between the precise karyotype and the form of congenital heart disease; 38% of patients with X0 had aortic valve anomalies and coarctation of the aorta, compared with 11% of individuals with mosaic X0 [34].

Fetuses with Turner's syndrome have been shown to have small hearts in 90% of the cases. Significant myocardial hypoplasia is thought to be associated with the high incidence of fetal death [32]. Neonatal diagnosis may be difficult but should be considered in females presenting with left-sided heart anomalies or lymphedema.

2.3. William's syndrome

The phenotype of Williams' syndrome is variable, but includes characteristic facies (flared eyebrows, bright stellate irides and wide mouth), specific personality and cognitive features, and infantile hypercalcaemia in addition to cardiac anomalies. The prevalence is 1 in 10,000–20,000. Children with Williams's syndrome can be diagnosed at different ages and present with a broad range of clinical features [35]. Early in life, feeding disorders and growth retardation are common. Hypercalcemia is seen in 15% of infants and usually resolves over time [36]. Cardiac anomalies are present in 55–80% of individuals with William's syndrome, which typically include supravalvar aortic stenosis and/or supravalvar pulmonary stenosis [37, 38]. The degree of the cardiovascular involvement and the relative involvement of the pulmonic or aortic vessels varies widely. By 1 year of age 41% of the pulmonary lesions will have improved, whereas 73% of the aortic lesions will have progressed [38].

Approximately 90% of patients with the clinical diagnosis of Williams's syndrome have a deletion at chromosome 7q11.23, which can be detected by fluorescence in situ hybridization (FISH), multiplex ligation- dependent probe amplification (MLPA) and microarray technologies. The gene mapping to this region has been defined and includes the gene ELN, whose product is elastin. The deletion of this gene results in the connective tissue abnormalities associated with the CHD of Williams' individuals [39, 40]. Prenatal genetic testing can be performed on Chorionic villus sampling or amniotic fluid samples in the few pregnancies considered to be at increased risk. Neonatal diagnosis is challenging, and full features become more apparent with time. William's syndrome is transmitted in an autosomal dominant manner. Most cases are de novo occurrence and recurrence risks are 50% if a parent is affected but otherwise low (<5%) [41, 42].

2.4. 22q11 deletion syndrome (DiGeorge syndrome, velocardiofacial syndrome, conotruncal anomaly face syndrome)

Molecular studies demonstrate that the vast majority of patients with clinical diagnosis of DiGeorge, velocardiofacial, conotruncal anomaly face syndromes share a common genetic cause, namely a 22q11.2 deletion [43–45]. The prevalence is 1 in 4000 to 6000 live births, but the severity of the phenotype is variable and in some the features may go unrecognized [46]. CHD are estimated to occur in 75–80% of patients with a 22q11.2 deletion. The most common CHDs associated with 22q11.2 deletion include tetralogy of Fallot (TOF) and aortic arch anomalies. Other conotruncal lesions include pulmonary atresia with ventricular septal defect (VSD), and truncus arteriosus [47, 48]. In cases of truncus arteriosus, the truncal valve tends to be more dysplastic when the 22q11 deletion is present [49].

Identifying the cardiac patient with a 22q11.2 deletion early in life can provide substantial benefits to the child and family. Currently, it is recommended that infant with interrupted aortic arch type B, truncus arteriosus, TOF and isolated aortic arch anomalies undergo testing for a 22q11.2 deletion [22]. Prenatal diagnosis can be performed using FISH technology on samples obtained from chorionic villus sampling or amniocentesis if cardiac defects are present. Non-cardiac lesions are not easily diagnosed but, absent fetal thymus has been reported [50]. Many children initially present without cardiac symptoms in the form of recurrent infections. This may point to an underlying immunodeficiency associated with 22q11.2 deletion [51]. The risk of recurrence is in 50% as this is transmitted in an autosomal dominant inheritance if either parent carries the deletion. If neither parent carries the deletion, there may still be germline mosaicism, but the risk of recurrence is small (1%) [22, 48].

2.5. CHARGE syndrome

The CHARGE syndrome was previously referred as an association, however this was resolved after the discovery of causative mutations in chromodomain helicase DNA-binding gene7 (CHD7) on chromosome 8q12.1 [52, 53]. The phenotype is described by its acronym:

colobomata (79%), heart defects (85%), choanal atresia (57%), growth and developmental retardation (100%), Genital hypoplasia (34%) and Ear anomalies (91%). Additional problems include renal anomalies, facial clefts and esophageal atresia [54]. CHD has been always been part of the core phenotype.

The frequency of the CHD range from 74–92% in CHD7 mutation-positive cases [55, 56], as compared to 71% in CHD7 mutation- negative individuals in one report [55]. A wide range of CHD has been reported in CHARGE syndrome, including conotruncal and aortic arch anomalies consistently over represented in clinical series [56]. The frequency of the CHARGE syndrome has been reported to range from 1 per 10,000 to 1 per 15,000 live births, although one population-based study estimated a frequency of 1 in 8500 live births [57]. Most of the cases of CHARGE syndrome are sporadic in occurrence, but autosomal dominant inheritance and germline mosaicism, have now been confirmed by molecular testing [55].

2.6. VACTERL association

The phenotype is described by its acronym: Vertebral defects, Anorectal anomalies, Cardiac anomalies, Tracheoesophageal fistula with Esophageal atresia, and Renal and upper Limb anomalies. A general diagnostic guideline requires three or more defects to establish the diagnosis [58]. It is usually a sporadic occurrence of unknown cause. In rare cases an association can occur in trisomy 18 [59], or trisomy 21 [60]. A cardiac anomaly is present in at least 73% of affected individuals and includes atrial septal defect (ASD), VSD, double-outlet right ventricle, TOF and dextrocardia [58].

No definitive prenatal testing is available, but the diagnosis should be considered if antenatal ultrasound demonstrates a vertebral anomaly, absence of the fetal stomach and a cardiac anomaly with or without polyhydramnios. The management involves a multidisciplinary approach [61]. VACTERL has a low recurrence risk of 2–3%, although there are rare reports of familial cases, including one of a mother and son, both with typical features [62].

2.7. Alagille syndrome

Alagille syndrome was originally defined as the presence of bile duct paucity on liver biopsy in conjunction with three of the following five findings: cholestasis, congenital heart disease, skeletal or ocular abnormalities or typical facial features which give the face an inverted triangle appearance (broad forehead, deep set eyes, rounded tip and pear like shape of the nose and pointed chin) [63, 64]. Alagille syndrome is an autosomal dominant condition with high penetrance (94%) and variable expressivity, which is the result of mutations or deletions in the JAG-1 gene (locus 20p11.2). De novo mutations occur in 50–60% of cases [65, 66]. Alagille syndrome is now recognized to be a genetically heterogeneous disorder. Approximately 5% of the patients with a chromosomal deletion involving one copy of the entire JAG1 gene, whereas most will have various intragenic JAG1 mutations [67].

The prevalence is 1 in 70,000 to 100,000 live births [68]. Cardiovascular anomalies are present 90% of the cases [68]. The most common cardiac lesion is pulmonary artery branch stenosis (PABS), tetralogy of Fallot (in up to 10% of cases), pulmonary stenosis and coarctation of the aorta [69]. If the mutation or deletion is identified in a parent, prenatal diagnosis is available on samples from chorionic villus sampling or amniocentesis. It is, however, not possible to predict the severity of the phenotype in an identified fetus [69]. The diagnosis needs to be considered in a baby with a cardiac defect and prolonged jaundice, and with at least three of the recognized features [61]. Alagille syndrome has a mortality rate around 10–20%. The risk of recurrence is low in the absence of a positive family history, but it is 50% if there is an affected parent [61, 68].

2.8. Holt-Oram syndrome

The phenotype is characterized by the bilateral, asymmetrical upper limb anomalies of variable severity and is estimated to occur in 1 per 100,000 live births. There is a variation in the severity of the phenotype even within a family, and in some the upper limb anomalies may be so mild that X-ray can only diagnose them. A thumb anomaly is usually present [70]. Approximately 75% of the patients diagnosed with Holt-Oram syndrome have CHD. Atrial septal defects (secundum type) are present in 58% of these patients, in addition 28% have VSD. Up to 40% have conduction defects including a long PR interval, sinus bradycardia, atrial fibrillation and complete heart block [71]. Other types of congenital heart diseases in the form of total anomalous pulmonary venous drainage, TOF and truncus arteriosus have been associated with this syndrome [72]. There appears to be a correlation between the severity of the upper limb anomaly and the cardiac lesion [73].

Holt-Oram syndrome is an autosomal dominant condition with 100% penetrance and variable expression. New mutations make up 30–40% of the inheritance pattern. The affected gene is TBX5 on chromosome locus 12q24 [74]. The diagnosis should be considered prenatally when a cardiac lesion occurs in the presence of an upper limb anomaly. The risk to the offspring of an affected individual is 50% [61].

2.9. Trisomy 21 (Down's syndrome)

The most familiar syndrome to cardiologists is Down's syndrome is trisomy 21 in which there is a complete extra copy of chromosome 21 in 94% of cases. Less commonly, partial trisomy of chromosome 21(6% overall), is present owing to a chromosomal translocation or mosaicism. Common findings include: hypotonia, global developmental delays and moderate intellectual disability, microbrachycephaly, small ears, mouth and nose, protruding tongue, up-slanting eyes with epicanthal folds, transverse palmar creases, and sparse hair. Skeletal anomalies include fifth finger clinodactyly, brachydactyly, a gap between first and second toes, atlantoaxial instability, hypoplastic pelvis, and joint laxity. Additional problems involve the visual, auditory, endocrine, hematologic, reproductive, and gastrointestinal systems. Almost half of live born Down's syndrome individuals have a CHD, approximately 40% of whom have a complete atrioventricular septal defect (also known as atrioventricular canal defect or endocardial cushion defect) [75]. The association of Down syndrome and atrioventricular septal defects is underscored by the fact that approximately 75% of patients with a complete atrioventricular septal defect have Down syndrome. Other common CHDs include secundum atrial septal defect, conoventricular and muscular ventricular septal defect, tetralogy of Fallot (with and without atrioventricular septal defect), and hemodynamically significant patent ductus arteriosus [75]. The overall prevalence of Down syndrome is 1 in 700 live births [76].

The risk of conceiving a child with aneuploidy (an extra chromosome), including Down's syndrome increases with maternal age. Overall survival has improved, although prenatally diagnosed CHDs and/or growth retardation may predict a poorer outcome [77]. The largest survey study to date reported that the frequency of CHDs in patients with Down syndrome mosaicism was similar to the complete trisomy 21 comparison group (~42 and 50%) [78]. Prenatal screening programs providing risk figures for Down's syndrome in individual pregnancies are widely available. Definitive testing involves an invasive procedure, either chorionic villus sampling or amniocentesis, and a rapid result can be obtained by FISH. The diagnosis is suspected clinically and confirmed by karyotyping. The risk of recurrence is about 1% for women aged 39 or less [61].

2.10. Trisomy 18 (Edward's syndrome)

It is a rare syndrome with a prevalence of 1 in 6000, and a male to female ratio of 1:4. Majority of this syndrome is caused by maternal meiotic non-disjunction. Greater than 90% of cases have trisomy 18, the remainder having trisomy 18-mosaicism or partial trisomy of 18q. All cases have cardiac anomalies: mal-aligned VSD is the most common finding; ASD and patent ductus arteriosus are also common findings in these patients. Polyvalvular dysplasia, usually without stenosis or regurgitation, is usually present [79, 80]. Karyotyping is indicated if prenatal screening detected structural anomalies on ultrasound. The risk of recurrence is low, at around 1 in 200 [61].

3. Counseling

3.1. Prenatal

The process of prenatal counseling and its recommendations, should be based on the best available current evidenced-based practice. This process may require more than one consultation due to its emotional nature of the situation and complexity of information being delivered. Any prenatal counseling should include the suspected cardiac diagnosis in detail based on the fetal ultrasound findings. The purpose of this is to give the most accurate and up to date information about the prognosis and outcome of the pregnancy and fetus. This will allow the parents to make the best-informed decision for them and the fetus.

In regards to the screening ultrasound, all relevant information available needs to be given prior to the examination. Ideally, all prescreening information should be made available to the referring hospital. It needs to be emphasized that not all cardiac defects can be detected in the initial ultrasound examination [81, 82]. Whenever a cardiac abnormalities is detected this will require prompt referral for specialist examination. The general screening detection rates for congenital heart disease (CHD) vary between 14–45% [83]. A standard 4-chamber view can detect 40–50% of major CHD [84], while a 4-chamber view and outflow tract detects 70–80% of major CHD [85]. In dedicated fetal cardiac centers the diagnostic accuracy is close to 100% [86, 87]. Thereafter a referral for specialized echocardiography and cardiology consultation should be done. If there are suspected cardiac abnormalities on the screening fetal ultrasound, there should be minimal time delay in referring the mother for a fetal echocardiogram and cardiology consultation. Delays in referral for further evaluation increase parental stress [88], and may prohibit the option of early termination of pregnancy. At the referral center, before the scan, the physician should make sure that the parents have consented to the examination and understand why they have been referred. A detailed review of past maternal history, including health wellbeing, previous pregnancies outcomes and similar conditions in the family need to be determined. In addition, any previous genetic screening has been performed or suspected in the family.

Ideally, the parents should be counseled by a pediatric cardiologist specialized in fetal cardiology, once the fetal echocardiogram is complete. The counselor needs to have full knowledge of the anatomy, physiology, gestational age, and association with extra-cardiac malformations and its natural history. In addition, the discussion should include the short and long-term management and possible outcomes. If possible a multidisciplinary meeting with the parents should be conducted. This conversation should include the most accurate information and include prenatal and postnatal management. Ideally this discussion should include fetal cardiologist, obstetrician, neonatologist, geneticist, pediatric cardiac surgeon and a psychologist or social worker. In addition to the physicians, a fetal nurse coordinator or midwife should be involved from the first counseling visit to delivery of the baby or termination of the pregnancy. This is to provide continuous support and ongoing resources for follow up with the family [89]. There is little research on performing prenatal counseling for CHD or determining the most effective strategies for providing family support. Therefore, it is important that counselors have good communication skills, show empathy, and be perceptive in assessing how the information is being received. The counselor must assess parental understanding and emotional status throughout the discussion.

A structured explanation focused on assessing the parents understanding is very important at this stage. Highlights of the counseling of session needs to repeated and the expected parent should be made to verbalize understanding in their own words. This may need to be repeated to ensure complete understanding of the situation and implication for treatment and intervention. Throughout this process, the counselor needs to assess and give feedback to the treating team on how the information is being received. Particularly at the first visit, the initial shock and grief reactions to an abnormal finding may inhibit the parents' ability to retain information. Therefore, it maybe necessary to repeat information on subsequent encounters and assess understanding. A common issue that complicates counseling in today technological age, is the access and availability of the vast amount of information on the Internet. At time such recourses can be beneficial, but more often than not, this information is misleading, biased and inappropriate for the precise circumstances. Unfortunately, none of this information is subject to review and can be a source of major confusion for the parent [90].

Complications of the cardiac abnormality and its progression in utero, and the results of surgery or any intervention also figure in to the discussion. There is a need to describe possible poor outcomes, so that they have been informed of all possible scenarios, even though unlikely to happen. This information allows the parents to decide how best to proceed with knowledge of the worst-case scenario [91]. One of the most important points which needs to be mentioned during the consultation is that the risk of intrauterine death is low in fetuses with CHD who are in sinus rhythm with good myocardial function [89]. Characterization of the cardiac defect and its association with genetic syndrome or not will guide the counselor on how best to give the information to the parent [92]. The parent should be counseled after each scan, and should be given enough time for questions and follow up information [89]. If the amniocentesis detects a chromosomal abnormality, advance cytogenetic testing may be warranted. These testing include FISH, chromosomal microarray and whole exome sequencing [93]. The next step in the counseling, should mention the possibility of chorionic villus sampling or amniocentesis, as this knowledge may help determine prognosis and guide postnatal care. The finding of an associated chromosomal abnormality may also strongly influence decisions about pregnancy termination [94, 95]. Whatever the parental decision is made, the counselor should express full support.

In the final step, the counselor needs to identify and discuss the prenatal options and parental decision-making. This stage is crucial, because the counselor will be discussing the management options with the parents in regards to the outcome of the pregnancy. The management options include: pregnancy continuation, pregnancy termination (if legally allowed) and prenatal intervention if available [96].

If the decision is to continue with the pregnancy, there will be further decisions to be made as to where the infant will to be delivered, mode of delivery and the need for postnatal care and intervention [97]. Delivery at a tertiary care facility with access to pediatric cardiac care is recommended for ductal-dependent lesions and any heart defect that is expected to require neonatal and surgical interventions. Transfer is usually between 30 and 34 weeks gestation to allow the mother to become familiar with the new obstetrician and hospital in the time of her delivery. At the same time, it can be useful to have parent meet the surgeon. The fetus can be delivered at the local hospital, depending on the nursery's comfort level in dealing with such newborns. However, continued communications between the referral hospitals is vital for optimal outcome [98]. Delivery after 39 weeks is typically recommended because of high morbidity, and mortality has been reported in babies born before 36 weeks. Particularly in those with extracardiac and genetic abnormalities [99]. Parents should be counseled that IUGR is associated with increased morbidity after cardiac surgery [100]. Similarly, lower weight (<2.5 kg) is associated with higher mortality after cardiac surgery [101]. Mode of delivery is not typically altered in the setting of fetal CHD, and high rates of vaginal delivery can be achieved [102]. Cesarean section is almost never indicated for cardiac reasons and should be avoided if possible if the cardiac malformation is associated with a high mortality [103]. When the parents make an informed decision to continue the pregnancy, it may be useful for them to meet and speak with parents who have had a child with similar cardiac abnormalities. This will allow for them to have a better understanding of what is to be expected of the journey ahead.

If the decision is to terminate the pregnancy, parents should be counseled and supported fully, as this can cause guilt and emotional stress. Counselor should appreciate the mixed feelings of the parents when it comes to such decisions. It is very important to highlight that termination of pregnancy is never recommended nor absolutely indicated in any circumstances. Termination of pregnancy is a legal option in most of the developed world, but the gestational age limit is variable. In general, it is allowed up to 24 weeks of gestation in most countries all over the world, but late termination, even up to term, can be obtained in some countries like the United States of America for fetal malformations. The counselor must be able to discuss the options of termination of pregnancy and its risks, regardless of their personnel beliefs. The earlier the diagnosis of fetal malformation can be reached (possible from as early as 12 weeks of gestation) the more safely termination of pregnancy can be accomplished. This will create the least amount of physical and emotional trauma for the mother and family [90, 96, 104]. In one center experience, over 2000 sets of parents were counseled, half of them chose termination and the other half continued with pregnancy. Those who accepted termination of pregnancy recovered from it and with time ended up as normal healthy family. However, many of those who continued with the pregnancy, eventually lost the affected child, which was associated with increase grief and agony. In addition, break- down of the whole family unit after many years was reported [90].

Outcomes in terms of rate of termination, after prenatal diagnosis of heart defects vary between countries and even between centers within the same country [105, 106]. The reason for this may be due to differences in social/religious elements and in the local laws and practices. Termination rates are greatly influenced by the gestational age at the time of diagnosis [107], by the presence of the chromosomal abnormalities and other extracardiac malformations [25]. Severity of the cardiac malformation also influences the termination rate like hypoplastic left heart syndrome [81, 105].

Intrauterine interventions may be available for some cardiac malformations like Balloon aortic and pulmonary valvuloplasty. Currently there is a conflict between American College of Obstetricians and Gynecologists and the American Academy of Pediatrics (AAP) regarding the issue of fetal interventions [108]. The AAP favors fetal intervention if available, and puts less weight in maternal decision that is recommended for fetal benefits. This approach may place the mother at greater risks and decrease autonomy [96, 109]. If the intervention considered are questionable and carry a high risks to the mother, it is prudent to respect the mothers autonomy and giving her priority [96], until further research and consensuses are definitive in this regards.

In case of multiple pregnancies with one fetus with a serious congenital anomaly need to be highlighted in this step of the counseling. These risks and benefits of continuing or terminating the pregnancy of affected twin needs to be considered and balanced. The expectant parents need to understand that the death of the normal twin can occur if the twin pregnancy is continued. This is particularly true when there is a monochorionic twin pregnancy [96, 110].

The prenatal counseling should discuss the anticipated postnatal course, intervention and outcome/survival. In most cases, the infant born with cardiac malformation will require immediate medical and/or surgical intervention. Medical intervention to ensure patency of the ductus arteriosus will include starting Prostaglandin for duct-dependent lesions for either pulmonary blood flow (e.g., severe TOF or pulmonary atresia) or systemic blood flow (e.g., HLHS, interrupted aortic arch). Once these patients are stable medically, they may require cardiac catheterization and/or surgical repair. Parents should be counseled on what to expect in the delivery room. Management will vary, depending on the severity of the cardiac defect. Decision such as, where the baby will be admitted and how much time they will have the baby, will be decided prior to the delivery date. Parent should be made aware that the postnatal cardiac diagnosis might be modified after birth. Emphasis on the possibility of modification of the postnatal course, including change in the interventions and length of stay needs to be discussed. Helping the parents understand and deal with changes that may occur and be contrary to what they might have been told [98].

The outcomes and long-term survival (20 years) are profoundly dependent on the type of defect in babies born with CHD. Majority of these babies, approximately 85% are expected to reach adult age. For example, infants with simple CHD such as VSD or ASD have survival rate of 95%, whereas moderate severity such as TOF reach 90%, and complex CHD such as single ventricle reach 80%.) [111]. A follow up study of 1000 Fontan patients by d'Udekem et al. showed 97% 10-year survival rate [112]. Although there are relatively good survival many of these patient may manifest other complications, including dysrhythmias, need for pacemaker and thromboembolic events [98]. Parents have to be informed about that there is an increased risk of neurodevelopmental delay in children with cardiac malformations. The severity of cardiac defect correlates with the degree of developmental delay [113]. In a recent meta-analysis, fetuses with severe cardiac malformation showed signs of impaired fetal cerebral development as shown by fetal MRI or ultrasound. However, correlations of fetal brain findings with neurodevelopmental outcome have been inconclusive and more long-term data are needed [114].

3.2. Postnatal

The advancement of cardiac diagnostic and therapeutic techniques in the past decade, with relatively low morbidity and mortality, has led to more and more children with congenital heart disease living to adulthood. Therefore, the role of genetic counseling becomes even more paramount as there is a higher likelihood of these patients living to reproduce and that they may have families of their own [22]. It is very important to help elucidate the genetic basis for patients' congenital cardiac malformation for the reason mentioned, as there may be important reproductive risks that the families need to know about [22, 115, 116]. Recent analysis indicate that adults now constitute roughly two-thirds of the congenital heart disease population, representing a nearly 60% increase in congenital heart disease among adult patients since the year 2000 [115, 116]. The greatest increase in congenital heart disease survival has occurred among the 18-year old to 40-year-old demographic, which has clear implications for heritability [116].

One of the obstacles, in performing genetic testing in patients with congenital heart disease is that there are no standardized recommendations or protocols incorporating, newer genetic testing technologies at present. The literature is sparse with guidelines, and there is evidence that there is under use even of those modalities of testing that are available [22, 115]. However, there has been an emphasis from the American Heart Association in the recent past, in obtaining genetic testing in these patients [117].

3.2.1. Genetics in congenital heart disease

Cardiac malformation present at birth are an important component of pediatric cardiovascular disease. Defects can range from simple ventricular septal defects to complicated cyanotic lesions, requiring complex interventions shortly after birth. With the possibility of myriad of presentations, it begets one to ask, what is the percentage of pediatric cardiac defects are a result of a genetic anomaly. CHD is estimated that the prevalence of cardiac malformation at birth ranges from 4 to 10 live born infants per 1000. The true incidence, perhaps maybe higher as there are silent cardiac malformations that are only found later on in life [115]. As most calculations do not include bicuspid aortic valves, mitral valve prolapse and conduction problems, such as prolonged QT syndrome and complete atrioventricular block [115, 116]. The care of the pediatric patient with cardiac malformation is multifaceted, ranging from simple reassurance and observation to advanced surgeries and interventional techniques shortly after birth. The primary focus of treatment of the patient with cardiac malformation is diagnosis and best course of treatment. However an important and integral part of the care of these patients is to have genetic counseling with their parents in regards to possible etiologies of the congenital heart disease. In the past, it was believed that the recurrence of congenital cardiovascular malformations in the same family was low, with expert quoting recurrence rate of only 3–5%. However currently it is known that for a family with autosomal-dominant 22q 11 deletion syndrome, the risk is up to 50% with a variable phenotypic expression [117, 118].

Etiology of some cardiac malformation that are known to have genetic components, where they make up approximately 5–17% are part of a genetic syndrome. Environmental factors need to be considered and a detailed family history needs to be elicited [119]. The role of the primary care giver is paramount, in detecting possible associated cardiac genetic syndromes. When genetic syndromes are a possibility, intervention requires referral to a genetic counselor for accurate diagnosis and possible future pregnancy. Since approximately, 75% of currently known cardiac malformations have no identifiable cause or underlying condition, the necessity for genetic counseling may appear unwarranted. However with the advent of advanced genetic testing such as whole exome sequencing, once unrecognized features are now being associated with syndromes [120–123]. Postnatal, the purpose of the genetic evaluation is to help establish a diagnosis and educate the family about future risk recurrence and expected outcomes. Parents need to be counseled and educated on both the numeric risk and the variable expressivity that makes predicting severity difficult.

3.2.2. Genetic evaluation of congenital heart disease

The role of genetic evaluation in patients with cardiac malformations, as patients live longer is becoming increasingly important. In the past, where genetic testing was limited to research laboratories, in today clinical practice this is no longer the case. The current clinical practice allows for the physician to obtain chromosomal analysis and request FISH testing when looking for specific deletions [22, 121–123]. The yields of these testing becomes higher when a genetic counselor is consulted prior to obtaining specific test. However even with the advancement on genetic testing, not all patients with congenital heart disease will be identified to have a genetic cause. The recommend approach for newly diagnosed patients with cardiac malformations includes the routine evaluation of all available relatives for a potential genetic contribution [22], and obtaining an accurate and complete medical history and documenting and extended pedigree. If from the information a syndrome if recognized, then evaluation and counseling of other family members becomes extremely important. Depending on the suspected diagnosis or syndrome, other consultation will need to be obtained such neurology, ophthalmology, and others subspecialties.

Cytogenetic testing should be obtained in the following situations (from AHA Scientific Statement):

1. Any child or infant with the phenotype of a recognizable chromosomal syndrome (e.g., Trisomy 21 or 18)

2. Because not all chromosomal abnormalities result in a clinically recognizable syndrome, any infant or child with congenital heart disease combined with (a) dysmorphic features (b) growth retardation that cannot be explained by the heart defect (c) developmental delay or mental retardation or (d) multiple congenital anomalies.

3. Infant or children with a family history of multiple miscarriage and/or sibling with birth defects

4. If major cardiac and/or other visceral organ malformations are documented by prenatal ultrasound and/or fetal echocardiogram.

   Review of the literature shows that chromosome abnormalities were present in 12% of patients with TOF, 26% in tetralogy of Fallot/pulmonary atresia, 44% in interrupted aortic arch, 12% in truncus arteriosus, 5% in double outlet right ventricle, and 60% in absent pulmonary valve. With certain cardiac defect, chromosomal analysis should be considered. In patients with conotruncal defects or interrupted aortic arch, FISH should be used looking for 22q11 deletion. Also analysis of the 8p region should be included [124].

3.2.3. *Types of genetic testing*

3.2.3.1. *Karyotype*

Prior to the advent of advanced cytogenetic testing, the standard chromosomal analysis (i.e., karyotype) was widely used. Chromosome testing using standard metaphase karyotype is the traditional method and remains standard for the detection of aneuploidy (Trisomy 13, 18 and 21 and Turners 45 XO) and detecting gross changes such translocation and duplications [22, 117, 125]. A more sensitive karyotype is also available, which allows for the visualizations of greater number of bands. However, standard karyotype has an estimated 3% detection rate for pathogenic chromosome abnormalities. Conventional chromosome analysis detects well-known chromosome aneuploidies in about 10% of cases of CHDs [126]. with the advent and feasibility of newer technology, karyotype maybe used less and become replaced.

3.2.3.2. *Florescence in situ hybridization (FISH)*

More advanced cytogenetic techniques such as FISH and chromosome microarray are required to diagnose more subtle structural abnormalities, such as microdeletions, tiny duplications and/or subtle translocations. This technology can be used to detect small deletions and duplications in chromosomes that cannot be detected with standard analysis as it looks specifically at the one area of the chromosome. A final FISH analysis will report on how many chromosomes of a certain type are present, in addition confirm suspected rearrangements. FISH technology uses probes of DNA that have been labeled with a fluorescent dye, that bind to complementary parts of a DNA, when it is heated. These probes are able to attach to their complementary DNA sequence [127]. The classic examples that uses this technology is the diagnosis of DiGeorge Syndrome with 22q11 deletion and William Syndrome with 7q11.23 deletion. The drawback of fluorescence in situ hybridization (FISH) lies in its targeted approach to detect chromosomal defects, rather than a genome-wide screening method like microarrays [128].

3.2.3.3. Chromosome microarray

Chromosomal microarray (CMA) testing looks for extra (duplicated) or missing (deleted) chromosomal segments, sometimes called copy number variants (CNVs). It refers to a microchip-based testing platform that allows high-volume, automated analysis of many pieces of DNA at once. CMA chips use labels or probes that bond to specific chromosome regions [129]. The resolution of conventional karyotype analysis is limited to 5 Mb or larger genomic imbalances. Chromosome Microarray Analysis (CMA) is a routine technique in clinical molecular testing nowadays, which contains two types of arrays: oligonucleotide arrays and Single Nucleotide Polymorphism arrays (SNP arrays). Computer analysis is used to compare a patient's genetic material to that of a reference sample. A difference between a patient's DNA and the reference sample is called a variant. These include chromosomal microdeletions and micro-duplications that are too small, abnormalities of chromosome number like the trisomies. In addition other variants include unbalanced rearrangements of chromosome structure such as translocations and triploidies.

Both the arrays could detect genome-wide CNVs. Moreover, SNP arrays can detect mosaicism, triploid, loss of heterozygosity and uniparental disomy. In 2010, the American College of Medical Genetics issued practice guidelines for CMA, and pointed out that CMA was recommended as a first-tier test for postnatal patients with multiple congenital anomalies, intellectual disabilities/developmental delay (ID/DD) and autism spectrum disorders [127, 129]. Recently, CMA has been successfully applied to detect CNVs in patients with CHD, which confirmed the relationship between chromosome microdeletion/microduplication and CHD [128].

3.2.3.4. Whole exome sequencing

Whole exome sequencing is part of next-generation sequencing. With this technology, it is now possible to sequence large amounts of DNA that provide genetic code for making proteins, which are called exons. All the exons in a genome are referred to as the exome, hence this method of sequencing them is known as whole exome sequencing, which allows for the identification of variations in the protein-coding region. It is known that most mutations that cause disease states, occur in these regions. Therefore, the use of this technology allows an efficient way to detect possible disease-causing mutations [130]. Whole exome sequencing has been successfully applied to patients with CHD. Many de novo mutations involved in cardiac related genes to the developing heart have been detected. [22, 130, 131]. This finding helped better elucidate understanding of overall CHD and its developmental pathways. However, more research needs to be done to determine a causal relation and best therapeutic interventions in these cohort of patient studied [130].

3.2.4. Preimplantation genetic diagnosis

In the current era of in vitro fertilization, preimplantation genetic diagnosis is possible. PGD provides chromosomal and mutational analysis of blastocyst that results from in vitro fertilization before implantation [22]. In assisted reproductive technology, PGD is becoming a treatment option for some inherited disorders. The application of PGD can be used in some conditions present at birth, in addition to prevent carrier states that may or may not present later on in life. Holt-Oram syndrome (HOS) was the first heart disease in which PDG was used successfully [125, 132]. The features of HOS include ASD and cardiac conduction disorder, which has a variable penetrance. Currently there is no treatment prospect as it may manifest later on in life. Clinical manifestations may be extremely variable, and may not be present at birth, or present subtly as a sinus bradycardia, as the only clinical sign. So PGD may provide a treatment option to prevent offspring with this genetic diagnosis [117, 125, 132].

3.2.5. Impact on patients and families

The identification of genetic cause in congenital heart disease can prove to be very beneficial. Firstly is allows for the physician to be confident of the diagnosis and explain the mechanism of disease and other prognostic factors.[1] When the cardiac malformation is part of a genetic syndrome, it allows for the care team to look for other associated anomalies in other organ system. A genetic basis for disease may also necessitate evaluation into other family members [22, 117]. This will help further characterize the extent of the disease in the family and monitor risks and assess ability to pass on to future offspring [117]. Patients and families need to be made aware of both the numeric risk, as in Marfan and William Syndrome, an affected person has a 50% risk. However when the cardiac malformation has variable expressivity, predicting severity becomes extremely difficult [118].

4. Conclusion

Since approximately, 75% of congenital heart diseases have no identifiable cause or underlying condition, the notion of formal genetic evaluation may appear unwarranted [123]. However with the development and feasibility of genetic evaluations improving, more and more cardiac malformation are being linked to underlying genetic anomalies. Therefore the need to look for a genetic link become more crucial, as more patient with congenital heart disease live into adult age, it is very important that families understand their recurrence risk [120–122]. Unfortunately genetic counseling is not an integral or compulsory part of the treatment plan for families at many centers. Too many times, parents are exhausted from the complex interventional procedures and surgeries and its subsequent complications, the need for such counseling is forgotten and pushed aside [22, 117]. There are likely to be approximately 400 genes involved in the causation of congenital heart disease, many of which are yet to be identified [119]. Therefore the role of genetic counselors, with specialized skills in cardiovascular genetics is of utmost importance in the adult patient with congenital heart disease. Such genetic counselors play a crucial role in providing accurate recurrence risk, facilitating appropriate genetic testing, interpreting of results and appropriate subspecialty referrals. Phenotypic heterogeneity and incomplete penetrance complicate our understanding of the genesis of congenital heart disease. However it seems more likely than ever that our gaps in understanding the causes of congenital heart disease are primarily genetic and that the mechanism are multifactorial [117].

It is know that the prenatal diagnosis of moderate to severe CHD is associated with improved outcomes and reduction in the morbidity in select cardiac defects. Prior knowledge of the cardiac lesion allows, the delivery room team to be prepared with appropriate resources to help minimize hypoxemia and metabolic acidosis. The likely need of invasive ventilation can be assed prior to delivery. Therefore the prenatal counseling allows for an accurate diagnosis of the cardiac defect, with parents educated on the possible interventions and expected outcomes after birth. Counseling and the availability of a multidisciplinary team will give the expectant parents support and allows for them to make informed decision before and after delivery.

Author details

Amal Zubani*, Irfan Asra and Amjad Kouatli

*Address all correspondence to: azubani@kfshrc.edu.sa

King Faisal Specialist Hospital and Research Center 'Gen.-Org.', Jeddah, Saudi Arabia

References

[1] Hoffman JI, Kaplan S. The incidence of congenital heart disease. Journal of the American College of Cardiology. 2002 Jun 19;**39**(12):1890-1900. Available from: https://doi.org/10.1016/S0735-1097(02)01886-7

[2] Chervenak FA, McCullough LB. Perinatal ethics: A practical method of analysis of obligations to mother and fetus. Obstetrics and Gynecology. 1985 Sep;**66**(3):442-446. Available from: http://hdl.handle.net/10822/727565

[3] American Academy of Pediatrics Committee on Bioethics. Fetal therapy: Ethical considerations. Pediatrics. 1988 Jun;**81**(6):898-899. Available from: http://pediatrics.aappublications.org/content/81/6/898

[4] Allan LD, Sharland GK, Milburn A, Lockhart SM, Groves AM, Anderson RH, et al. Prospective diagnosis of 1,006 consecutive cases of congenital heart disease in the fetus. Journal of the American College of Cardiology. 1994 May;**23**(6):1452-1458. Available from: https://doi.org/10.1016/0735-1097(94)90391-3

[5] Donofrio MT, Moon-Grady AJ, Hornberger LK, Copel JA, Sklansky MS, Abuhamad A, et al. Diagnosis and treatment of fetal cardiac disease: A scientific statement from the American Heart Association. Circulation. 2014 May 27;**129**(21):2183-2242. Available from: https://doi.org/10.1161/01.cir.0000437597.44550.5d

[6] Brown KL, Sullivan ID. Prenatal detection for major congenital heart disease: A key process measure for congenital heart networks. Heart. 2014 Mar;**100**(5):359-360. Available from: https://doi.org/10.1136/heartjnl-2013-305161

[7] Kipps AK, Feuille C, Azakie A, Hoffman JI, Tabbutt S, Brook MM, et al. Prenatal diagnosis of hypoplastic left heart syndrome in current era. The American Journal of Cardiology. 2011 Aug 1;**108**(3):421-427. Available from https://doi.org/10.1016/j.amjcard.2011.03.065

[8] Levey A, Glickstein JS, Kleinman CS, Levasseur SM, Chen J, Gersony WM, et al. The impact of prenatal diagnosis of complex congenital heart disease on neonatal outcomes. Pediatric Cardiology. 2010 Jul;**31**(5):587-597. Available from: https://doi.org/10.1007/s00246-010-9648-2

[9] Landis BJ, Levey A, Levasseur SM, Glickstein JS, Kleinman CS, Simpson LL, et al. Prenatal diagnosis of congenital heart disease and birth outcomes. Pediatric Cardiology. 2013 Mar;**34**(3):597-605. Available from: https://doi.org/10.1007/s00246-012-0504-4

[10] Wright LK, Ehrlich A, Stauffer N, Samai C, Kogon B, Oster ME. Relation of prenatal diagnosis with one-year survival rate for infants with congenital heart disease. The American Journal of Cardiology. 2014 Mar 15;**113**(6):1041-1044. Available from: https://doi.org/10.1016/j.amjcard.2013.11.065

[11] Oster ME, Kim CH, Kusano AS, Cragan JD, Dressler P, Hales AR, et al. A population-based study of the association of prenatal diagnosis with survival rate for infants with congenital heart defects. The American Journal of Cardiology. 2014 Mar 15;**113**(6):1036-1040. Available from: https://dx.doi.org/10.1016%2Fj.amjcard.2013.11.066.

[12] Wan AW, Jevremovic A, Selamet Tierney ES, McCrindle BW, Dunn E, Manlhiot C, et al. Comparison of impact of prenatal versus postnatal diagnosis of congenitally corrected transposition of the great arteries. The American Journal of Cardiology. 2009 Nov 1;**104**(9):1276-1279. Available from: https://doi.org/10.1016/j.amjcard.2009.06.047

[13] McBrien A, Sands A, Craig B, Dornan J, Casey F. Major congenital heart disease: Antenatal detection, patient characteristics and outcomes. Journal of Maternal-Fetal and Neonatal Medicine. 2009 Feb;**22**(2):101-105. Available from: https://doi.org/10.1080/14767050802483106

[14] Fuchs IB, Muller H, Abdul-Khaliq H, Harder T, Dudenhausen JW, Henrich W. Immediate and long-term outcomes in children with prenatal diagnosis of selected isolated congenital heart defects. Ultrasound in Obstetrics & Gynecology. 2007 Jan;**29**(1):38-43. Available from: https://doi.org/10.1002/uog.3900

[15] Chung ML, Lee BS, Kim EA, Kim KS, Pi SY, YM O, et al. Impact of fetal echocardiography on trends in disease patterns and outcomes of congenital heart disease in a neonatal intensive care unit. Neonatology. 2010 Jun;**98**(1):41-46. Available from: https://doi.org/10.1159/000264673

[16] Morris SA, Ethen MK, Penny DJ, Canfield MA, Minard CG, Fixler DE, et al. Prenatal diagnosis, birth location, surgical center, and neonatal mortality in infants with hypoplastic left heart syndrome. Circulation. 2014 Jan 21;**129**(3):285-292. Available from: https://doi.org/10.1161/CIRCULATIONAHA.113.003711

[17] Rychik J, Szwast A, Natarajan S, Quartermain M, Donaghue DD, Combs J, et al. Perinatal and early surgical outcome for the fetus with hypoplastic left heart syndrome: A 5-year single institutional experience. Ultrasound in Obstetrics & Gynecology. 2010 Oct;**36**(4):465-470. Available from: https://doi.org/10.1002/uog.7674

[18] Raboisson MJ, Samson C, Ducreux C, Rudigoz RC, Gaucherand P, Bouvagnet P, et al. Impact of prenatal diagnosis of transposition of the great arteries on obstetric and early postnatal management. European Journal of Obstetrics, Gynecology, and Reproductive Biology. 2009 Jan;**142**(1):18-22. Available from: https://doi.org/10.1016/j.ejogrb.2008.09.001

[19] Swanson TM, Selamet Tierney ES, Tworetzky W, Pigula F, McElhinney DB. Truncus arteriosus: Diagnostic accuracy, outcomes, and impact of prenatal diagnosis. Pediatric Cardiology. 2009 Apr;**30**(3):256-261. Available from: https://doi.org/10.1007/s00246-008-9328-7

[20] Holland BJ, Myers JA, Woods CR Jr. Prenatal diagnosis of critical congenital heart disease reduces risk of death from cardiovascular compromise prior to planned neonatal cardiac surgery: A meta-analysis. Ultrasound in Obstetrics & Gynecology. 2015 Jun;**45**(6):631-638. Available from: https://doi.org/10.1002/uog.14882

[21] Jenkins KJ, Correa A, Feinstein JA, Botto L, Britt AE, Daniels SR, et al. Noninherited risk factors and congenital cardiovascular defects: Current knowledge: A scientific statement from the American Heart Association Council on cardiovascular disease in the young: Endorsed by the American Academy of Pediatrics. Circulation. 2007 Jun 12;**115**(23):2995-3014. Available from: https://doi.org/10.1161/CIRCULATIONAHA.106.183216

[22] Pierpont ME, Basson CT, Benson DW Jr, Gelb BD, Giglia TM, Goldmuntz E, et al. Genetic basis for congenital heart defects: Current knowledge: A scientific statement from the American Heart Association congenital cardiac defects committee, council on cardiovascular disease in the young: Endorsed by the American Academy of Pediatrics. Circulation. 2007 Jun 12;**115**(23):3015-3038. Available from: https://doi.org/10.1161/CIRCULATIONAHA.106.183056

[23] Williams IA, Shaw R, Kleinman CS, Gersony WM, Prakash A, Levasseur SM, et al. Parental understanding of neonatal congenital heart disease. Pediatric Cardiology. 2008 Nov;**29**(6):1059-1065. Available from: https://doi.org/10.1007/s00246-008-9254-8

[24] Jones KL. Smith's Recognizable Pattern of Human Malformation. 6th ed. Philadelphia, PA: Elsevier Sanders; 2006. pp. 1-62. Available from: https://www.amazon.com/Smiths-Recognizable-Patterns-Human-Malformation/dp/0721606156/ref=pd_lpo_sbs_14_t_0?_encoding=UTF8&psc=1&refRID=73KJQGRMPXAPD38BSQ3C&dpID=41QY2NQ44HL&preST=_SY344_BO1,204,203,200_QL70_&dpSrc=detail

[25] Romano AA, Allanson JE, Dahlgren J, Gelb BD, Hall B, Pierpont ME, et al. Noonan syndrome: Clinical features, diagnosis and management guideline. Pediatrics. 2010 Oct;**126**(4):746-759. Available from: https://doi.org/10.1542/peds.2009-3207

[26] Noonan JA et al. Hypertelorism with turner phenotype. A new syndrome with associated congenital heart disease. American Journal of Diseases of Children. 1968 Oct;**116**(4):373-380. Available from: https://jamanetwork.com/journals/jamapediatrics/fullarticle/502812

[27] Allanson JE. Noonan syndrome. In: Cassidy SB, Allanson JE, editors. Management of Genetic Syndromes. 2nd ed. Hoboken, NJ: Wiley Liss; 2005. p. 385. DOI: 10.1002/0471695998.mgs032

[28] Chakraborty A. Noonan syndromes: A brief overview. Hospital Medicine. 2002 Dec;**63**(12):743-745. Available from: https://www.ncbi.nlm.nih.gov/pubmed/12512201

[29] Tramboo NA, Iqbal K, Dar MA, Malik RA, Naikoo BA, Andrabi MA. Unusual dysmorphic features in five patients with Noonan's syndrome: A brief review. Journal of Paediatrics and Child Health. 2002 Oct;**38**(5):521-525. DOI: 10.1046/j.1440-1754.2002.00027.x

[30] Gelb BD. Genetic basis of congenital heart disease. Current Opinion in Cardiology. 2004 Mar;**19**(2):110-115. Available from: https://www.ncbi.nlm.nih.gov/pubmed/15075735

[31] Menashe M, Arbel R, Raveh D, Achiron R, Yagel S. Poor prenatal detection rate of cardiac anomalies in Noonan syndrome. Ultrasound in Obstetrics & Gynecology. 2002 Jan;**19**(1):51-55. Available from: https://doi.org/10.1046/j.0960-7692.2001.00485.x

[32] Barr M Jr, Oman-Ganes L. Turner syndrome morphology and morphometrics: Cardiac hypoplasia as a cause of midgestation death. Teratology. 2002 Aug;**66**(2):65-72. Available from: https://doi.org/10.1002/tera.10064

[33] Sybert VP, McCauley E. Turner's syndrome. The New England Journal of Medicine. 2004 Sept;**351**:1227-1238. Available from: https://doi.org/10.1056/NEJMra030360

[34] Gotzsche CO, Krag-Olsen B, Nielsen J, Sorensen KE, Kristensen BO. Prevalence of cardiovascular malformations and association with karyotypes in Turner's syndrome. Archives of Disease in Childhood. 1994 Nov;**71**(5):433-436. Available from: https://www.ncbi.nlm.nih.gov/pmc/articles/PMC1030059/

[35] Morris CA, Mervis CB. William syndrome and related disorders. Annual Review of Genomics and Human Genetics. 2000 Sept;**1**:461-484. Available from: https://doi.org/10.1146/annurev.genom.1.1.461

[36] Kruse K, Pankau R, Gosch A, Wohlfahrt K. Calcium metabolism in Williams-Beuren syndrome. The Journal of Pediatrics. 1992 Dec;**121**(6):902-907. Available from https://www.ncbi.nlm.nih.gov/pubmed/1333009

[37] Kececioglu D, Kotthoff S, Vogt J. Williams-Beuren syndrome: A 30-year follow-up of natural and postoperative course. European Heart Journal. 1993 Nov;**14**(11):1458-1464. Available from https://doi.org/10.1093/eurheartj/14.11.1458

[38] Eronen M, Peipo M, Hiippala A, Raatikka M, Arvio M, Johansson R, et al. Cardiovascular manifestations in 75 patients with Williams syndrome. Journal of Medical Genetics. 2002 Aug;**39**(8):554-558. Available from: https://www.ncbi.nlm.nih.gov/pmc/articles/PMC1735199/

[39] Curran ME, Atkinson DL, Ewart AK, Morris CA, Leppert MF, Keating MT. The elastin gene is disrupted by a translocation associated with supravalvular aortic stenosis. Cell. 1993 Apr 9;**73**(1):159-168. Available from: https://doi.org/10.1016/0092-8674(93)90168-P

[40] Metcalfe K, Rucka AK, Smoot L, Hofstadler G, Tuzler G, Mckeown P, et al. Elastin: mutational spectrum in supravalvular aortic stenosis. European Journal of Human Genetics. 2000 Dec;**8**(12):955-963. Available from: https://doi.org/10.1038/sj.ejhg.5200564

[41] Wu YQ, Sutton VR, Nickerson E, Lupski JR, Potocki L, Korenberg JR, et al. Delineation of the common critical region in Williams syndrome and clinical correlation of growth, heart defects, ethnicity, and parental origin. American Journal of Medical Genetics. 1998 Jun 16;**78**(1):82-89. Available from. DOI: 10.1002/(SICI)1096-8628(19980616)78:1<82::AID-AJMG17>3.0.CO;2-K

[42] Stromme P, Bjornstad PG, Ramstad K. Prevalence estimation of Williams syndrome. Journal of Child Neurology. 2002 Apr;**17**(4):269-271. Available from: https://doi.org/10.1177/088307380201700406

[43] Driscoll DA, Spinner NB, Budarf ML, Mcdonald- McGinn DM, Zackai EH, Goldberg RB, et al. Deletion and micodeletion of 22q11.2 in velo-cardio- facial syndrome. American Journal of Medical Genetics. 1992 Sept;**44**:261-268. DOI: 10.1002/ajmg.1320440237

[44] Greenberg F. DiGeorge syndrome: An historical review of clinical and cytogenetic features. Journal of Medical Genetics. 1993 Oct;**30**(10):803-806. Available from: https://www.ncbi.nlm.nih.gov/pmc/articles/PMC1016558/

[45] Burn J, Takao A, Wilson D, Cross I, Momma K, Wadey R, et al. Conotruncal anomaly face syndrome is associated with a deletion within chromosome 22q11. Journal of Medical Genetics. 1993;**30**(10):822-824. Available from: DOI: 10.1136/jmg.30.10.822

[46] Botto LD, May K, Fernhoff PM, Correa A, Coleman K, Rasmussen SA, et al. A population- based study of the 22q11.2 deletion: Phenotype, incidence and contribution to major birth defects in the population. Pediatrics. 2003 Jul;**112**(1 Pt 1):101-107. Available from: http://pediatrics.aappublications.org/content/112/1/101.short

[47] Ryan AK, Goodship JA, Wilson DI, Philip N, Levy A, Seidel H, et al. Spectrum of clinical features associated with interstitial chromosome 22q11 deletion. A European collaborative study. Journal of Medical Genetics. 1997 Oct;**34**(10):798-804. Available from: https://www.ncbi.nlm.nih.gov/pmc/articles/PMC1051084/

[48] McDoland-McGinn DM, LaRossa D, Goldmuntz E, Sullivan K, Eicher P, Gerdes M, et al. The 22q11.2 deletion: Screening, diagnostic workup and outcome of results; report of 181 patients. Genetic Testing. 1997;**1**(2):99-108. Available from: https://doi.org/10.1089/gte.1997.1.99

[49] McElhinney DB, Driscoll DA, Emanuel BS, Goldmuntz E. Chromosome 22q11 deletion in patients with truncus arteriosus. Pediatric Cardiology. 2003 Nov-Dec;**24**(6):569-573. Available from: https://doi.org/10.1007/s00246-003-0441-3

[50] Barrea C, Yoo SJ, Chitayat D, Valsangiacomo E, Winsor E, Smalhorn JF, et al. Assessment of the thymus at echocardiography in fetuses at risk for 22q11.2 deletion. Prenatal Diagnosis. 2003 Jan;**23**(1):9-15. Available from: https://doi.org/10.1002/pd.508

[51] McElhinney DB, McDonald-McGinn D, Zackai EH, Goldmuntz E. Cardiovascular anomalies in paticnts diagnosed with chromosome 22q11 deletion beyond 6 month of age. Pediatrics. 2001;**108**(6):E104. Available from: https://doi.org/10.1542/peds.108.6.e104

[52] Graham JM Jr et al. A recognizable syndrome within CHARGE association: Hall- Hittner syndrome. American Journal of Medical Genetics. 2001 Mar 1;**99**(2):120-123. Available from https://www.ncbi.nlm.nih.gov/pubmed/11241469

[53] Vissers LE, van Ravenswaaij CM, Admiraal R, Hurst JA, de Vrias BB, Janssen IM, et al. Mutations in a new member of the chromodomain gene family cause CHARGE syndrome. Nature Genetics. 2004 Sep;**36**(9):955-957. Available from: https://doi.org/10.1038/ng1407

[54] Verloes A. Update diagnostic criteria for CHARGE syndrome: A proposal. American Journal of Medical Genetics. Part A. 2005 Mar 15;**133A**(3):306-308. Available from: https://doi.org/10.1002/ajmg.a.30559

[55] Lalani SR, Safiullah AM, Fernbach SD, Harutyunyan KG, Thaller C, Peterson LE, et al. Spectrum of CHD7 mutations in 110 individuals with CHARGE syndrome and genotype-phenotypr correlation. American Journal of Human Genetics. 2006 Feb;**78**(2):303-314. Available from: https://doi.org/10.1086/500273

[56] Corsten-Janssen N, Kerstijens-Frederikse WS, du Marchie Sarvaas GJ, Baardam ME, Bakker MK, Bergman JE, et al. The cardiac phenotype in patients with a CHD7 mutation. Circulation: Cardiovascular Genetics. 2013 Jun;**6**(3):248-254. Available from https://doi.org/10.1161/CIRCGENETICS.113.000054

[57] Issekutz KA, Graham JM Jr, Prasad C, Smith IM, Blake KD. An epidemiological analysis of CHARGE syndrome; preliminary results from a Canadian study. American Journal of Medical Genetics. Part A. 2005 Mar 15;**133A**(3):309-317. Available from: https://doi.org/10.1002/ajmg.a.30560

[58] Botto LD, Khoury MJ, Mastroiacovo P, Castilla EE, Moore CA, Skjaerven R, et al. The spectrum of congenital anomalies of the VATER association: An international study. American Journal of Medical Genetics. 1997 Jul 11;**71**(1):8-15. Available from: https://www.ncbi.nlm.nih.gov/pubmed/9215761

[59] Weaver DD, Mapstone CL, Yu PL. The VATER association. Analysis of 46 patients. American Journal of Diseases of Children. 1986 Mar;**140**(3):225-229. Available from: https://www.ncbi.nlm.nih.gov/pubmed/3946352

[60] Solomon BD, Pineda-Alvarez DE, Raam MS, Bous SM, Keaton AA, Velez JI, et al. Analysis of component findings in 79 patients diagnosed with VACTERL association. American Journal of Medical Genetics. Part A. 2010 Sep;**152A**(9):2236-2244. Available from: https://doi.org/10.1002/ajmg.a.33572

[61] Manning N, Kaufman L, Roberts P. Genetic of cardiological disorders. Seminars in Fetal & Neonatal Medicine. 2005 Jun;**10**(3):259-269. Available from: https://doi.org/10.1016/j.siny.2005.04.010

[62] Nezarati MM, McLeod DR. VACTERL manifestations in two generations of a family. American Journal of Medical Genetics. 1999 Jan 1;**82**(1):40-42. Available from: https://www.ncbi.nlm.nih.gov/pubmed/9916841

[63] Watson GH, Miller V. Arteriohepatic dysplasia: Familial pulmonary arterial stenosis with neonatal liver disease. Archives of Disease in Childhood. 1973 Jun;**48**(6):459-466. Available from: https://www.ncbi.nlm.nih.gov/pmc/articles/PMC1648450/

[64] Alagille D, Odievre M, Gautier M, Dommergues JP. Hepatic ductular hypoplasia associated with characteristic facies, vertebral malformations, retarded physical, mental,

and sexual development, and cardiac murmur. The Journal of Pediatrics. 1975 Jan;**86**(1): 63-71. Available from: https://doi.org/10.1016/S0022-3476(75)80706-2

[65] Byrne JL, Harrod MJ, Friedman JM, Howard-Peebles PN. del(20p) with manifestations of arteriohepatic dysplasia. American Journal of Medical Genetics. 1986 Aug;**24**(4):673-678. Available from: https://doi.org/10.1002/ajmg.1320240411

[66] Krantz ID, Rand EB, Genin A, Hunt P, Jones M, Louis AA, et al. Deletion of 20p12 in Alagille syndrome: Frequency and molecular characterization. American Journal of Medical Genetics. 1997 May 2;**70**(1):80-86. DOI: 10.1002/humu.20310

[67] Warthen DM, Moore EC, Kamath BM, Morrissette JJ, Sanchez-Lara PA, Krantz ID, et al. Jagged 1 (JAG1) mutations in Alagille syndrome: Increasing the mutation detection rate. Human Mutation. 2006 May;**27**(5):436-443. Available from: https://doi.org/10.1002/humu.20310

[68] Krantz ID, Piccoli DA, Spinner NB, et al. Alagille syndrome. Journal of Medical Genetics. 1997 Feb;**34**(2):152-157. Available from: https://www.ncbi.nlm.nih.gov/pmc/articles/PMC1050871/

[69] McElhinney DB, Krantz ID, Bason L, Piccoli DA, Emerick KM, Spinner MB, et al. Analysis of cardiovascular phenotype and genotype-phenotype correlation in individuals with a JAG1 mutation and/ or Alagille syndrome. Circulation. 2002 Nov 12;**106**(20):2567-2574. Available from: https://doi.org/10.1161/01.CIR.0000037221.45902.69

[70] Bossert T, Walther T, Gummert J, Hubald R, Kostelka M, Mohr FW. Cardiac malformations associated with the Holt-Oram syndrome e report on a family and review of the literature. The Thoracic and Cardiovascular Surgeon. 2002;**50**(5):312-314. DOI: 10.1055/s-2002-34573

[71] Bruneau BG, Logan M, Davis N, Lavi T, Tabin CJ, Seidman JG, et al. Chamber-specific cardic expression of Tbx5 and heart defects in Holt-Oram syndrome. Developmental Biology. 1999 Jul 1;211(1):100-108. Available from: https://doi.org/10.1006/dbio.1999.9298

[72] Huang T. Current advances in Holt-Oram syndrome. Current Opinion in Pediatrics. 2002 Dec;**14**(6):691-695. Available from https://www.ncbi.nlm.nih.gov/pubmed/12436037

[73] Newbury-Ecob RA, Leanage R, Raeburn JA, Young ID. Holt-Oram syndrome: A clinical genetic study. Journal of Medical Genetics. 1996 Apr;**33**(4):300-307. Available from: https://www.ncbi.nlm.nih.gov/pmc/articles/PMC1050579/

[74] Bonnet D, Pelet A, Legeai-Malle L, Sidi D, Mathieu M, Parent P, et al. A gene for Holt-Oram syndrome maps to the distal long arm of chromosomal 12. Nature Genetics. 1994 Apr;**6**(4):405-408. Available from: https://doi.org/10.1038/ng0494-405

[75] Freeman SB, Bean LH, Allan EG, Tinker SW, Locke AE, Druschel C, et al. Ethnicity, sex, and the incidence of congenital heart defect: A report from the national down syndrome project. Genetics in Medicine. 2008 Mar;**10**(3):173-180. Available from: https://doi.org/10.1097/GIM.0b013e3181634867

[76] Freeman SB, Taft LF, Dooley KJ, Allran K, Sherman SL, Hassold TJ, et al. Population-based study of congenital heart defects in down syndrome. American Journal of Medical Genetics. 1998 Nov 16;**80**(3):213-217. Available from: https://www.ncbi.nlm.nih.gov/pubmed/9843040

[77] Wessels MV, Los FJ, Frohn-Mulder JM, Niermeijer MF, Willems PJ, Wladimiroff JW. Poor outcome in down syndrome fetuses with cardiac anomalies or growth retardation. American Journal of Medical Genetics. Part A. 2003 Jan 15;**116A**(2):147-151. Available from: https://doi.org/10.1002/ajmg.a.10823

[78] Papavassilious P, York TP, Gursoy N, Hill G, Nicely LV, Sundaram U, et al. The phenotype of persons having mosaicim for trisomy 21/ down syndrome reflects the percentage of trisomic cells present in different tissues. American Journal of Medical Genetics. 2009 Feb 15;(4):573-583. Available from: https://dx.doi.org/10.1002%2Fajmg.a.32729

[79] Musewe NN, Alexander DJ, Teshima I, Smallhorn JF, Freedom RL. Echocardiographic evaluation of the spectrum of cardiac anomalies associated with trisomy 13 and trisomy 18. Journal of the American College of Cardiology. 1990 Mar 1;**15**(3):673-677. Available from: https://doi.org/10.1016/0735-1097(90)90644-5

[80] Balderton SM, Shaffer EM, Washington RL, Sondheimer HM. Congenital polyvalvular disease in trisomy 18: Echocardiographic diagnosis. Pediatric Cardiology. 1990 Jul;**11**(3):138-142. Available from: https://doi.org/10.1007/BF02238843

[81] Bull C. Current and potential impact of fetal diagnosis on prevalence and spectrum of serious congenital heart disease at term in the UK. British Paediatric Cardiac Association. Lancet. 1999 Oct 9;**354**(9186):1242-1247. Available from: http://dx.doi.org/10.1016/S0140-6736(99)01167-8

[82] Garne E, Stoll C, Clementi M. Evaluation of prenatal diagnosis of congenital heart diseases by ultrasound: Experience from 20 European registries. Ultrasound in Obstetrics & Gynecology. 2001 May;**17**(5):386-391. Available from: https://doi.org/10.1046/j.1469-0705.2001.00385.x

[83] Grandjean H, Larroque D, Levi S. The performance of routine ultrasonographic screening of pregnancies in the Eurofetus study. American Journal of Obstetrics and Gynecology. 1999 Aug;**181**(2):446-454. Available from: http://dx.doi.org/10.1016/S0002-9378(99)70577-6

[84] Montana E, Khoury MJ, Cragan JD, Sharma S, Dhar P, Fyfe D. Trends and outcomes after prenatal diagnosis of congenital cardiac malformations by fetal echocardiography in a well defined birth population, Atlanta, Georgia, 1990-1994. Journal of the American College of Cardiology. 1996 Dec;**28**(7):1805-1809. Available from https://doi.org/10.1016/S0735-1097(96)00381-6

[85] Chew C, Stone S, Donath SM, Penny DJ. Impact of antenatal screening on the presentation of infants with congenital heart disease to a cardiology unit. Journal of Paediatrics and Child Health. 2006;**42**:704-708. DOI: 10.1111/j.1440-1754.2006.00955.x

[86] Menahem S, Grimwade J. Counseling strategies in the prenatal diagnosis of major heart abnormality. Heart, Lung & Circulation. 2004;**13**(3):261-265. Available from: https://doi.org/10.1016/j.hlc.2004.06.009

[87] Stiimpflen I, Stumpflen A, Wimmer M, Bernaschek G. Effect of detailed fetal echocardiography as part of routine prenatal ultrasonographic screening on detection of congenital heart disease. Lancet. 1996 Sep 28;**348**(9031):854-857. Available from: https://doi.org/10.1016/S0140-6736(96)04069-X

[88] Lalor JG, Devane D, Begley CM. Unexpected diagnosis of fetal abnormality: women's encounters with care-givers. Birth. 2007 Mar;**34**(1):80-88. Available from: https://doi.org/10.1111/j.1523-536X.2006.00148.x

[89] Mellander M. Perinatal management, counselling and outcome of fetuses with congenital heart disease. Seminars in Fetal & Neonatal Medicine. 2005 Dec;**10**(6):586-593. Available from: https://doi.org/10.1016/j.siny.2005.08.002

[90] Allan LD, Huggon IC. Counselling following a diagnosis of congenital heart disease. Prenatal Diagnosis. 2004 Dec 30;**24**(13):1136-1142. Available from: https://doi.org/10.1002/pd.1071

[91] Menahem S, Gillam L. Fetal diagnosis—Obligations of the clinician: Case studies in the prenatal diagnosis of major heart abnormality. Fetal Diagnosis and Therapy. 2007;**22**:233-237. Available from: https://doi.org/10.1159/000098725

[92] Mone F, Walsh C, Mulcahy C, McMahon CJ, Farrell S, MacTiernan A, et al. Prenatal detection of structural cardiac defects and presence of associated anomalies: A retrospective observational study of 1262 fetal echocardiograms. Prenatal Diagnosis. 2015 Jun;**35**(6):577-582. Available from: https://doi.org/10.1002/pd.4575

[93] Practice bulletin no. 162: Prenatal diagnostic testing for genetic disorders. Obstetrics and Gynecology. 2016 May;**127**(5):e108-e122. Available from: https://doi.org/10.1097/AOG.0000000000001405

[94] Bratt EL, Jarvholm S, Ekman-Joelsson BM, Mattson LA, Mellander M. Parent's experiences of counselling and their need for support following a prenatal diagnosis of congenital heart disease—A qualitative study in a Swedish context. BMC Pregnancy and Childbirth. 2015 Aug;**15**:171. Available from: https://dx.doi.org/10.1186%2Fs12884-015-0610-4

[95] Zyblewski SC, Hill EG, Shirali G, Atz A, Forbus G, Gonzalez J, et al. Chromosomal anomalies influence parental treatment decisions in relation to prenatally diagnosed congenital heart disease. Pediatric Cardiology. 2009 Nov;**30**(8):1105-1111. Available from: https://doi.org/10.1007/s00246-009-9514-2

[96] Malhotra A, Menahem S, Gillam L. Ethical issues in Fetal management: A cardiac perspective. International Journal of Pediatrics;**2010**:6, Article ID 857460. Available from: http://dx.doi.org/10.1155/2010/857460. Review article

[97] Menahem S, Grimwade. Pre-natal counselling-helping couples make decisions following the diagnosis of severe heart disease. Early Human Development. 2005 Jul;**81**(7):601-607 Epub 2005 Apr 13. Available from: https://doi.org/10.1016/j.earlhumdev.2005.02.001

[98] Lee CK. Prenatal counseling of fetal congenital heart disease. Current Treatment Options in Cardiovascular Medicine. 2017 Jan;**19**(1):5. Available from: https://doi.org/10.1007/s11936-017-0502-1

[99] Andrews RE, Simpson JM, Sharland GK, Sullivan ID, Yates RW. Outcome after preterm delivery of infants antenatally diagnosed with congenital heart disease. The Journal of

Pediatrics. 2006 Feb;**148**(2):213-216. Available form: https://doi.org/10.1016/j.jpeds.2005.10.034

[100] Graf R, Ghanayem NS, Hoffmann R, Dasgupta M, Kessel M, Mitchell ME, et al. Impact of intrauterine growth restriction on cardiac surgical outcomes and resource use. The Annals of Thoracic Surgery. 2015 Oct;**100**(4):1411-1415. Available from: https://doi.org/10.1016/j.athoracsur.2015.05.064

[101] Curzon CL, Milford-Beland S, Li JS, O'Brien SM, Jacobs JP, Jacobs ML, et al. Cardiac surgery in infants with low birth weight is associated with increased mortality: Analysis of the Society of Thoracic Surgeons congenital heart database. The Journal of Thoracic and Cardiovascular Surgery. 2008 Mar;**135**(3):546-551. Available from: https://doi.org/10.1016/j.jtcvs.2007.09.068

[102] Jowett VC, Sankaran S, Rollings SL, Hall R, Kyle PM, Sharland GK. Foetal congenital heart disease: Obstetric management and time to first cardiac intervention in babies delivered at a tertiary centre. Cardiology in the Young. 2014 Jun;**24**(3):494-502. Available from: https://doi.org/10.1017/S1047951113000681

[103] Sanapo L, Moon-Grady AJ, Donofrio MT. Perinatal and delivery management of infants with congenital heart disease. Clinics in Perinatology. 2016 Mar;**43**(1):55-71. Available from: https://doi.org/10.1016/j.clp.2015.11.004

[104] Shinebourne EA, Carvalho JS. Ethics of fetal echocardiography. Editorial. Cardiology in the Young. 1996;**6**:261-263. Available from: https://doi.org/10.1017/S1047951100003875

[105] Garne E, Loane M, Dolk H. Prenatal diagnosis of severe structural congenital malformations in Europe. Ultrasound in Obstetrics & Gynecology. 2005 Jan;**25**(1):6-11. Available from: https://doi.org/10.1002/uog.1784

[106] Khoshnood B, De Vigan C, Vodovar V. Trends in prenatal diagnosis, pregnancy termination, and perinatal mortality of newborns with congenital heart disease in France, 1983e2000: A population-based evaluation. Pediatrics. 2005 Jan;**115**(1):95-101. Available from: https://doi.org/10.1542/peds.2004-0516

[107] Carvalho JS. Fetal heart scanning in the first trimester. Prenatal Diagnosis. 2004 Dec 30;**24**(13):1060-1067. Available from: https://doi.org/10.1002/pd.1063

[108] Brown SD, Truog RD, Johnson JA, Ecker JL. Do differences in the American Academy of Pediatrics and the American College of Obstetricians and Gynecologists positions on the ethics of maternal-fetal interventions reflect subtly divergent professional sensitivities to pregnant women and fetuses. Pediatrics. 2006 Apr;**117**(4):1382-1387. Available from: https://doi.org/10.1542/peds.2004-2724

[109] Simpson M, Sharland GK. Natural history and outcome of aortic stenosis diagnosed prenatally. Heart. 1997 Mar;**77**(3):205-210. Available from: https://www.ncbi.nlm.nih.gov/pmc/articles/PMC484683/

[110] Malhotra A, Menahem S, Shekleton P, Gillam L. Medical and ethical considerations in twin pregnancies discordant for serious cardiac disease. Journal of Perinatology. 2009 Oct;**29**(10):662-667. Available from: https://doi.org/10.1038/jp.2009.88

[111] Warnes CA, Liberthson R, Danielson GK, Dore A, Harris L, Hoffman JI, et al. Task force 1: The changing profile of congenital heart disease in adult life. Journal of the American College of Cardiology. 2001 Apr;**37**(5):1170-1175. Available from: https://doi.org/10.1016/S0735-1097(01)01272-4

[112] d'Udekem Y, Iyengar AJ, Galati JC, Forsdick V, Weintraub RG, Wheaton GR, et al. Redefining expectations of long-term survival after the Fontan procedure: Twenty-five years of follow-up from the entire population of Australia and New Zealand. Circulation. 2014 Sep 9;**130**(11 Suppl 1):S32-S38. Available from https://doi.org/10.1161/CIRCULATIONAHA.113.007764

[113] Marino BS, Lipkin PH, Newburger JW, Peacock G, Gerdes M, Gaynor JW, et al. Neurodevelopmental outcomes in children with congenital heart disease: Evaluation and management: A scientific statement from the American Heart Association. Circulation. 2012 Aug 28;**126**(9):1143-1172. Available from: https://doi.org/10.1161/CIR.0b013e318265ee8a

[114] Jansen FA, Everwijn SM, Scheepjens R, Stijnen T, Peeters-Scholte CM, van Lith JM, et al. Fetal brain imaging in isolated congenital heart defects—A systematic review and meta-analysis. Prenatal Diagnosis. 2016 Jul;**36**(7):601-613. Available from: https://doi.org/10.1002/pd.4842

[115] Zeigler VL. Congenital heart disease and genetics. Critical Care Nursing Clinics of North America. 2008 Jun;**20**(2):159-169. Available from: https://doi.org/10.1016/j.ccell.2008.01.008

[116] Cowan JR, Ware SM, et al. Genetics and genetic testing in congenital heart disease. Clinics in Perinatology. 2015 Jun;**42**(2):373-393. Available from: https://doi.org/10.1016/j.clp.2015.02.009

[117] Edwards JJ, Gelb BD, et al. Genetics of congenital heart disease. Current Opinion in Cardiology. 2016 May;**31**(3):235-241. Available from: https://doi.org/10.1097/HCO.0000000000000274

[118] Hoess K, Goldmuntz E, Pyeritz RE. Genetic counseling for congenital heart disease: New approaches for a new decade. Current Cardiology Reports. 2002 Jan;**4**(1):68-75. Available from: https://doi.org/10.1007/s11886-002-0129-y

[119] Blue GM, Kirk EP, Giannoulatou E, Sholler GF, Dunwoodie SL, Harvey RP, et al. Advances in the genetics of congenital heart disease. Journal of the American College of Cardiology. 2017 Feb 21;**69**(7):859-870. Available from: https://doi.org/10.1016/j.jacc.2016.11.060

[120] Connor JA, Hinton RB, Miller EM, Sund KL, Ruschman JG, Ware SM, et al. Genetic testing practices in infants with congenital heart disease. Congenital Heart Disease. 2014 Mar-Apr;**9**(2):158-167. Available from: https://doi.org/10.1111/chd.12112

[121] Richards AA, Garg V, et al. Genetics of congenital heart disease. Current Cardiology Reviews. 2010 May;**6**(2):91-97. Available from: https://dx.doi.org/10.2174%2F157340310791162703

[122] Fesslova V, Brankovic J, Lalatta F, Villa L, Meli V, Piazza L, et al. Recurrence of congenital heart disease in cases with familial risk screened prenatally by echocardiography. Journal of Pregnancy. 2011;**2011**:9, Article ID 368067. Available from: http://dx.doi.org/10.1155/2011/368067

[123] Goldmuntz E, Crenshaw M. Genetic Aspect of Congenital Heart Disease. Moss & Adams' Heart Disease in Infants, Children, and Adolescents: 87-115 (textbook). Available from: https://thoracickey.com/genetic-aspects-of-congenital-heart-defects/

[124] Johnson MC, Hing A, Wood MK, Watson MS. Chromosome abnormalities in congenital heart disease. American Journal of Medical Genetics. 1997 Jun 13;**70**(3):292-298. Available from: https://www.ncbi.nlm.nih.gov/pubmed/9188669

[125] Gatzoulis MA, Webb GD, Daubeney PE. Diagnosis and Management of Adult Congenital Heart Disease. 3rd ed. pp. 26-30. Available from: https://www.elsevier.com/books/diagnosis-and-management.../978-0-7020-6931-4

[126] Helm BM, Freeze SL. Genetic evaluation and use of chromosome microarray in patients with isolated heart defects: Benefits and challenges of a new model in cardiovascular care. Frontiers in Cardiovascular Medicine. 2016 Jun;**3**:19. Available from: https://dx.doi.org/10.3389%2Ffcvm.2016.00019

[127] Chromosome Disorder Support Group. Whales England. Understanding Chromosome Disorders: Florescence in situ hybridization. Unique 2013. Available from: www.rarechromo.org/information/Other/FISH%20FTNW.pdf.

[128] Wu X, Li R, Fu F, Pan M, Han J, Yang X, et al. Chromosome microarray analysis in the investigation of children with congenital heart disease. BMC Pediatrics. May 4;**17**(1):117. Available from: https://doi.org/10.1186/s12887-017-0863-3

[129] The Jackson Laboratory. What you Need to Know before Ordering Chromosomal Microarray. The Jackson Laboratory 1017. Available from: https://www.jax.org/education-and-learning/clinical-and-continuing-education/cancer-resources/deciding-to-test

[130] Blue GM, Winlaw DS. Next generation sequencing in congenital heart disease: Gene discovery and clinical application. Journal of Next Generation Sequencing and Applications;**2**(1). DOI: 10.4172/2469-9853.1000113

[131] LaHaye S, Corsmeier D, Basu M, Bowman JL, Fitzgerald-Butt S, Zender G, et al. Utilization of whole exome sequencing to identify causative mutations in familial congenital heart disease. Circulation. Cardiovascular Genetics. 2016 Aug;**9**:320-329. Available form: https://dx.doi.org/10.1161%2FCIRCGENETICS.115.001324

[132] Kuliev A, Pakhalchuk T, Rechitsky S. Preimplantation genetic diagnosis (PGD) for heart disease determined by genetic factors. Arrhythm Open Access. 2016;**1**(1). DOI: 10.4172/atoa.1000103

2

Congenital Abdominal Anomalies

Ples Liana and Anca Lesnic

Abstract

Introduction: Abdominal anomalies that appear during intrauterine life are complex due to many organs that are affected. In cases, the ultrasound appearance is a cystic image with different content and the differential diagnosis is often difficult. Body—research methods: the organs affected by abdominal congenital anomalies involve the gastrointestinal tract (stomach, duodenum, small bowel or colon, and gall bladder), the kidney and urinary tract, the peritoneal cavity (ascites), suprarenal glands, and tumors of the reproductive system (especially the ovaries). In order to identify the affected structures, it is mandatory to know the normal aspect of the abdominal content at different gestational ages. The diagnosis may be very difficult, but its accuracy is important, considering the need of further counseling the couple. In minor conditions, without chromosomal anomalies or associations, the outcome is usually good, and there are even possibilities of in utero treatment. In severe conditions, with poor outcome, the couple can choose to terminate the pregnancy, after counseling is provided. Conclusion: abdominal congenital anomalies are common findings in ultrasound screenings for anomalies in all the trimesters of pregnancy and their recognition is important for subsequent management.

Keywords: gastrointestinal anomalies, cystic anomalies, congenital anomalies of the kidney and urinary tract

1. Introduction

The chapter will be structured on four main sections: the normal ultrasonographic appearance of the fetal abdominal cavity and abdominal wall, the absence of the normal abdominal structures, abnormal structures present in the abdomen (cysts, tumors, etc.), and abdominal wall anomalies.

Abdominal anomalies that appear during intrauterine life are complex due to the number of different organs that are affected. In most cases, the ultrasound appearance is of a cystic image with different content, and the differential diagnosis is often difficult.

2. Congenital anomalies overview

Congenital anomalies of the abdominal contents involve organs of the gastrointestinal tract, kidneys and urinary tract, suprarenal glands, and genital organs (mainly the ovaries).

Anomalies in the fetal abdomen are diagnosed either by the lack of visualization of normal structures or evidence of abnormal images during the anomalies screening ultrasound examination. Therefore, obtaining and documenting standard normal images of the abdomen is of crucial importance.

This chapter is structured in 4 subsections:

2.1. Normal aspect of the fetal abdomen.

2.2. Anomalies consisting of absent structures.

2.3. Abnormal structures present in the abdomen: cystic or echoic masses.

2.4. Abdominal wall anomalies.

2.1. Normal ultrasound images of the abdomen

At the midtrimester routine ultrasound scan, there are a couple of images that must be obtained according to ISUOG guidelines [1], images that can rule out most of the abdominal pathological conditions.

First step of the examination should be visceral situs assessment, by demonstrating the position of the stomach, liver veins, abdominal aorta, and superior cava vein as seen in **Figures 1** and **2**.

The abdominal transverse section at the umbilical vein–portal sinus is the level for abdominal circumference measurement and a standard image to identify some important structures:

- fetal stomach-an anechoic structure of bean-like form. It can be seen from 9 weeks, but at 14 weeks, the different parts of the stomach can be seen and gastric peristalsis can be detected

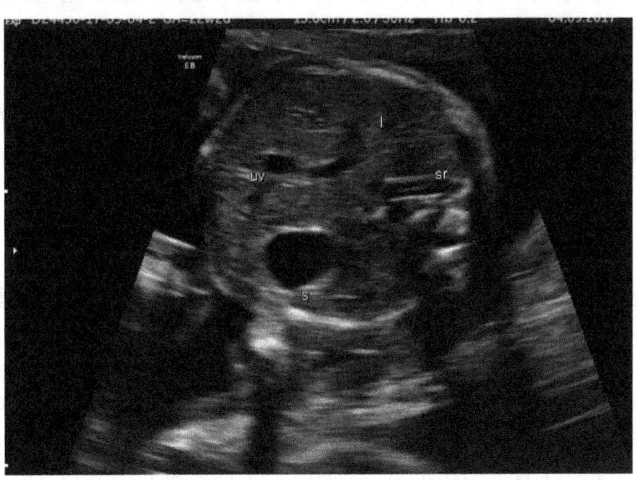

Figure 1. Transverse section of the fetal abdomen—the structures that can be seen are: stomach (s), umbilical vein (uv), liver (l), and suprarenal gland (sr).

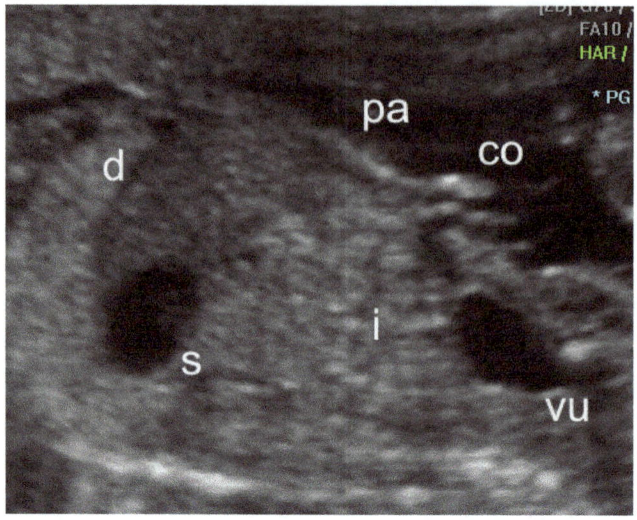

Figure 2. Sagittal section of the fetal abdomen—the continuity of the anterior abdominal wall is obvious (pa), the cord insertion (co), stomach (s), urinary bladder (vu), diaphragm (d), and bowel (i).

after 16 weeks of gestation. Nomograms of stomach size have been imagined at different gestational age [2]. Hyperechoic mass of uncertain origin may be seen inside the stomach and may disappear at the following examinations without pathological significance [3].

- fetal liver is an hypoechogenic structure that occupies the section on the right of the stomach.
- gall bladder is an ovoid, hypoechoic structure on the right and under the intrahepatic part of the umbilical vein.
- the umbilical vein has a caudal trajectory, penetrates the liver and connects with the left portal vein. Actually, the umbilical vein is the left portal vein, because the right portal vein regresses at 6–7 weeks.
- the anterior abdominal—skin, subcutaneous cellular tissue, and muscles.

The sagittal section at the abdominal level is essential for assessing the integrity of the anterior abdominal wall, because the insertion of the umbilical cord and the wall above and below the insertion can be visualized. Differentiating between the internal structures of the abdomen can be difficult, because the liver and intestinal loops have similar echogenicity. Between 8 and 10 weeks of gestation, the physiological gut herniation can be visualized by ultrasound, as a hyperechoic mass at the base of the umbilical cord. Reintegration occurs between 10 and 12 weeks and it is complete at approximately 11 weeks and 5 days.

At a lower transverse section of the abdomen, the kidneys, small bowel, and colon can be seen as the following:

- the kidneys are located on both sides of the spine; their adult similar shape can be recognized from 12 weeks but the medular/cortical differentiation is obvious starting from 15 weeks of gestation. The fluid filled structure of the calyces is a useful landmark to identify the kidneys. Corticomedullary differentiation (CMD) is determined according to echogenicity of the cortex and the medulla, considering that during the prenatal period, the normal renal cortex is as echogenic as the liver or spleen and that the normal renal medulla is relatively hypoechogenic, which leads to a well-defined CMD [4].

- the small bowel is visible as a uniform, echogenic mass that can be differentiated from the colon by its central layout, aspect, and peristaltic changes, until the third trimester when its aspect is of round anechoic image with peristalsis (large intestinal loops filled with meconium) [5].
- the colon appears as a tubular structure located at the periphery of the abdomen, meanwhile the small intestine is centrally placed. The haustration of the wall serves to differentiate from other anechoic or hypoechoic structures. Meconium production begins at 16 weeks of pregnancy, giving the ultrasound-like appearance of the intestinal wall.

The echogenicity of the colon is established in comparison to other structures such as the liver or bladder:

- grade 0: the abdomen is uniformly homogeneous and the colon cannot be visualized.
- grade 1: the colon is hypoechogenic, isoechoic with the stomach and the bladder, haustrations being present.
- grade 2: the colon's echogenicity is higher than the bladder, but lower than the liver and occurs after 29 weeks.
- grade 3: echogenicity is similar to the liver's and occurs after 34 weeks.

Coronal or sagittal section of the fetal abdomen allows the visualization of the urinary bladder. It can be identified starting at 11–12 weeks of gestation as an anechoic mass with a thin wall, delineated by two umbilical arteries.

2.2. Absence of normal abdominal structures

The most common condition is the nonvisualization of the stomach, kidneys, or urinary bladder.

Nonvisualization of the gall bladder occurs in rare chromosomal diseases, mucoviscidosis, and in 20% of the fetuses with biliary atresia [6].

Absent stomach or small stomach can be associated with mechanical or functional absence of stomach filling:

- absent or reduced fetal swallowing: facial clefts, neuromuscular conditions, infections, SNC conditions, and fetal hydrops.
- mechanical obstruction or compression: esophageal atresia, diaphragmatic hernia, and thoracic tumors.
- reduced amniotic fluid production: oligohydramnios of any cause.

2.2.1. Esophageal atresia

There are five types of esophageal atresia, but the most common one after de Jong is the type with esophageal stump and trachea-esophageal connection below the interruption. In such cases, it is important to look after other indirect signs, like polyhydramnios and small for gestational age. Many of the anomalies are nonisolated [7]. Still, 44% of the anomalies are not diagnosed during the prenatal period [7].

Esophageal atresia is a condition defined by the lack of continuity between the proximal and the distal esophagus. The missing portion is the middle one and the main cause is poor blood flow. The anomaly appears during the 8th week of pregnancy when the primitive intestine fails to divide forming the trachea anteriorly and esophagus posteriorly. According to de Jong, in 90% of cases, esotracheal fistulae are associated. There are five types of esophageal atresia considering the anatomical location of the defect and the existence of the tracheoesophageal fistula [7]:

- type A: without fistula
- type B: proximal fistula
- type C: distal fistula (88% of cases)
- type D: double fistula, proximal, and distal
- type E: existing fistula without concomitant atresia

The incidence of this anomaly is 1:3500 live born and usually is nonisolated, being associated with CNS anomalies, VACTERL association, T21, T18, diaphragmatic hernia, and abdominal wall anomalies. [7]. Twenty percent of cases of the associations are with chromosomal anomalies (trisomy 13, 18, 21) [8] and cardiac defects may be present in 50% of cases. VACTERL syndrome is comprised of vertebral defects, ventricular septal defect, anal atresia, esotracheal fistula, renal anomalies, radial aplasia, and single umbilical artery [9].

Ultrasound diagnosis of esophageal atresia can be missed in pregnancy according to Brandberg and 44% of the cases cannot be diagnosed.

The prenatal diagnosis of esophageal atresia is difficult due to the absence of specific signs. The rate of detection varies between 8 and 24% [10, 11], and the lack of detection is due in 85% of cases to the tracheoesophageal fistulae association.

Prenatal esophageal atresia must be suspected if polyhydramnios is present after the 25th week of gestation and if the gastric pouch is absent. Sometimes, gastric secretions are sufficient to distend the gastric pouch, and make the diagnosis more difficult; if an esotracheal fistula is present, the gastric pouch may appear normal. Sometimes, the distal dilated portion of the esophagus may be observed as a hypoechoic area in the mediastinum, behind the heart (blind pouch aspect). Although the sign has a great diagnostic value, it is rarely present before 25 weeks of gestation [8, 12, 13]. The detection rate is improved if an antenatal MRI is performed.

The differential ultrasound diagnosis can be made with other conditions with absent stomach, the most frequent are:

- facial cleft;
- congenital diaphragmatic hernia;
- neuromuscular conditions [9].

The risk of association with other anomalies, chromosomal and nonchromosomal, is high rising to 30–40% of cases: trisomy 21 and 18, VACTERL association. Perinatal approach implies karyotype analysis when the diagnosis is made. The birth should take place in a tertiary center with a neonatal intensive department considering the high risk of fetal hypotrophy (40% of cases) and prematurity (due to polyhydramnios). Surgical reconstruction of the esophagus is possible. The prognosis depends on the association with other congenital anomalies and on the gestational age at birth. After 32 weeks of gestation, if the prenatal diagnosis is achieved, reflux and aspiration pneumonia can be prevented and the survival rates are over 95%. Long time prognosis is affected by the high rate of postoperative complications [9]. The postoperative mortality is approximately 9%, with a intrauterine fetal mortality of 22%. Retrospective studies have shown a neonatal mortality of 75%.

2.2.2. *Absence of the kidney in the renal fossa*

It can be caused by renal agenesis or ectopic kidney. True isolated renal agenesis is confirmed by the absence of renal artery and is associated with oligoamnios if it is bilateral. Unilateral renal agenesis can be isolated but association as VACTERL is common [14]. Failing to visualize the urinary bladder can be caused more frequently by bilateral renal agenesis or exstrophy.

2.2.3. *Renal agenesis*

It is defined as bilateral absence of kidneys with an incidence variable from 1 to 3/10000 births and it is more frequent in male fetuses—**Figures 3** and **4**. Renal agenesis can be sporadic (due to teratogens or diabetes mellitus), isolated, or part of syndrome association, the most frequent found being:

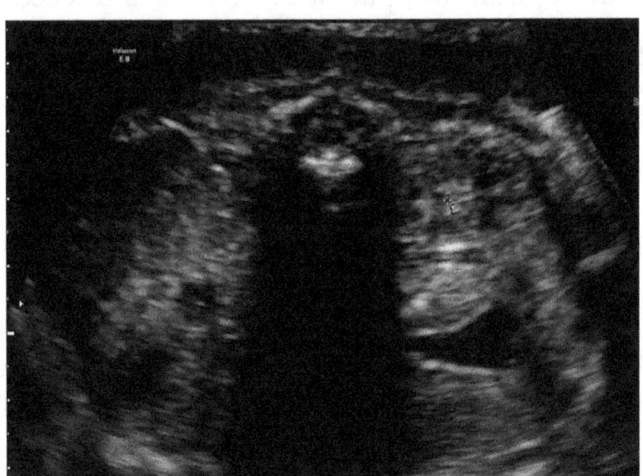

Figure 3. Renal agenesis—transverse abdominal section—no renal structure on the right side.

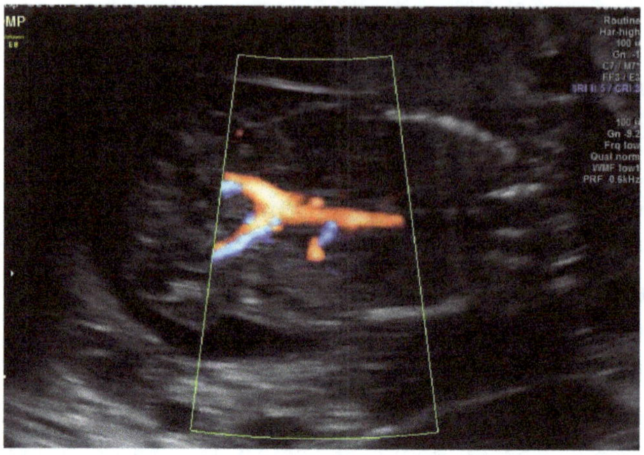

Figure 4. Unilateral renal agenesis—coronal section depicting only one renal artery.

- Cat's eye syndrome, characterized by iris coloboma, anal atresia, preauricular tags, and renal anomalies.
- 4p-Syndrome is characterized by multiple heterotopies of cells (in adrenals, brain, pancreas, and skin), renal agenesis, cardiac, facial, and genital anomalies.
- Fraser syndrome with: cryptophthalmos, syndactyly, auditory canal atresia, cleft palate, renal agenesis, and genital anomalies.
- a very severe syndrome: cerebro-oculo-facio-skeletal syndrome, characterized by: microcephaly, microphthalmia, narrow palpebral fissures, high nasal bridge, large ears, micrognathia, kyphosis, scoliosis, flexion contraction of the extremities, and rocker-bottom foot.
- in some cases, Müllerian duct anomalies can be associated.

Oligohydramnios is a constant finding in bilateral renal agenesis, and it can be seen from 14 weeks of gestation. "Potter syndrome" associates the following abnormalities:

- pulmonary hypoplasia.
- typical face—low set ears, epicanthus, parrot-beak nose, and receding chin.
- abnormal position of the hand and foot and bowed legs, clubbed feet, hip dislocation.
- intrauterine growth retardation.
- absence of urinary bladder visualization.

Ultrasound diagnosis of bilateral renal agenesis is based on three main elements:

- oligohydramnios.
- bilateral absence of the fetal kidney (sometimes the adrenal glands can be confused with the kidneys therefore the visualization of the normal cortical and medular structures is useful for exclusion).
- absence of the urinary bladder. If the urinary bladder is present the bilateral adrenal agenesis is excluded.

The differential diagnosis should include other anomalies of the kidney, associated with oligohydramnios as polycystic kidney disease, multicystic kidneys, etc.

When bilateral renal agenesis is suspected, a detailed examination of the fetal anatomy should be performed considering the high risk of other anomalies association [15]:

- Cardiovascular malformations (14%): tetralogy of Falloch, ventricular septal defect, atrial septal defect, hypoplastic left ventricle, coarctation of the aorta, dextrocardia, single ventricle, transposition of the great vessels, total anomalous pulmonary venous drainage, tricuspid atresia, and hypoplastic aorta.
- Musculoskeletal malformations (40%): absent radius and fibula, digital anomalies, lumbar hemivertebrae, cleft palate, sacral agenesis, and diaphragmatic hernia.
- Central nervous system malformations (11%) include hydrocephaly, microcephaly, meningocele, cephaloceles, holoprosencephaly, and iniencephaly.
- Gastrointestinal malformations (19%): duodenal atresia, imperforate anus, esotracheal fistula, intestinal malrotations, absent stomach or gallbladder, and omphalocele.
- Single umbilical artery.

The prognosis is usually lethal due to the association of pulmonary hypoplasia and growth retardation, the fetuses die in utero or in the first days of life.

2.2.4. *Bladder exstrophy*

Bladder exstrophy as well as cloacal exstrophy arise from the abnormal growth of the caudal fold, resulting in a anterior abdominal wall defect. The absence of the anterior abdominal wall and the anterior bladder wall will expose the posterior bladder wall to the amniotic fluid. Small defects result in epispadias, but a larger one might expose the posterior bladder wall. The incidence of bladder exstrophy is 1:30,000 births, with male fetuses being more affected [16]. These anomalies are frequently sporadic, although familial transmissions have been reported [16].

Positive and differential ultrasonographic diagnosis of bladder exstrophy should be suspected whenever the bladder cannot be visualized, even though the amniotic fluid volume is normal (the cycle of the bladder filling is 15 min)—**Figure 5**. Others ultrasound signs useful are:

- a solid hyperechoic mass that comes in close contact with the umbilical arteries.
- the absence of the bladder within the fetal pelvis.
- normal volume of the amniotic fluid.
- genital ambiguity (duplication and division of the penis).

Bladder exstrophy must be differentiated from gastroschisis and omphalocele. In those conditions, despite the abdominal wall defects, the bladder is still present within the fetal pelvis [17]. The risk of association with chromosomal and nonchromosomal syndromes is low. Perinatal counseling depends on the association with other anomalies. If the prenatal diagnosis of bladder exstrophy is made, therapeutic abortion must be offered as an option.

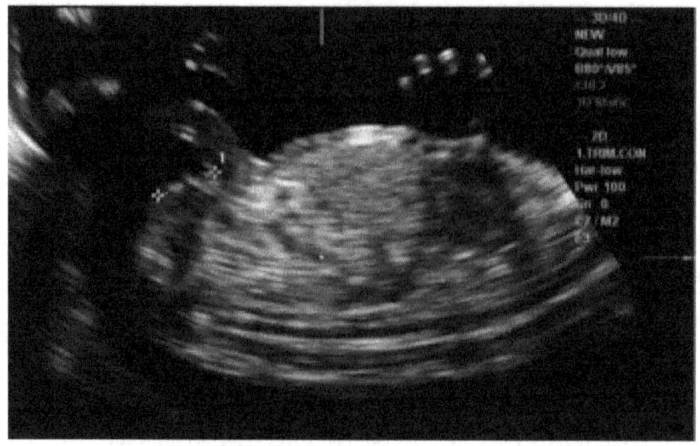

Figure 5. Bladder exstrophy—no urinary bladder can be seen.

The prognosis depends on the grade of urinary incontinence and the associated genital anomalies [17] with a survival rate of 80% in the cases where surgery interventions are needed to reconstruct the bladder wall and the genitalia. Although, it has been suggested that in the case of genital ambiguity, the sex should be deemed female, later follow-up has shown that the patients, male or female, can lead a normal life with a normal IQ and in some cases, corrective and fertility surgery can improve the quality of life.

2.3. Abnormal structures present in the abdomen: cystic or hypoechoic masses

The presence of cystic lesions in the fetal abdomen can have many underlying conditions. The diagnosis can be made upon their appearance: unique or multiple, the situs of the abnormal structure, and its relations with the abdominal viscera, the aspect of the wall and content. In most cases, the correct prenatal diagnosis of these structures is difficult to make and their origin can be determined only after birth.

Single cystic masses can be:

- megacystis,
- ovarian cysts,
- intestinal cysts (mesenteric or duplication intestinal cysts),
- choledocal cysts,
- hepatic cysts,
- kidney solitary cyst.

Multiple cystic lesions can be more frequent:

- double bubble image in duodenal atresia,
- bowel dilatations in obstruction conditions,
- multiple intestinal cysts,

- bowel volvulus,
- polycystic kidney,
- hydronephrosis,
- dilated megaureter in uretero-pelvic junction obstruction,

Other complex aspects involving hypo and hyperechoic structures can be found in:

- ascites,
- meconium peritonitis,
- liver calcification.

The differential diagnosis of the cystic abdominal proliferations includes:

- mesenteric cysts,
- omental cysts,
- choledochal cysts,
- renal cysts,
- intestinal obstruction,
- intestinal duplication,
- meconium peritonitis-related cysts,
- anterior meningomyelocele,
- ovarian cysts,
- hydrometrocolpos,
- megacystis,
- the persistence of the cloaca.

2.3.1. Duodenal atresia

It is defined as the obstruction of the bowel produced by a degenerated middle segment of the duodenum. It can be also extrinsic due to a malformed annular pancreas or fibrous peritoneal bands that cause compression. The most frequent affected segments are the 2nd and the 3rd segment of the duodenum. With an incidence is 1:10,000 births, it is the second main cause of small bowel obstruction [18].

The diagnosis is suspected in the presence of polyhydramnios and it is based on the "double bubble" sign (**Figure 6**) formed by the stomach and the proximal part of the duodenum, both appearing dilated. This sign may be present from 19 weeks, but usually it is seen in the second part of the pregnancy or even later due to the fetal capacity of swallowing small amounts

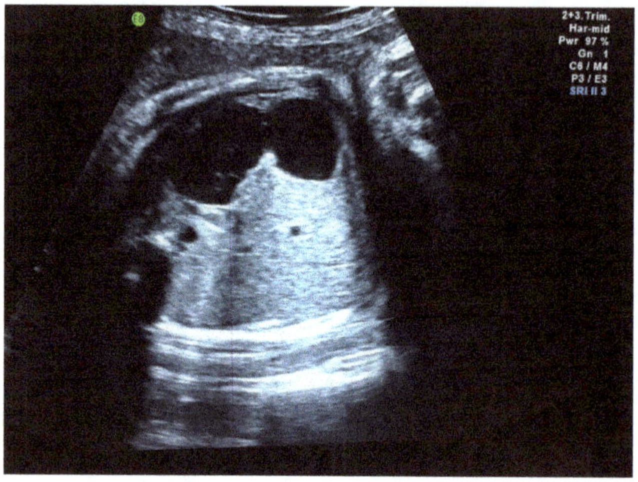

Figure 6. Duodenal atresia—double bubble sign.

of liquid and delaying the dilatation of the intestine. Sometimes, the only consistent sign at repeated scans is a dilated stomach. Differential ultrasonographic diagnosis should be made with other cystic structures present in the upper or inferior abdomen:

- persistent right umbilical vein or varicose veins pertaining to the umbilical vein.
- choledocal cyst.
- hepatic cyst.
- intestinal duplication cyst.
- ovarian cysts.
- kidney cyst or multicystic dysplastic kidney.
- mesenteric cysts.
- urachal cyst.
- ureterocele.
- pyelectasis.

Duodenal atresia has a high risk (62%) of association with chromosomal anomalies and associated anomalies mainly with Down syndrome. Duodenal atresia is a sporadic anomaly, but it has been demonstrated that it can be transmitted in an autosomal recessive manner. Almost half of the fetuses with duodenal atresia manifest other anomalies: skeletal defects (vertebral and rib abnormalities, sacral agenesis, esotracheal fistula, intestinal malrotation, Meckel's diverticulum, and anorectal atresia), renal and cardiac defects. Because of the close vicinity with the Vater Ampulla, in 1% of cases biliary duct anomalies are present. Gall bladder atresia is impossible to diagnose before birth, but it can be suspected, if duodenal atresia is present and the gall bladder cannot be visualized [18].

The prognosis of isolated duodenal atresia is favorable, the rate of survival after corrective surgery is over 95%. The incidence of early postoperative mortality is between 3 and 5%, and the long term postoperative mortality rate is 6%. Considering the high risk of chromosomal anomalies association, the karyotype analysis is mandatory whenever duodenal atresia diagnosis is made prenatally, and also a careful examination of the fetus anatomy. Polyhydramnios can cause preterm birth and although vaginal delivery is allowed, it must take place in a tertiary unit to assure proper care for the neonate.

2.3.2. Intestinal obstruction

Intestinal obstruction is defined by the total or partial intestinal obstruction, which can occur in an intrinsic or extrinsic manner. The intrinsic lesions are caused by intestine stenosis or atresia. In the case of atresia, the two intestinal segments can be completely separated or tied by a fibrous band. In the case of intestinal stenosis, the two segments can be separated by a septum or a central diaphragm or the intestinal lumen is very narrow. "Apple-peel" atresia is characterized by the absence of an important intestinal segment that can include the distal duodenum, the entire jejunum, or the proximal ileum—**Figure 7**. Conditions that can produce extrinsic obstruction are most frequently represented by:

- intestinal malrotations with volvulus,
- peritoneal adherences,
- meconium ileus.
- Hirschsprung's disease.

The intestinal areas affected in the order of frequency are: the distal ileum (35%), the proximal jejunum (30%), distal jejunum (20%), proximal ileum (15%), or it can be multicentric in approximately 5% of cases. Anorectal atresia results from an abnormal cloacal division in the 9 weeks of gestation [5]. The incidence of intestinal obstruction is 1:2000 births. In half of the cases, obstruction of the small intestine is present, and the other half is made up by anorectal atresia.

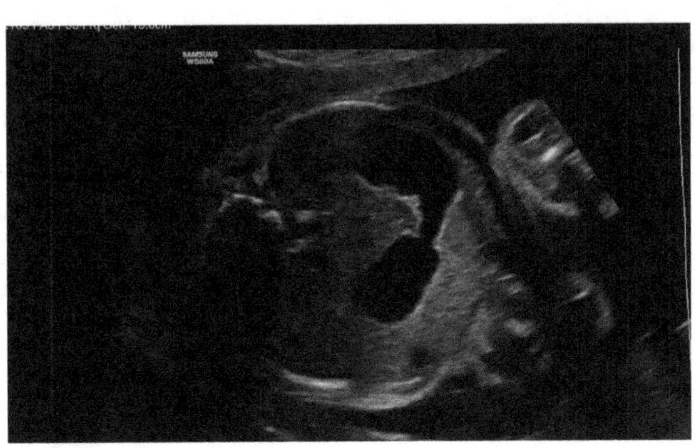

Figure 7. Duodenal stenosis—in utero image.

Intestinal obstruction is usually sporadic, but it can have a genetic transmission when the affected areas are multiple. Anorectal atresia is associated in 80% of cases with vertebral defects, genitourinary, cardiac and other gastrointestinal abnormalities. The association with chromosomal or other anomalies is rare.

Ultrasound diagnosis is usually possible beyond 25 weeks of gestation, due to the slowly dilation progression. The size of the intestinal lumen does not exceed 2–7 mm. The jejunum and ileum obstructions aspect is of dilations of the intestinal loops with active peristalsis. The fetal abdomen is fully distended and the majority of cases also present polyhydramnios, especially in the case of proximal obstructions. Similar images of the fetal abdomen can be found in Hirschsprung's disease. Transitory ascites or meconium peritonitis can appear when intestinal perforations occur [5]. When intestinal obstruction is diagnosed, the work-up to exclude other intestinal tract anomalies, ovarian cysts, mesenteric cysts, or intestinal duplication cysts is mandatory. Anorectal atresia is difficult to diagnose prenatally due to the great distension of the proximal bowel and the normal amount of amniotic fluid. Occasionally, calcification of the fetal meconium may be present within the fetal pelvis.

The prognosis depends on the type and location of the obstructed site and on the association of other anomalies. Considering that polyhydramnios that can occur, preterm births are common and the birth should take place in a tertiary unit. After birth, the affected babies develop emesis and abdominal distention, and can require immediate surgery repair. For isolated obstructions, requiring small resections of the intestine, the survival rates are over 95%. The resection of a large intestinal segment can lead to a lethal syndrome—short gut syndrome.

2.3.3. Hirschsprung's disease

It is caused by the congenital absence of intramural parasympathetic ganglia of the colon. The deficiency is caused by the lack in neuroblast migration from the neural crest, which occurs between the 6th and the 12th week of development. Also, the degeneration of the already migrated neuroblasts, which can occur before or after birth, may be involved. The incidence is approximately 1:3000 births. This disease is usually sporadic, but in 5% of cases there is a familial transmission. In a small number of cases, Hirschsprung's disease is associated with Down syndrome.

Ultrasound diagnosis can be suspected in the presence of the dilatation of the intestinal lumen produced by abnormal peristaltic movements. At the ultrasound scan, images are similar to those found in anorectal atresia, in which the colon is also affected. Similarly, when the small intestine loops are affected, the images are of an obstruction with dilated intestinal loops and polyhydramnios. The prognosis depends on the postnatal postoperative evolution, which aims to resect the affected intestinal segment, and can include a temporary colostoma with a neonatal mortality rate of 20%. Considering the prematurity risk due to associated polyhydramnios and the need for postnatal surgery, the birth must take place in a tertiary unit, but cesarean birth is not mandatory.

2.3.4. Choledochal cysts

They are defined as cystic dilatations of the common bile duct; they are rare and are usually of unknown etiology. The diagnosis is made in the presence of a transonic image located in the upper right abdominal quadrant. The differential diagnosis includes intestinal duplication cysts, hepatic cysts, situs inversus, and duodenal atresia. The absence of polyhydramnios and the presence of intestinal peristalsis are useful for excluding intestinal obstruction. Common complications that intervene after birth are: biliary cirrhosis, hypertension, lithiasis, and rarely—adenocarcinoma. The complications can be prevented by early postnatal diagnosis and surgical resection. Surgical mortality rate is about 10% [19].

2.3.5. Mesenteric and omentum cysts

They are usually an accumulation of lymphatic fluid produced by lymphatic hamartomas or blockage of the lymphatic drainage. Ultrasound diagnosis can be suspected in the presence of a hypoechoic lesion located usually on the midline. The cysts can vary in size, their content can be unilocular or multilocular, or filled with echoic masses with solid content caused by secondary hemorrhage. The cysts can be filled with serous, hemorrhagic, or chylous fluid.

The prognosis of the cyst depends on the possible complications: intestinal obstruction, torsion, and hemorrhage. Malignant transformation of the cysts is rare. Prenatally, the cysts require drainage by puncture, only when they are of important size and can cause compression and secondary hydrops. After birth, the management is surgical but a complete resection of the cysts is difficult because of the close vicinity with large vessels and because of the 20% rate of recurrence.

2.3.6. Hepatic cysts

Hepatic cysts are a rare finding in the prenatal life. Usually, they are located in the right hepatic lobe and can produce obstruction of the intrahepatic biliary system. Their ultrasound aspect is of a unilocular anechoic round structure. Even after birth, they are asymptomatic and complications like infections and hemorrhage rarely occur. In approximately 30% of cases, hepatic cysts are associated with polycystic renal disease [19].

2.3.7. Duplication intestinal cysts

Duplication intestinal cysts are rare but located throughout the entire gastrointestinal tract. They appear in the form of tubular-like structures of variable sizes, and can occur singularly or associated with renal malformations, adenomatous cystic lung malformations, and lung sequestration. The thickening of the cystic wall and the peristaltic movements make the diagnostic process easier. The surgical excision of the cysts is the only therapeutic choice.

2.3.8. Ovarian cysts

Ovarian cysts are the most frequent fetal tumors and they are a relatively frequent finding during fetal autopsy (approximately 1/3 of fetuses). The cysts are usually asymptomatic and small. Ovarian fetal cysts are hormone-dependent (influenced by the human chorionic gonadotropin hormone, estrogens, and placenta hormones) and appear after 25 weeks of gestation [20].

Ovarian cysts (**Figure 8**) appear as anechoic round images located laterally to the urinary bladder. They are unilateral and unilocular and appear most frequently in isoimmunization-affected fetuses or those coming from pregnancies associated with diabetes, probably due to placental hyperplasia.

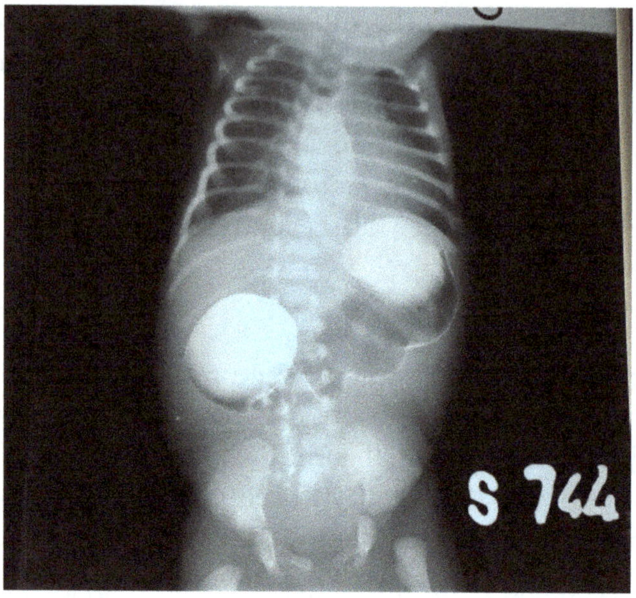

Figure 8. Duodenal stenosis—same case after birth.

The clear majority of the ovarian cysts is benign and resolves spontaneously after birth. The differential diagnosis has to be made with hydrocolpos, a condition that manifests itself as a hypoechoic or hyperechoic pelvic mass in a female fetus [20]. The prognosis is usually good but complications may appear like: torsion of the cysts, ascites, intracystic hemorrhage, rupture of the cysts, or cyst infarction. In such cases, the inner aspect of the cyst can change and speckles or hyperechoic structures inside the cyst can appear. When the cysts are large, intestinal compression could induce polyhydramnios. In such cases, cyst puncture and amnio-drainage should be considered. There is no need for cesarean section, but when the risk of premature birth is high due to polyhydramnios, birth should take place in a tertiary unit.

2.3.9. Congenital hydronephrosis

It is defined by a dilatation of the renal pelvis and calyceal system that exceeds the normal size according to the age of gestation (anteroposterior diameter of the renal pelvis over 4 mm at 20 weeks and over 7 mm at 32 weeks)—**Figures 9** and **10**. The most frequent cause is the ureteropelvic junction obstruction. When dilatation of the ureter occurs, the obstruction is lower usually at the vesicoureteral junction [21]. It is more common in males than in females, with a sex ratio of 5:1. Ureteropelvic junction obstruction is usually sporadic, but can also be inherited.

Anatomic causes that produce ureteropelvic junction obstruction are: fibrous adhesions, bands, kinks, ureteral valves, aberrant lower pole vessels, abnormal ureteral insertion, and unusual shapes of the pyeloureteral outlet. They can be associated with urinary anomalies and extraurinary anomalies: vesicoureteral reflux, bilateral ureteral duplication, bilateral obstructed megaureter, contralateral nonfunctioning kidney, contralateral renal agenesis, Hirschsprung's disease, cardiovascular abnormalities, neural tube defects, sagittal synostosis, mandibular hypoplasia, esophageal atresia and distal fistula, imperforate anus, syndactyly, congenital hip dislocation, and adrenogenital syndrome.

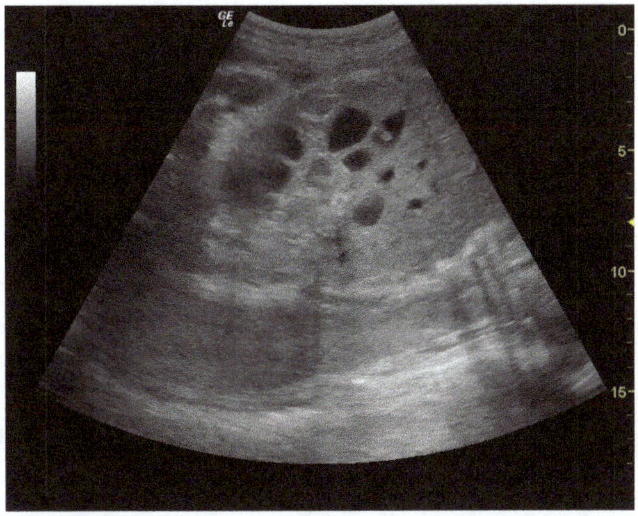

Figure 9. Intestinal obstruction—small bowel dilatations above the obstruction level.

Ultrasound diagnosis is based on the evidence of the dilated renal pelvis and on the measurement of the anteroposterior diameter of the dilatation on transverse abdominal section. Former criteria of hydronephrosis dilatation included also the ratio between the maximum transverse pelvic diameter and the renal diameter at the same level with ratios above 50% being the cut-off for hydronephrosis. Most UPJ obstructions are unilateral and bladder should fill normally. In case of severe oligohydramnios, association of unilateral hydronephrosis contralateral renal agenesis or dysplasia should be suspected. Differential diagnosis includes multicystic dysplastic kidneys, polycystic kidneys, and other condition associated with anechoic abdominal masses [22].

The prognosis of ureteropelvic obstruction is generally good, but requires serial ultrasound scans to evaluate the progress of the dilatation. In most cases, the surgery is not needed, but the postsurgery mortality is absent [23].

Concerning the prenatal management, there is no need for premature intervention and vaginal birth is preferred (**Figures 11** and **12**).

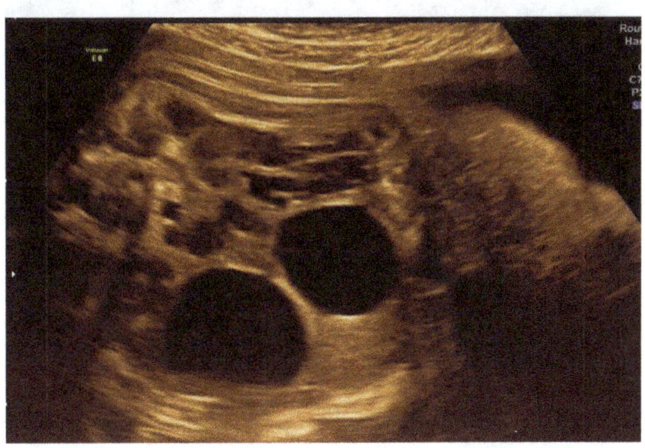

Figure 10. Ovarian cyst—two anechoic round structures in the fetal pelvis with no Doppler signal.

2.3.10. Multicystic kidney disease

It is a congenital disorder characterized by cystic lesions that correspond primarily to dilated collecting tubules. The disease can be bilateral, unilateral, or segmental and it is known also as Potter's type II syndrome, cystic kidney disease, and multicystic dysplastic kidneys.

It can be isolated or associated with urinary or extraurinary disorders such as: malrotations, ureteropelvic junction obstruction, horseshoe kidney, cardiovascular malformations, CNS abnormalities (anencephaly, hydrocephalus, iniencephaly, spina bifida, occipital meningocele), diaphragmatic hernia, cleft palate, microphthalmia, duodenal stenosis and imperforate anus, esotracheal fistula, and bilateral absence of radius and thumb. Association with liver cysts or pancreatic cysts is not characteristic for Potter II syndrome [24].

Ultrasound diagnosis of multicystic kidneys (**Figure 11**) is made in the presence of an enlarged unilateral or bilateral kidney with multiple round anechoic structures peripheral located and variable in size. In some cases, the kidneys can be small but the renal sinus cannot be identified. Oligohydramnios is a common association, but in some cases, when the lesion is unilateral or the obstruction is incomplete, amniotic fluid may have normal volume.

Differential diagnosis includes infantile polycystic kidney disease, single cyst, ureteropelvic junction obstruction, Wilms tumor and hamartoma that has undergone necrosis, but can be difficult to diagnose prenatally.

The prognosis of bilateral disease is poor and termination of pregnancy can be offered. Unilateral isolated disease prognosis can be favorable, but delivery should take place in a tertiary unit (**Figures 13** and **14**).

2.3.11. Autosomal dominant polycystic kidney disease (ADPKD)

Adult polycystic kidney disease (APKD) is an autosomal dominant condition characterized by the presence of multiple cysts of variable size in the renal parenchyma. The cysts can replace the parenchyma and are produced by the dilatation of the collecting tubules and other tubular segments

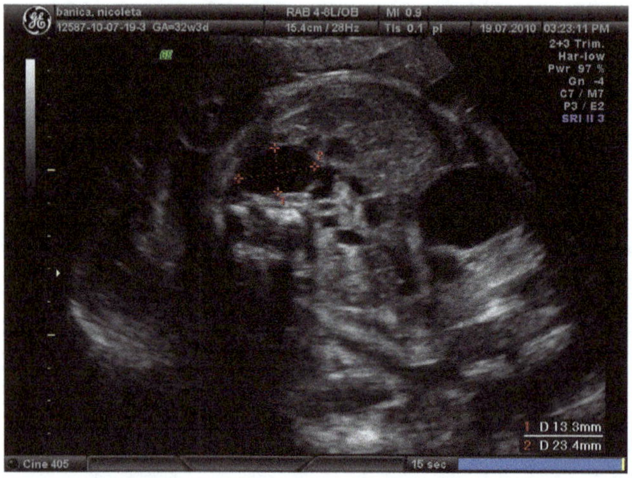

Figure 11. Hydronephrosis—significant dilatation of the renal pelvis and reduced thickens of the renal functional tissue.

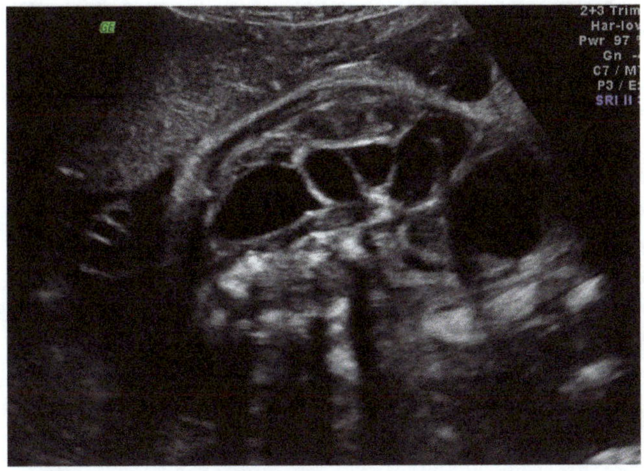

Figure 12. Ureteral dilatation consecutive to uretro-vesical obstruction.

of the nephrons. Potter's type III polycystic is one of the entities responsible for ADPKD in which cysts of variable sizes (some up to several centimeters) coexists with normal renal structure. Being an autosomal dominant disease, the risk of transmission to the off springs of the altered gene on chromosome 16 is 1/2 pregnancies. APKD is one of the most common genetic disorders and the third most prevalent cause of chronic renal failure [25]. Epigenetic factors and penetrance of the gene determine the variability in symptoms, the disease manifesting late in the fourth decade. Intrauterine manifestation of the disease is not uncommon [26]. APKD is associated with cysts affecting other organs: liver, pancreas, spleen, lungs, testes, ovaries, and epididymis.

Prenatal diagnosis is difficult and often late due to the nonspecific appearance of the kidneys; only a few of these diagnoses can be recognized in the prenatal period, by family history, amniotic fluid volume, associated abnormalities, and genetic testing [4].

Ultrasound diagnosis of the APKD can be suspected in the presence of moderately enlarged hyperechogenic kidneys, with increased corticomedullary differentiation (CMD), in association with a normal amount of amniotic fluid. The diagnosis is usually late and should prompt investigation of both parents.

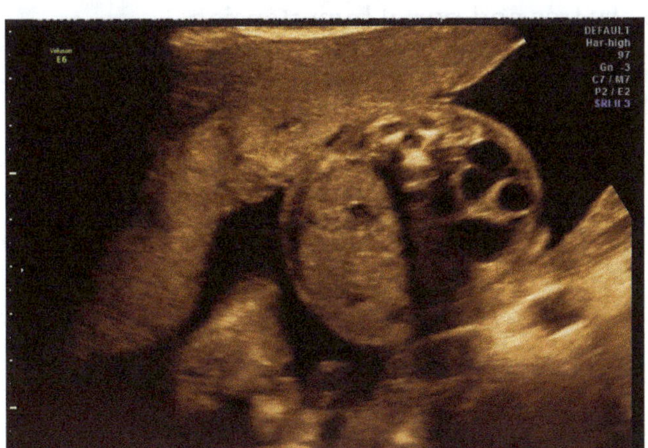

Figure 13. Multicystic kidney—multiple anechoic round structures occupying the whole renal aria with no remaining normal renal structure.

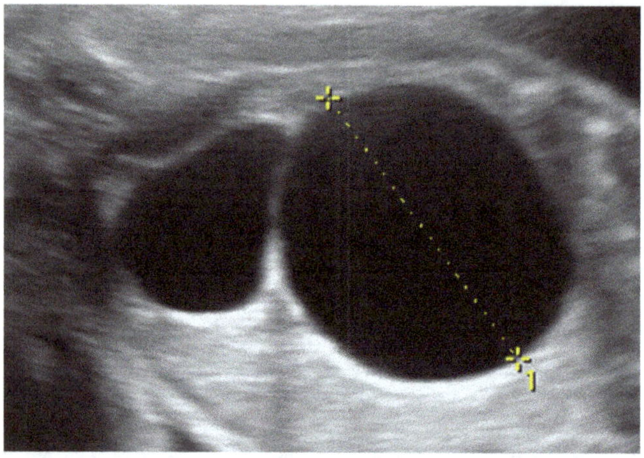

Figure 14. Giant kidney cyst.

The prognosis depends on other associated anomalies. The parents must be informed that the immediate outcome can be good, but the natural history of the disease includes the following: from completely asymptomatic to lower abdominal pain, renal enlargement, renal insufficiency, uremia and hypertension, with a mean age of onset of symptoms in the fourth decade of life.

Obstetrical management is based on the gestational age at diagnosis; in the first trimester, pregnancy termination can be offered. Family members should undergo ultrasound examination as well. The fetus must be thoroughly scanned to exclude other anomalies. Otherwise, the obstetrical attitude is not altered and vaginal birth is the first choice (**Figure 15**).

2.3.12. Infantile polycystic kidney disease

Infantile polycystic kidney disease (IPKD) is an autosomal recessive disorder characterized by bilateral and symmetrical enlargement of the kidneys. The disease is known also as polycystic kidney disease type I, infantile polycystic disease of the liver and kidney. Unlike the adult polycystic kidney disease, there is no renal parenchyma, only dilated collecting tubules [27]. As a recessive autosomal inherited condition, the risk of transmission is 25%. The disease is always bilateral. Other anomalies that can be associated: liver cysts, biliary duct hyperplasia, and dilatation of the biliary tree and portal hypertension.

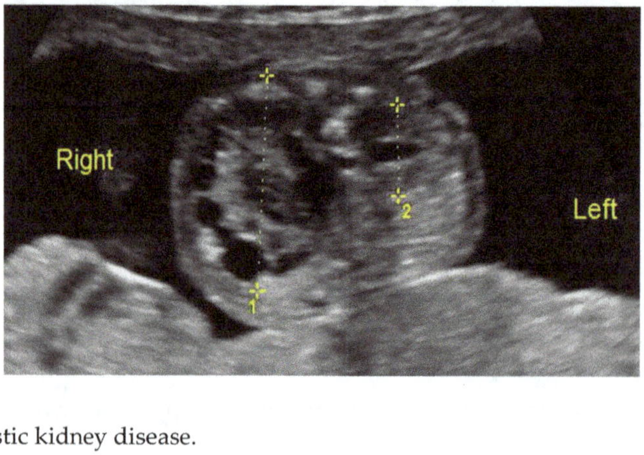

Figure 15. Autosomal polycystic kidney disease.

Ultrasound diagnosis is based on three elements:

- bilaterally enlarged kidneys of typical hyperechogenic texture.
- oligohydramnios.
- absent fetal bladder.

The disease can be diagnosed late in pregnancy or may progress gradually during pregnancy; therefore, repeated scans are mandatory.

The prognosis depends on the clinical variety of IPKD, which can vary from mild to severe with intrauterine death. After birth, the most important complications are respiratory, as a consequence of the pulmonary hypoplasia. Death later in life is the result of renal failure.

The management depends on the diagnosis age; if the diagnosis is made before viability, termination of pregnancy should be offered to the parents. Also in cases with severe oligohydramnios and absent bladder, the termination of pregnancy can be offered even in the third trimester.

2.3.13. Megacystis

It represents an enlarged urinary bladder usually due to a bladder outlet obstruction [lower urinary tract obstruction (LUTO)], which may appear also in nonobstructive conditions (megacystis-microcolon-intestinal hypoperistalsis syndrome). It can be detected from the first trimester scan in about 1 in 1500 pregnancies [28].

Prognosis, management, prediction of resolution, and postnatal outcome depend on the subsequent cause. Fetal lower urinary tract obstruction (LUTO) has an incidence of 2.2/10000 births and it is usually diagnosed during the late first or early second trimester of pregnancy [28, 29]. The most common condition in the LUTO spectrum includes urethral valves, urethral atresia, and urethral stenosis.

2.3.14. Posterior urethral valves

It is a condition that causes lower urinary tract obstruction due to a membrane-like structure in the posterior urethra of male fetuses. The disease is usually sporadic, and has a heterogeneous embryologic origin. Young type I syndrome valves seem to result from an exaggerated development of the urethrovaginal folds with an abnormal insertion of the distal end of the Wolffian ducts. Other valves, like in Young type III, develop because of abnormal canalization of the urogenital membrane [30]. Distention of the bladder (megacystis) leads to vesicoureteral reflux and hydronephrosis and can cause renal dysplasia [30].

Posterior urethral valves can be associated with other anomalies of the urinary tract (sequence) megacystis, megaureter, hydronephrosis, paraureteral diverticula, and dilatation of proximal urethra, cryptorchidism, and hypospadias. There are also extraurinary anomalies that can be associated: tracheal hypoplasia, patent ductus arteriosus, total anomalous pulmonary vein drainage, mitral stenosis, scoliosis, skeletal anomalies in lower extremities, and imperforate anus. The most frequent chromosomal abnormalities that can be associated are: trisomies 18 and 13, del 2q, and 69 XXY.

Ultrasound diagnosis can be made in the presence of megacystis, hydroureter, and hydronephrosis in a male infant. In female fetus, lower urinary tract obstruction includes agenesis of the urethra, megacystis-microcolon-intestinal hypoperistalsis syndrome, and variants of the caudal regression syndrome. When the rupture of the megacystis intervenes, urine can extravasate into the peritoneal cavity. Oligohydramnios can also occur.

The differential diagnosis is difficult in prenatal life, and includes ureteropelvic junction obstruction, ureterovesical junction obstruction, primary megaureter, and massive vesicoureteral reflux, absence of the urethra or detrusor hypertrophy.

Prognosis depends on the renal reserve, which can be difficult to assess prenatally. Another factor that can influence the outcome is the timing of the occurrence of urinary obstruction, and this is a critical factor: the earlier its appearance–the worse the prognosis. Complications include: pneumomediastinum and pneumothorax, related to pulmonary hypoplasia, associated congenital anomalies, renal failure, and surgical complications after decompressive surgery. Termination of pregnancy can be offered if the prognosis is poor and if other anomalies are associated. In utero vesicoamniotic shunts are possible, but the results at 2 years of life are not very encouraging [31].

2.3.15. Meconium peritonitis

Intestinal perforation in fetuses during pregnancy can lead to a sterile, chemical, and localized type of peritonitis. At the site of the perforation, a reactive process of calcification and fibrosis occurs in order to stop the progression. The etiology is in over 50% of cases due to intestinal stenosis, atresia, or meconium ileus. Other cited situations are volvulus or Meckel's diverticulitis. Meconium ileus is associated with cystic fibrosis and results from the blockage of the distal ileum with compacted meconium. The incidence is 1:3000 births.

The diagnosis is suggested by the dilatation of the intestinal loops or the presence of hyperechoic areas situated in the abdomen of the fetus. Over 80% of the fetuses that developed meconium peritonitis also have intra-abdominal calcifications. Ascites is an important sign of intestinal peritonitis. Other ultrasonographic signs suggesting meconium peritonitis include: polyhydramnios, meconial pseudocysts, thickening of the abdominal wall or pleural effusions.

The differential diagnosis of hyperechoic abdominal masses include: intra-amniotic hemorrhage, early ascites, fetal hypoxia, meconium peritonitis, and cystic fibrosis.

Meconium ileus and hyperechoic images of the intestinal loops at 16–18 weeks of gestation can be present in over 75% of cystic fibrosis affected fetuses. The incidence of cystic fibrosis in fetuses diagnosed before birth with intestinal obstruction is approximately 10%, consequently when other causes of intestinal blockage have been excluded, a genetic cystic fibrosis test is recommended.

The prognosis is poor in this case; approximately, 50% of fetuses suffering from meconium peritonitis pass away in the neonatal period.

2.3.16. Liver calcifications

Most of them are idiopathic, but can be associated with congenital infections and chromosomal anomalies. The incidence rate is 1:2000 fetuses, especially in the 3rd trimester. The ultrasonographic image is of hyperechoic nodules situated in the liver parenchyma or liver capsule. The diagnosis is easy in the presence of solitary or multiple hyperechoic images (size between 1 and 2 mm) situated in the liver parenchyma or capsule. The prognosis depends on the association with infections or chromosomal anomalies. Isolated calcifications do not have pathological significance.

2.4. Abdominal wall anomalies

The evaluation is the integrity of the abdominal wall is part of routine midtrimester scan, although it can be performed starting with the first trimester examination. Conditions as: oligoamnios, placenta, or uterine wall proximity, excessive movement of the fetus can obstruct the proper visualization of the abdominal anterior wall. It is very important that the integrity of the abdominal wall is assessed by showing the insertion of the umbilical cord and visualization of the bladder in the pelvis, so that that bladder and cloacal exstrophy can be excluded.

The abdominal wall anomalies will be discussed separately in a subsequent chapter.

Author details

Ples Liana[1*] and Anca Lesnic[2]

*Address all correspondence to: plesliana@gmail.com

1 UMF Carol Davila, Bucharest, Romania

2 Bucur Maternity, Bucharest, Romania

References

[1] Salmon LJ, Alfirevic Z, Berghella V, Bilardo C, Hernandez-Andrade E, Johnsen SL, Kalache K, Leung K-Y, Malinger G, Munoz H, Toi A. Practice guidelines for performance of the routine mid-trimester ultrasound scan. Ultrasound in Obstetrics & Gynecology. 2011;**37**:111-126

[2] Goldstein I, Reece EA, Yarkoni S, et al. Growth of the fetal stomach in normal pregnancies. Obstetrics and Gynecology. Oct 1987;**70**(4):641-644

[3] Fakhry J, Shapiro LR, Schechter A, et al. Fetal gastric pseudomasses. Journal of Ultrasound in Medicine. 1987;**6**:177

[4] Brun M, Maugey-Laulom B, Eurin D, Didier F, Avni EF. Prenatal sonographic patterns in autosomal dominant polycystic kidney disease: A multicenter study. Ultrasound in Obstetrics & Gynecology. 2004;**24**:55-61. DOI: 10.1002/uog.1098

[5] Nyberg DA, Mack LA, Patten RM, Cyr DR. Fetal bowel: Normal sonographic findings. Journal of Ultrasound in Medicine. 1987;**6**:3

[6] Shen O, Rabinowitz R, Yagel S, Gal M. Absent gallbladder on fetal ultrasound: Prenatal findings and postnatal outcome. Ultrasound in Obstetrics & Gynecology. Jun 2011;**37**(6): 673-677

[7] de Jong EM, Felix JF, de Klein A, Tibboel D. Ethiology of the esopagheal atresia and tracheoesopahean fistula: Mind the gap. Current Gastroenterology Reports. 2010;**12**:215-222

[8] Kalache KD, Chaoui R, Mau H, Bollmann R. The upper neck pouch sign: A prenatal sonographic marker for esophageal atresia. Ultrasound in Obstetrics & Gynecology. 1998;**11**: 138-140

[9] Malinger G, Levine A, Rotmenschi S. The fetal esophagus: anatomical and physiological ultrasonographic characterization using a high-resolution linear transducer. Ultrasound Obstet Gynecol. 2004;**24**:500-505

[10] Sparey C, Jawaheer G, Barret A, Robson S. Oesophageal atresia in the northern region 1985±1997: Prenatal diagnosis and outcome. American Journal of Obstetrics and Gynecology. Feb 2000;**182**(2):427-431

[11] Spitz L. Esophageal atresia: Past, present, and future. J Pediatric Surg. 1996;**31**:19-25

[12] Engum S, Grosfeld J, West K, Rescorla F, Scherer LT. Analysis of morbidity and mortality in 227 cases of oesophageal atresia and/or tracheo-oesophageal ® stula over two decades. Archives of Surgery. 1995;**130**:502-508

[13] Vijayaraghavan SB. Antenatal diagnosis of oesophageal atresia with tracheo-oesophageal ® stula. Journal of Ultrasound in Medicine. 1996;**15**:417-419

[14] Brantberg A, Blaas H-GK, Haugen SE, Eik-Nes SH. Esophageal obstruction-prenatal detection rate and outcome. Ultrasound in Obstetrics & Gynecology. 2007;**30**:180-187

[15] Ryckewaert-D'Halluin A, Le Bouar G, Odent S, Milon J, 'Hervé D, D, Lucas J, Rouget F, Loget P, Poulain P, Le Gall E, Taque S. Diagnosis of fetal urinary tract malformations: Prenatal management and postnatal outcome. Prenatal Diagnosis. November 2011;**31**(11): 1013-1020

[16] Baird PA, MacDonald EC. An epidemiologic study of congenital malformations of the anterior abdominal wall in more than half a million consecutive live births. American Journal of Human Genetics. 1981;**33**:470

[17] David AL, Tan A, Curry J. Gastroschisis: Sonographic diagnosis, associations, management and outcome. Prenat Diagn. 2008;**28**:633-644. Published online 13 June 2008 in Wiley InterScience

[18] Brantberg A, Blaas H-GK, Salvesen KÅ, Haugen SE, Møllerløkken G, Eik-Nes Fetal SH. Duodenal obstructions: Increased risk of prenatal sudden death. Ultrasound in Obstetrics & Gynecology. 2002;**20**:439-446

[19] Leombroni M, Buca D, Celentano C, Liberati M, Bascietto F, Gustapane S, Marrone L, Manzoli L, Rizzo G, D'Antonio F. Outcomes associated with fetal hepatobiliary cysts: Systematic review and meta-analysis. Ultrasound in Obstetrics & Gynecology. 2017; **50**(2):167-174

[20] Heling K-S, Chaoui R, Kirchmair F, Stadie S, Bollmann R. Fetal ovarian cysts: Prenatal diagnosis, management and postnatal outcome. Ultrasound in Obstetrics & Gynecology. 2002;**20**(1):47-50

[21] Sohn YK, Han SY, Chun DW, Park JS, Jun JK, Yoon BH, Syn HC, Lee HP. Fetal hydronephrosis—Natural history and predictors of postnatal outcome. Ultrasound in Obstetrics & Gynecology. October 2001;**18**(s1):64

[22] Ouzmanian JG, Castro MA, Fusquez M, al-Sulyman OM, Kovacz BW. Prognostic significance of antenatally detected fetal pyelectasis. Ultrasound in Obstetrics & Gynecology. 1996;**7**:424-428

[23] Corteville JE, Gray DL, Crane JP. Congenital hydronephrosis correlation of fetal ultrasonograpic findings with infant outcome. American Journal of Obstetrics and Gynecology. 1991;**165**:384-388

[24] Damen-Elias HAM, Stoutenbeek PH, Visser GHA, Nikkels PGJ, de Jong TPVM. Concomitant anomalies in 100 children with unilateral multicystic kidney. Ultrasound in Obstetrics & Gynecology. 2005;**25**(4):384-388

[25] Demetriou K, Tziakouri C, Anninou K, Eleftheriou A, Koptides M, Nicolaou A, Deltas CC, Pierides A. Autosomal dominant polycystic kidney disease-type 2. Ultrasound, geneticand clinical correlations. Nephrology, Dialysis, Transplantation. 2000;**15**:205-211

[26] MacDermot KD, Saggar-Malik AK, Economides DL, Jeffery S. Prenatal diagnosis of autosomal dominant polycystic kidney disease (PKD1) presenting in utero and prognosis for very earlyonset disease. Journal of Medical Genetics. 1998;**35**:13-16

[27] Bronshtein M, Bar-Hava I, Blumenfeld Z. Clues and pitfalls in the early prenatal diagnosis of 'late onset' infantile polycystic kidney. Prenatal Diagnosis. 1992;**12**(4):293-298

[28] Sebire NJ, Von Kaisenberg C, Rubio C, Snijders RJ, Nicolaides KH. Fetal megacystis at 10-14 weeks of gestation. Ultrasound in Obstetrics & Gynecology. Dec 1996;**8**:387-390

[29] McHugo J, Whittle M. Enlarged fetal bladders: Aetiology, management and outcome. Prenatal Diagnosis. Nov 2001;**21**:958-963

[30] Kelalis, King, Belman, editors. Clinical Pediatric Urology. 2nd ed. Philadelphia: Saunders; 1985;**1**:527-558

[31] Nassr AA, Shazly SAM, Abdelmagied AM, Araujo Júnior E, Tonni G, Kilby MD, Ruano R. Effectiveness of vesicoamniotic shunt in fetuses with congenital lower urinary tract obstruction: an updated systematic review and meta-analysis. Ultrasound in Obstetrics & Gynecology. 2017;**49**(6):696-703

3

Congenital Anomalies of Urinary Tract and Anomalies of Fetal Genitalia

Sidonia Maria Sandulescu, Ramona Mircea Vicol, Adela Serban, Andreea Veliscu Carp and Vaduva Cristian

Abstract

Congenital anomalies of the kidney, urinary tract and genitalia anomalies are among the most frequent types of congenital malformations. Many can be diagnosed by means of ultrasound examination during pregnancy. Some will be discovered after birth. Kidney and urinary malformations represent 20% of all birth defects, appearing in 3–7 cases at 1000 live births. Environmental factors (maternal diabetes or intrauterine exposure to angiotensin-converting enzyme inhibitors) and genetic factors (inherited types of diseases) seem to be among causes that lead to the disturbance of normal nephrogenesis and generate anomalies of the reno-urinary tract. It is very important to diagnose and differentiate between the abnormalities incompatible with life and those that are asymptomatic in the newborn. The former requires interruption of pregnancy, whereas the latter could lead to saving the renal function if diagnosed antenatally. In many cases, the congenital anomalies of the urinary and genital tract may remain asymptomatic for a long time, even up until adulthood, and can be at times the only manifestation of a complex systemic disease. Some can manifest in more than one member in the family. This is the reason why the accurate genetic characterization is needed; it can help give not only the patient but also her family the appropriate genetic counseling, and also, in some cases, the management may prevent severe complications.

Keywords: genital, urinary, kidney, anomalies, fetal, malformation

1. Introduction

The congenital anomalies of the urinary tract include a large number of diseases caused by anomalies in the morphogenesis of the urinary system. These anomalies include obstructive and nonobstructive dilatation of the urinary tract that can be associated with alterations in the number, size and/or position of the kidneys [1, 2].

We will discuss the congenital anomalies of the urinary and genital tract, with a short review of kidney abnormalities. These malformations may coexist within the same case, and this is due to their common embryonic origin [3].

The reno-urinary anomalies occur more frequently in males than in females, the ratio being 2.5:1 (M-F), and there are many cases with family aggregation. The incidence is 3–4 at 1000 lives or 1–5% of all pregnancies [4, 5]. If including all cases detected at post-mortem fetal autopsies, the prevalence of these malformations is much higher [2].

2. Congenital anomalies of urinary tract

2.1. Relevant embryology

The urogenital system is represented by two major components: the urinary system and the genital system. Embryological and fetal kidneys, genital tract and the urinary system develop from intermediate mesoderm. The rhythm of growth and development of the collector tubes differs greatly during pregnancy. Until 15 weeks of gestation, the rhythm of development is very rapid and later decreases [1, 2].

The urinary tract is almost entirely developed from the intermediate mesoderm. The evolution implies different stages in development: pronephros, mesonephros and metanephros. These stages will appear successively in the craniocaudal direction and coexist over time. Intermediate mesoderm is divided in the upper cervical and thoracic region, resulting in nephrotomes [2, 3].

The mesonephric duct will give rise to the ureteral bud after the formation of the pronephros. This, after 15 generations of divisions, will lead to the formation of the ureter, the calves, the collector tubes and the kidney pelvis. The lack of formation or agenesis of the pronephros or of the mesonephric duct can lead to the total or partial absence of the kidney or to other anomalies of the reno-urinary tract [4, 5].

CAKUT (congenital anomalies of kidney and urinary tract) may be part of multi-organ processes in single-gene disorders, with dominant or recessive inheritance, as we can find in Fraser syndrome, the branchiootorenal syndrome, Kallmann syndrome, Ehlers-Danlos syndrome and others [5, 6].

The genitalia differentiation, which leads to female or male gender, starts at 7–8 weeks of pregnancy and finalizes at 12–13 weeks. Every fetus will develop female characteristics, because at the beginning of gestational period, the Mullerian and Wolffian structures coexist. If the Mullerian structure will suffer atrophy, due to testosterone and anti-Mullerian hormone effects, male sex structures will develop from the Wolffian structure, and the fetus will become a male. In the opposite circumstance, the fetus will become a female. In conclusion, from the embryological point of view, an individual could be a female if the masculine features will not develop [7, 8].

2.2. Classification

Congenital urinary abnormalities are often associated with the kidney anomalies, and there is a wide range of malformations resulting from disorders in the normal development process [9].

Malformations of renal parenchyma may occur due to the abnormal nephron development—in cases of renal dysplasia, renal agenesis and renal polycystic disease. The migration abnormalities of kidney embryo buds are found in renal ectopy and in the mismatched malformations [10].

Abnormalities in the development of the urinary tract system cause duplicated collective systems, posterior urethral valves and obstructions of the pyeloureteral junction. Defects may be unilateral or bilateral, and several types of defects may be associated [1–3, 6, 7].

The anomalies of the urinary system can be divided into nephropathies and uropathies:

a. Nephropathy involves the renal parenchyma and refers to multicystic kidney disease (MCDK), renal dysplasia disease, renal agenesis defect, congenital polycystic kidney disease and other anomalies (nephromegaly, trisomy 13, Meckel syndrome, Beckwith-Wiedemann syndrome) [6–8].

b. Uropathies represent the pathology of the urinary tract, and by the site of the defect, they can be pyeloureteral and ureterovesical, or they can refer to the vesicoureteral reflux and to the posterior urethral valve. Many authors also consider here the urachal fistula, the urachal cyst and the exstrophy of the urinary bladder [10–12].

For a better understanding of urinary tract abnormalities, we will summarize the classification of kidney malformations that may accompany these anomalies:

I. Anomalies in number

a. *Complete bilateral renal agenesis* is a rare condition, not compatible with extrauterine life. The physical appearance of the babies is very characteristic (the so-called Potter syndrome). The absence of the kidneys may be suspected before conventional postmortem autopsy. Fetal ultrasound examination is very difficult, due to the absence of amniotic fluid.

b. *Unilateral renal agenesis* or the 'congenital solitary kidney' is probably the most difficult diagnosis of renal malformations. There is a consensus in terms of a definitive diagnosis, autopsy being the only conclusive method.

c. *Renal aplasia*—there is a fetal bud, but it does not develop into a normal functioning organ. The pelvis and ureter are usually absent or are rudimentary.

d. *Supernumerary kidney* is the rarest anomaly and consists of a third kidney with excretory cavities and its own vascularity, completely separated from the other kidney [1–8].

II. Renal size abnormalities

a. *Renal hypoplasia.* There are small congenital kidneys, located next to the median line and excretory cavities. The renal function is normal or low.

b. *Kidney hyperplasia.* There is a large kidney, after ruling out any other cause [5–7].

III. Kidney's shape abnormalities

a. *Lobular kidney.* There is a persistence of fetal lobulation.

b. *Kidney fusion.* There are bilateral symmetrical or asymmetrical mergers or unilateral asymmetry.

c. *The kidney in the horseshoe.* In 90% of the cases, kidneys join at the lower pole through a parenchymal or fibrous bridge.

d. *Bilateral asymmetric mergers.* One of the kidneys is smaller than the other.

e. *Unilateral asymmetric fusions.* There is a single kidney mass with a crossed ectopic kidney, known as 'the sigmoid kidney', usually located in the pelvis [7–10].

VI. Renal position abnormalities

a. *Ectopic kidney.* A birth defect given by an abnormal (unilateral or bilateral) kidney position. The ectopic kidney is more often located on the left side. There are several ectopic kidney types: the caudal (lumbar, iliac, sacral) kidney, the cranial kidney and the crossed kidney.

b. *Renal dystopia.* Initially, in embryonic life, the hill and pelvis are located in the anterior part, and then they undergo a rotation around the longitudinal axis, until they reach the median side [1–4, 7].

V. Multicystic renal dysplasia

These are large and hyperechogenic kidneys, including renal ciliopathies. These conditions may be divided into autosomal dominant diseases and autosomal recessive disorders, including the polycystic kidney disease, renal dysplasia, glomerulocystic kidney disease (trisomy 13 and trisomy 18, Beemer syndrome), multicystic dysplastic kidneys (MCDK), medullary cystic dysplasia (Meckel-Gruber and Beckwith-Wiedemann syndromes, as well as congenital infections) [10–13].

2.3. Diagnosis

Nowadays, the fetal bladder and kidneys may be visualized starting with 11 weeks (by transvaginal echography) or 12 weeks (by means of transabdominal echography). The fetal bladder and kidneys are located near the spine, having an elliptical shape [1, 2].

In the first trimester of pregnancy, the kidneys appear as an ovoid structure located on both sides of the spine (**Figure 1**) [1–4].

Renal urine production begins during week 9 of embryonic life, making it possible to visualize the bladder, as a fluid collection in the fetal pelvis. The bladder appears spherical and transonic and is located between the iliac bone centers of ossification, in the lower pelvis. It can be visualized starting with the ninth week of pregnancy, and the umbilical arteries can be visualized laterally next to the bladder. Beyond the first trimester, the bladder will fill and empty in an intermittent manner, every 25–30 minutes, due to the influence of hormonal factors on the bladder (**Figure 2**) [2, 3].

Normal ureters cannot be visualized by means of echography. The ratio of renal circumference to abdominal circumference is 0.27–0.30 and remains constant during pregnancy [8].

Evaluation of the urinary tract also requires the evaluation of the amniotic fluid volume. After the 14th week of intrauterine life, the amniotic fluid comes mainly from the production of fetal urine and only one-third of its quantity comes from the pulmonary fluid [2, 5].

For a correct diagnosis, the clinician has to perform a complete examination in all of the three planes, the coronal, the sagittal and the longitudinal plane, using 2D grayscale and color Doppler. The examination should be complete. Sometimes, the ultrasound examination has to be completed by another screening method. Due to the association between renal malformations and other congenital defects or chromosomal anomalies, performing an invasive diagnosis method may be required [14].

The renal pelvic dilatation (RPD) is the most common of the abnormalities that can be detected during antenatal ultrasonography and is probably the most frequent sign of a reno-urinary

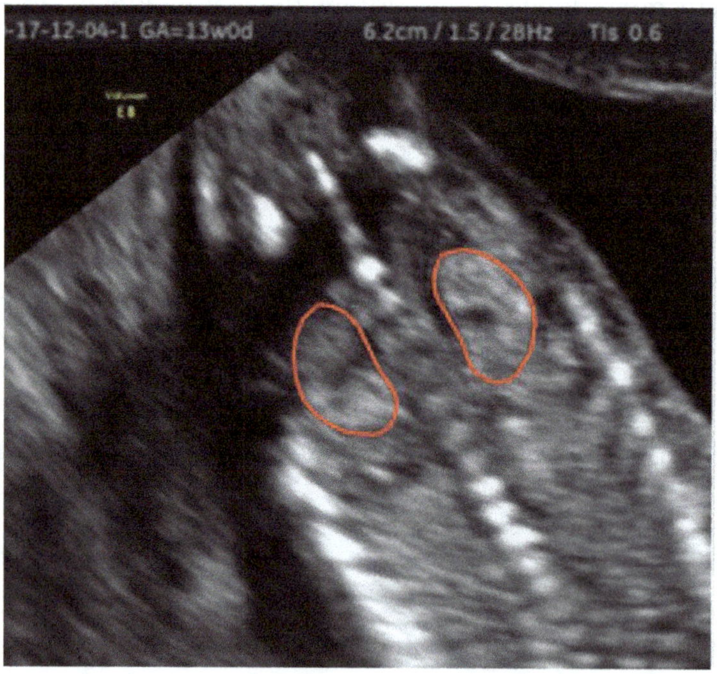

Figure 1. Fetal kidneys in the first trimester of pregnancy.

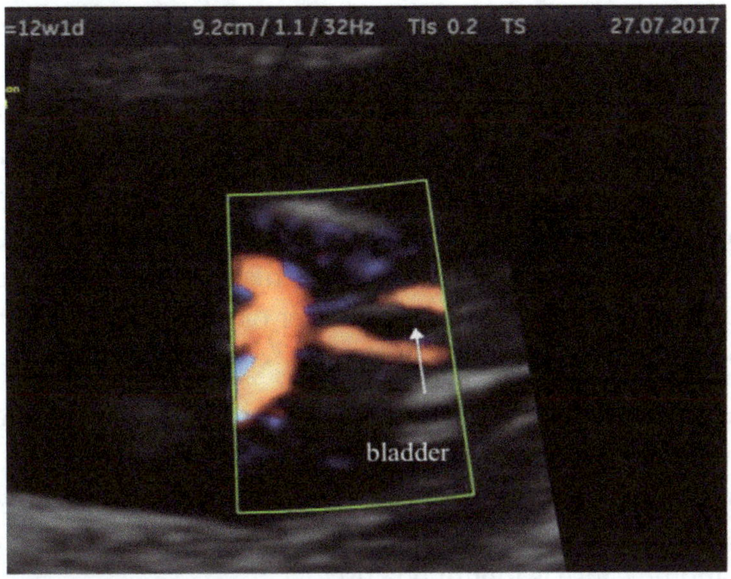

Figure 2. The bladder in the first trimester of pregnancy.

anomaly. The diagnosis of the RPD is based on an increased anteroposterior diameter of the renal pelvis in the transverse plane, and the value allows classification: severe, moderate or mild RPD. Normal values of anteroposterior diameter of the kidney pelvis are up to 4 mm at week 16 of pregnancy, less than 7 mm at 28 weeks of pregnancy and less than 10 mm postnatal [15].

In many cases a transient dilatation occurs. This situation is caused by narrowing or natural folds of the urinary tract that may occur during the early stages of development. Transient dilatation is usually less than 6 mm in the second trimester and less than 8 mm in the third trimester. It usually resolves spontaneously or disappear postnatally [16].

- Many authors concluded that for an accurate diagnosis, the assessment of the renal and urinary function may be performed by ultrasound [5, 6]. The following statements gained acceptance:
- The amount of amniotic fluid is an indirect indicator of the kidney function.
- The bladder filling indicates the normal functioning of at least one kidney.
- The absence of the bladder filling may indicate renal agenesis and bilateral ureteral obstruction.
- The bladder distension may hide a urethral reflux problem.
- The ureteral dilatation may be caused by a lower obstruction of the inferior urinary tract.
- The echogenicity of renal parenchyma cannot be considered for the renal function assessment.
- The increasing rebound pressure in the renal artery may cause renal function [5–12].

2.4. Uropathies

Uropathies are the most common reno-urinary abnormalities diagnosed during the prenatal period and may be caused by obstructive or nonobstructive factors [10–13]. The most common urinary malformations encountered in children are vesicoureteral reflux (VUR), obstructive megaureter, posterior urethral valve and megacystis [11].

Fetal hydronephrosis may result in a number of conditions, like pelvic or vesicoureteral junction obstruction, posterior urethral valves, vesicoureteral reflux, pelvic-ureteric junction obstruction and other rare congenital anomalies [12, 13]. A clear definition of hydronephrosis would be that it is a dilatation of the calyces and the renal pelvis of over 10 mm or more than 50% of the anteroposterior diameter of the kidney. This dilatation of the urinary system may occur at the upper urethral segment, ureters, bladder or kidney pelvis. Pyelectasis is the dilatation of the renal pelvis only (**Figure 3**) [6, 15].

By some authors, the clinician can diagnose hydronephrosis if the renal pelvic AP diameter is increased over 4 mm in the second trimester and 7 mm in the third trimester [3, 11, 15] (**Figure 4**). A renal pelvic AP diameter > 15 mm is strongly associated with a pathology of the urinary tract that requires treatment after birth. However, in the majority of cases, the renal pelvis is mildly or moderately dilated, and no cause is identified [16].

There is no clear consensus on the follow-up and management of mild or moderate hydronephrosis observed on antenatal ultrasound, although it is generally accepted that a postnatal assessment should be performed if the AP diameter of the renal pelvis exceeds 10 mm at any point in gestation [17].

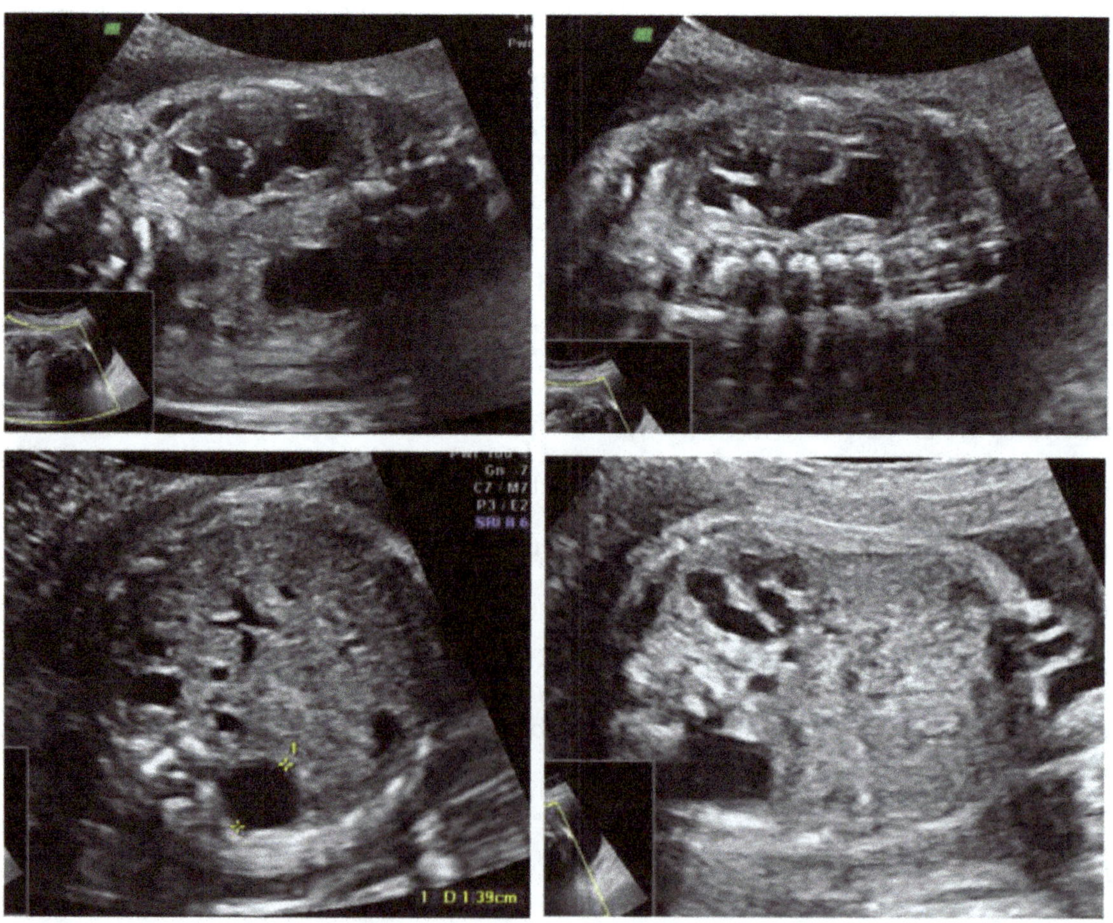

Figure 3. Second trimester: different aspects in hydronephrosis cases.

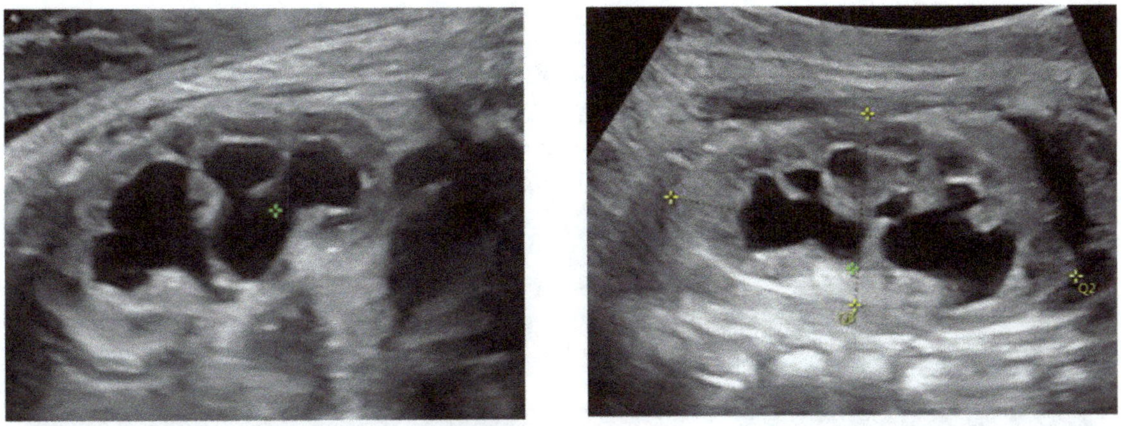

Figure 4. Hydronephrosis in the third trimester of pregnancy.

Many studies show that a right or left prenatal AP renal pelvic diameter > 4 mm is associated with a higher risk of postnatal hydronephrosis compared with a right and left prenatal AP renal pelvic diameter ≤ 4 mm [15, 16]. Male neonates have a higher risk of postnatal hydronephrosis than females. These results can assist in establishing the appropriate follow-up method and evaluation of fetuses with renal pelvic dilatation [18, 19].

2.5. Ureteral malformations

In medical practice many abnormalities can occur, like:

- Number abnormalities
- Structure abnormalities
- Calibration abnormalities
- Vesicoureteral reflux (VUR)
- Abnormalities of the pyeloureteral junction
- Position and opening abnormalities [1, 2, 14]

a. Ureteral abnormalities

- Ureteral agenesis is accompanied by the absence of the ipsilateral kidney. It may be uni- or bilateral, the latter being incompatible with life.
- Incomplete ureteral duplication (ureter fissus or ureter bifid)—a double-sided pyeloureteral system: the ureters bend before opening into the bladder through a single orifice.
- Complete ureteral duplication (duplex ureter)—a double-sided pyeloureteral collection system: the ureters open through separate boreholes in the bladder, one in orthoposition and the other in the ectopic position (**Figure 5**) [15–17].

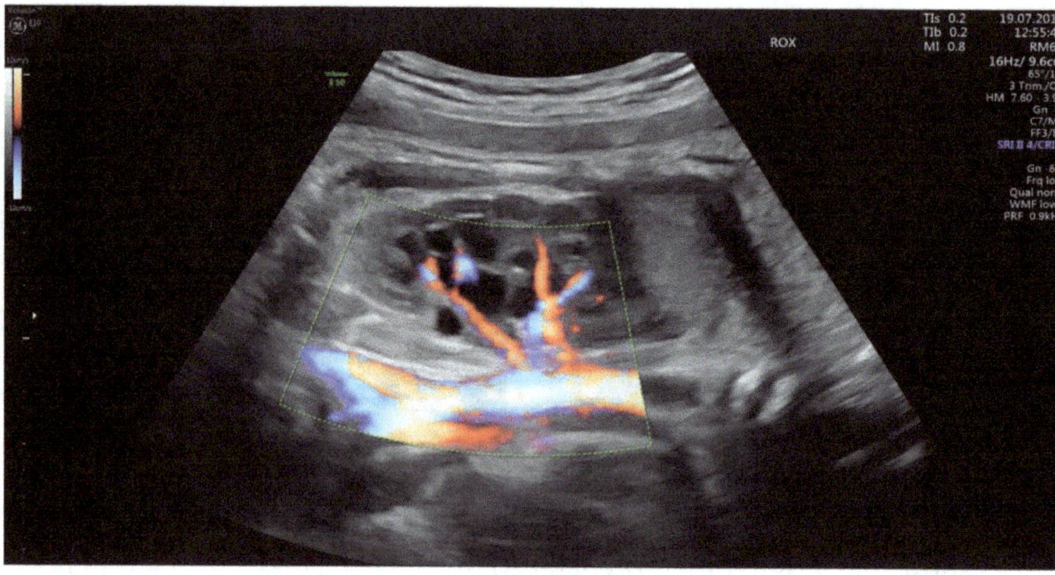

Figure 5. Coronal section and high-definition power color Doppler, in a supernumerary kidney cases. Visualization of the double renal artery.

b. The ureteropelvic junction obstruction

Obstruction of the ureterobladder junction (obstructive megaureter) or obstruction on pyeloureteral junction is one of the most common causes of hydronephrosis found in children, its incidence being 1 case in 1000–2000 newborns. In this situation, hydronephrosis may be caused by an abnormal shape of the ureteral junction—the existence of the ureteral valves and the mucosal fold at this level. Like many other abnormalities, this pathology occurs much more frequently in males, usually unilaterally and especially on the left side [10, 14].

The ultrasound diagnosis is based on the observation of the increase of the anteroposterior diameter of the kidney, a degree of kidney pyelectasis. If the obstruction is unilateral and the filling of the bladder is normal, the normal amount of amniotic fluid will be preserved. When the damage is bilateral, the oligoamnios/oligohydramnios may appear.

In most cases this condition does not produce symptoms after birth; in 10–15% of the cases, it regresses spontaneously, but sometimes repeated evaluation is needed [1–8].

c. Obstruction of the ureterobladder junction

This condition is the cause of approximately 5–10% of all cases of dilatation of the urinary tract. Ultrasound diagnosis is based on dilated urethra, with renal pelvis dilatation and normal bladder image. The cause of the disease is the dysfunction of the lower ureter, the outcome is favorable and the pathologic aspects disappear postnatally in many cases [16] (**Figure 6**).

The normal ureter size in children is up to 5 mm. Normal ureter cannot be detected during prenatal ultrasound examination. It can only be detected if it is dilated to a size greater than 7 mm and is observed like a translucent structure. The dilated ureter should be differentiated from full intestinal loops. Pathological dilatation of the ureter is more common in male patients, usually appearing to be unilateral (**Figure 7**) [15–17].

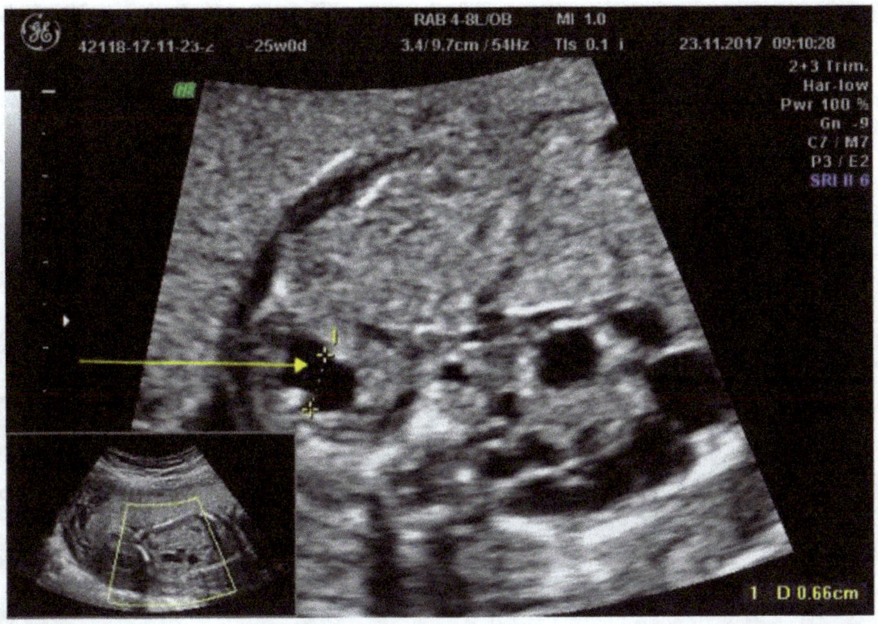

Figure 6. Contralateral pyelectasis in a unilateral MCDK case.

The dilatation of the ureter may be partial or total, and this pathology can be classified into the following conditions:

- Obstructive-type megaureter
- Reflux-type megaureter
- Megaureter without reflux and without obstruction
- Obstructive- and reflux-type megaureter

d. Vesicoureteral reflux

Vesicoureteral reflux (VUR) is characterized by the return of urine from the bladder to the kidney which often causes hydronephrosis and sometimes even abnormalities in kidney development (renal dysplasia). Causes include transient obstruction of bladder discharge, delayed maturation of the vesicoureteral junction and high bladder evacuation pressure. Patients with vesicoureteral reflux have a high risk of pyelonephritis, hypertension and progressive renal failure. Vesicoureteral reflux is represented by the retrograde passage of urine from the bladder to the ureter and subsequently to the kidneys, due to the incompetence of antireflux mechanisms [17, 19, 20].

This condition is usually easy to diagnose prenatally, when visualizing renal pelvis and calyces dilatations that vary in size, associated with unilateral or bilateral ureteral dilatations. RVU reveals a nonprogressive hydronephrosis with normal amniotic fluid index [10–13, 18].

VUR classification:

- Grade I reflux: reflux is only present in the ureter that has various degrees of dilatation.

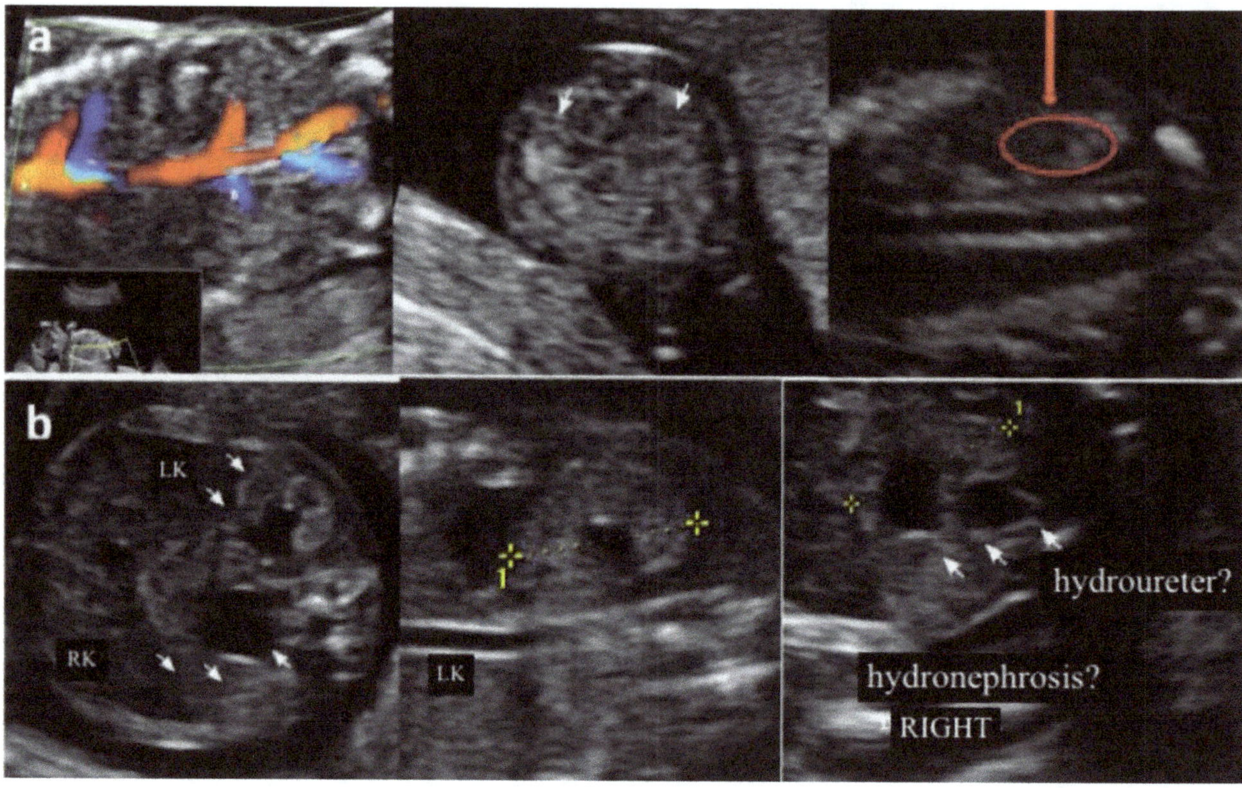

Figure 7. (a) First trimester: both renal arteries visualized in color Doppler, normal kidney images on both sides of the cross section and a kidney highlighted in the coronal section. (b) Second trimester (same case): asymmetrical bilateral pyelectasis, left kidney longitudinal diameter and hydroureter on the right side.

- Grade II reflux: reflux reaches the renal pelvis, without dilatation of the collector system, the papillae being normal.
- Grade III reflux: moderate dilatation of the ureter, with or without sinusitis; moderate dilatation of the collector system.
- Grade IV reflux: moderate dilatation of the ureter with or without sinuosity; moderate dilatation of the collector system; calyces are flattened but with the impression of the papilla still visible.
- Grade V reflux: severe dilatation with ureter sinuosity and marked dilatation of the collector system; reflux in the parenchyma, with parenchymal thinning [10–15, 18].
- The prognosis is good. The prenatal diagnosis is important. Forty percent of the newborns develop severe kidney damage [2].

e. Ureterocele

As many other kidney abnormalities, ureterocele is more common in male patients. This pathology appears as a thin wall cyst or sept on the bladder wall [1, 16]. In many cases the diagnosis may be omitted when the bladder is full, the filling masking the cyst. There have been described cases of ureterocele shed in the urethra. This phenomenon may lead to acute obstruction of the lower urinary tract [1, 2]. The prognosis is favorable, but its evolution must be assessed postnatally, by residual renal function testing and reflux tests (**Figure 8**) [20].

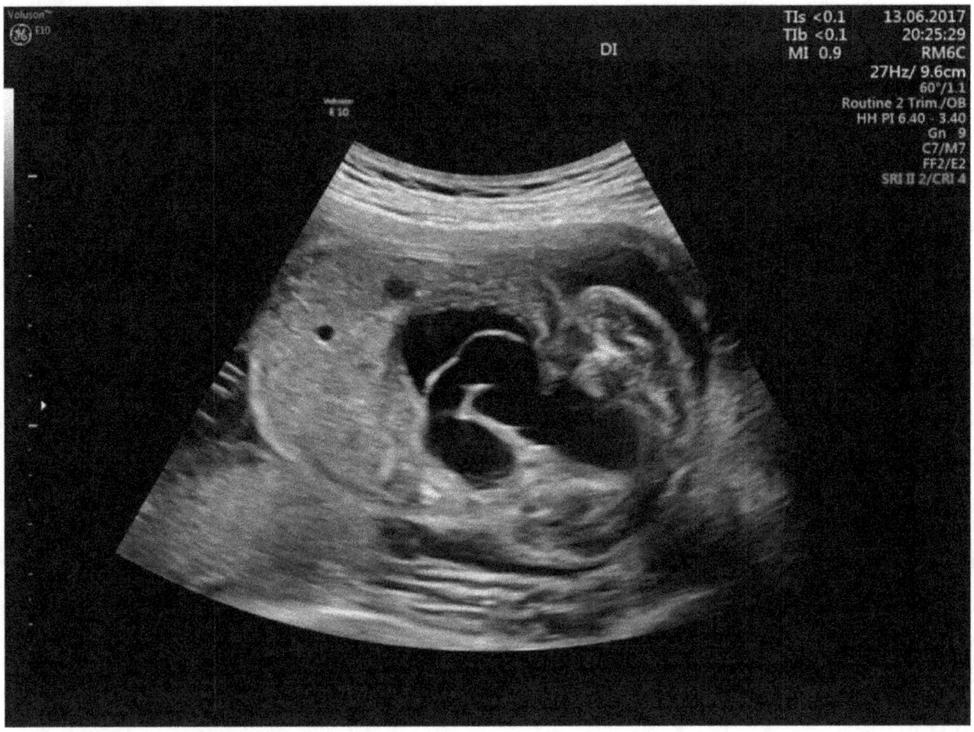

Figure 8. Ureterocele and hydroureter.

3. Bladder anomalies

The bladder is a very important element in antenatal fetal examination. Clinicians may suspect anomalies of the bladder when not visualized on prenatal examination or when enlarged. From the pathological point of view, we may encounter various anomalies as well:

a. Megacystis is a neurodysplastic disease, due to the anomaly of innervation. This leads to bladder dilatation (over 7 cm in diameter). It may be associated with small, short and dilated bowels, as well as a low-caliber colon. At ultrasound, the striking signs are polyhydramnios, enlarged ureters and kidneys [17].

b. Congenital bladder diverticulitis. A septum can be observed.

c. Bladder exstrophy. It is commonly associated with other urogenital malformations and is constantly accompanied by epispadias. This pathology is characterized by many anomalies and lesions, such as:

- Abdominal anterior wall injuries: inguinal hernia is common.
- Lesion of pelvic bones: shortening and defects of rotation of pubic bones.
- Lesions of the genitalia: micropenis and cryptorchidism appear in boys; in girls, the vagina is short and has various degrees of stenosis, the clitoris is bifid and the small labia are divergent.
- The anterior bladder wall is absent, and the posterior wall is the submuscular segment of the anterior abdominal wall.

- The bladder mucosa is exposed to the external environment, with the ureteric holes and the inner urethra opening visible.
- Vesicoureteral reflux is present in all cases.
- Some patients have rectal prolapse and anal incontinence; this phenomenon is due to the malposition of sphincter structures [1–4, 15–17, 19, 20].

4. Urethral malformations

The most common obstructive cause of the lower urinary tract is the posterior urethral valve (PUV). PUV is due to the existence of membranes in the posterior urethra. Echography shows dilated bladder and urethral dilatation, giving a classic echographic sign—'the keyhole sign'. Dystriation of ureters and troughs also occurs [14]. In advanced forms, oligohydramnios-associated pulmonary hypoplasia and urinary ascites may also appear. These fetuses require prenatal intervention to avoid kidney damage. Some authors tried to demonstrate that creating a vesicoamniotic passage may lead to a better outcome, but this has not yet been fully demonstrated [16].

In the prenatal life, other malformations may be seen:

1. Urethral agenesis (absence of urethra) is a rare malformation, incompatible with life unless an alternative communication between the bladder and amniotic sac exists. The urine is discharged through abnormal communication with other organs (between bladder and bowels or by umbilical fistula).
2. Congenital structures.
3. Rear urethral valves: mucosal lining located in the posterior urethra originating from the seminal colonic and insertion on the anterior wall of the urethra [14–17].
4. Epispadias: abnormality characterized by opening the urethra on the dorsal face of the penis at variable distance of the gland, dorsal curvature of the penis and foreskin abnormalities. There are many forms of epispadias:
    - Balanic: distal incomplete defect.
    - Penian: incomplete proximal defect.
    - Penopubian: a complete defect, often associated with bladder exstrophy. In this situation, a distinct pathological condition appears: the exstrophy-epispadias complex [19].
    - Hypospadias: the anomaly is characterized by opening the urethra on the ventral side of the penis, at any level between the gland and the perineum, causing a ventral penis (chord). Patients with hypospadias have often abnormalities of the foreskin and cryptorchidic scrotum, inguinal hernia and hydrocele. Studies have shown a higher presence of hypospadias in patients with fetal growth restriction (**Figures 9** and **10**) [19]

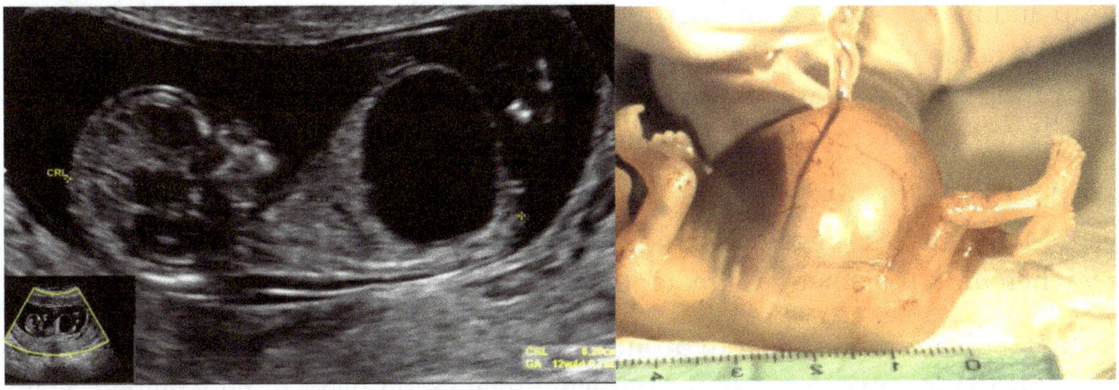

Figure 9. Isolated megacystis: the right-side image is the sagittal plane of the fetus and the CRL (crown-rump length) measurement; the left-side image (same case) is the pathological specimen after medical termination of pregnancy.

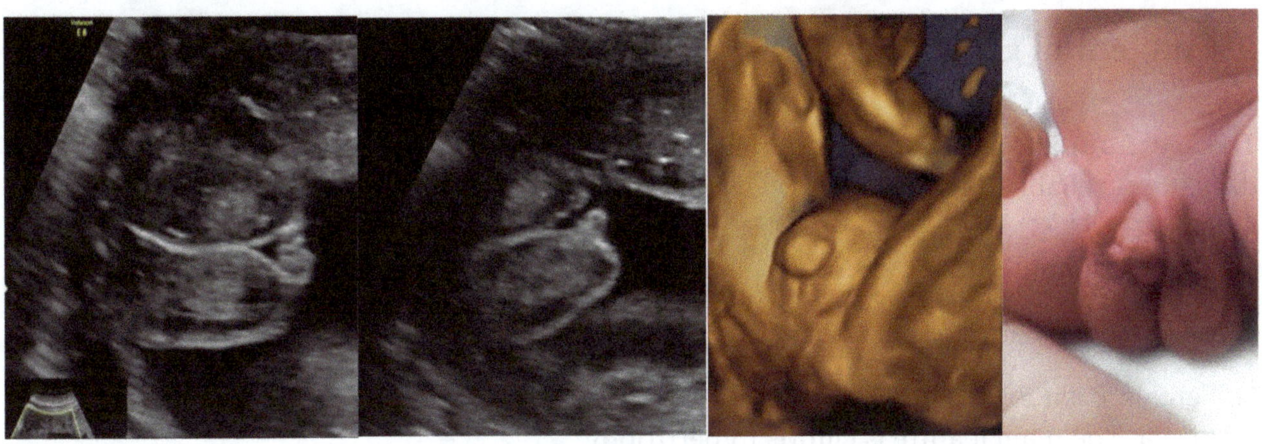

Figure 10. Grade III hypospadias (perineal) is the most severe form, with the opening of the urethra at the penoscrotal junction.

The diagnosis of hypospadias with prenatal ultrasound is based on several important criteria:

- A blunter bulbous tip to the penile shaft rather than the normal.
- A 'tulip' sign formed by the ventral-bent penis located between the two scrotal folds.
- Abnormal curvature of the penis.
- A short penile shaft.
- Ventral deflection of the urinary stream which can be studied by color Doppler [20].

5. Evolution and treatment

Renal pelvic dilatation is commonly seen during antenatal ultrasound examinations, and its management remains a clinical dilemma. Although it is proven that severe antenatal hydronephrosis requires postnatal clinical and ultrasound evaluation, there is no consensus on the follow-up and management of mild or moderate hydronephrosis observed during antenatal ultrasound examinations [15]. The prenatal diagnosis may improve the prognosis and the outcome of the fetus. An early diagnosis and treatment of urinary obstruction may prevent the renal damage or loss of renal function [5, 21].

Most of the cases will spontaneously resolve after delivery. Thus, some assurance should be given. Many studies suggest follow-up when the AP diameter is 4–7 mm and antibiotic therapy when the AP diameter is greater than 7 mm [14, 18].

The postnatal assessment of fetal hydronephrosis may be invasive and lengthy [6–8]. Thus, the risks and the inconvenience of a protracted evaluation need to be weighed against the probability that milder degrees of renal pelvic dilatation will decrease without resulting in any renal damage [17].

6. Congenital genital anomalies

The spectrum of congenital genital malformation is very broad, and the diagnosis is usually difficult. A reliable classification reveals four main types of genital anomalies:

1. True hermaphroditism: an individual has both ovarian and testicular tissues.
2. Male pseudohermaphroditism.
3. Female pseudohermaphroditism: adrenogenital syndrome or congenital adrenal hyperplasia. The main feature is clitoris hypertrophy.
4. Gonadal dysgenesis [5, 19, 20].

Fetal gender abnormality is diagnosed by ultrasound or by finding a discrepancy between fetal phenotype and sex chromosomes. The ultrasound diagnosis is late, usually accessible in the second or third trimesters [5, 20–24].

I. Male genital malformations

Due to improved ultrasound technology and increased experience in this area, the fetal sex can be established with high accuracy beyond 13 weeks of pregnancy [5]. Determination of fetal sex is based on the 'sagittal sign'. During the first trimester, in the sagittal plane, the penis is oriented upwards and the clitoris downwards. In the third trimester, the genitalia can be described with high accuracy [21].

Penian malformations (abnormal phallic structure)

1. Micropenis or penian hypoplasia
2. Penian agenesis
3. Megalopenia or hyperplasia of the penis [1–3, 22]

Testicular malformations.

1. Number abnormalities

    - Anorchia (or anorchism): the absence of both testicles in the presence of a normal male phenotype (46XY)
    - Monorchism (or monorchidism): the absence of a testicle
    - Polyorchism: the presence of more than two testicles
    - Testicular fusion: the fusion of the two testicles in the same scrotum [2, 5, 20–24]

2. Development abnormalities

    - Microorchidism: small, hypoplastic testicles.
    - Macroorchidism may be secondary to contralateral testicular damage and may be bilateral in congenital syndromes (fragile X syndrome) or other disorders (hypophysis adenoma, aromatase deficiency).
    - Cystic dysplasia of the testicle: benign, congenital tumor, frequently associated with other testicular malformations [5, 20–24].

3. Migration abnormalities

    - Cryptorchidism: the process of descensus testis is affected by anatomical and mechanical factors, such as a poor connection between the gubernaculum and testis and endocrine factors (**Figure 11**) [5, 22].

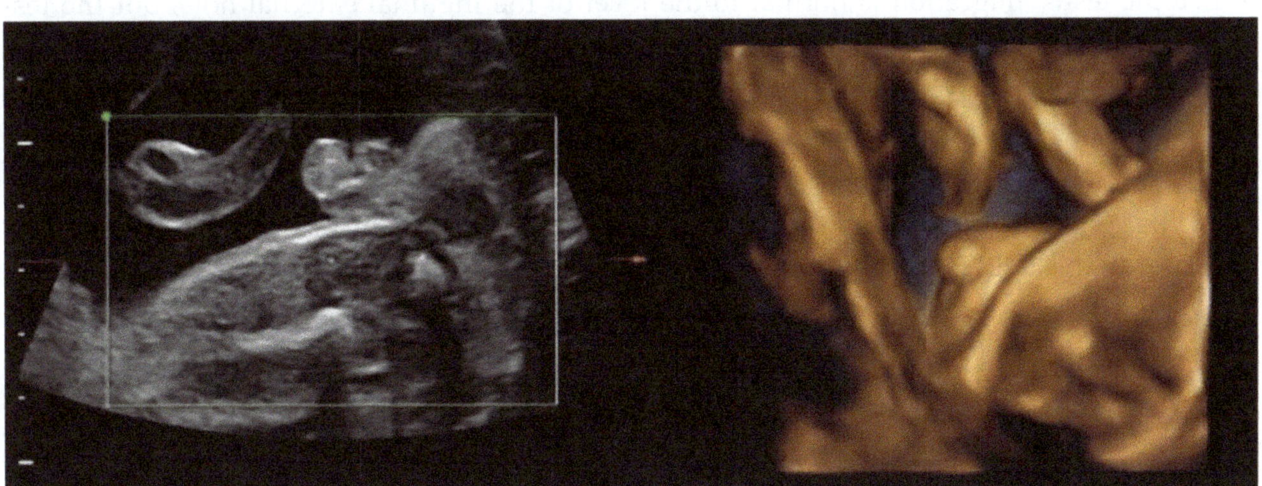

Figure 11. Hypospadias: the left-side image is the 'tulip sign' in 2D conventional ultrasound; the right-side image is a 3D reconstruction, surface rendering technique.

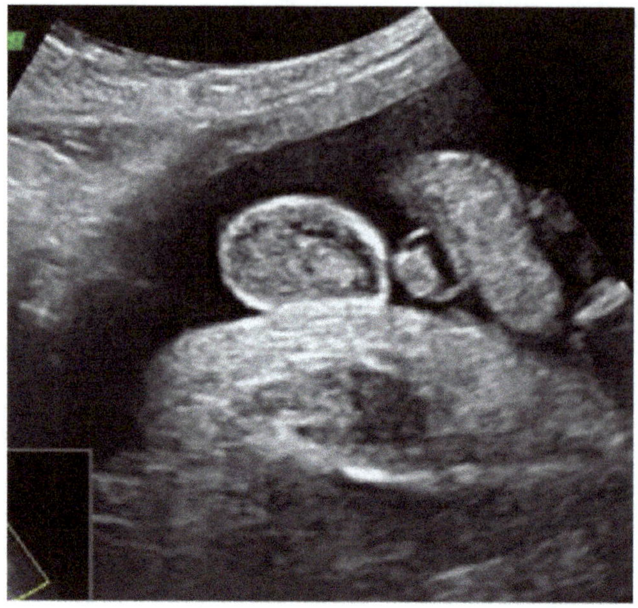

Figure 12. Unilateral cryptorchidism (in association with penian anomaly).

Classification:

- Intraabdominal: above or at the internal inguinal opening
- Intracanalicular: in the inguinal canal, between the inguinal inlet and the external groove
- Extracanalicular:
- Suprapubian: just above the external inguinal opening above the pubic symphysis level
- Infrapubian: in retroscrotal space, inferior to pubic symphysis [1, 5] (**Figure 12**)

- Ectopic testis: migration is normal to the level of the inguinal external hole, but the testicle follows an abnormal tract. Possible localizations are between aponeurosis of external oblique muscle and subcutaneous or femoral, etc. [24].

It is recommended that information about the fetal abnormalities, postnatal and prenatal options of treatment and prognosis should be presented to the parents by a multidisciplinary team that includes neonatologists, urologists, perinatologists and medical geneticists with expertise in this field [5].

7. Female genital malformations

7.1. Ovarian cysts

Ovarian cysts are the most frequently abdominal tumors that may be seen in female fetuses and newborns. The incidence of fetal ovarian cysts has increased lately, due to the improvement

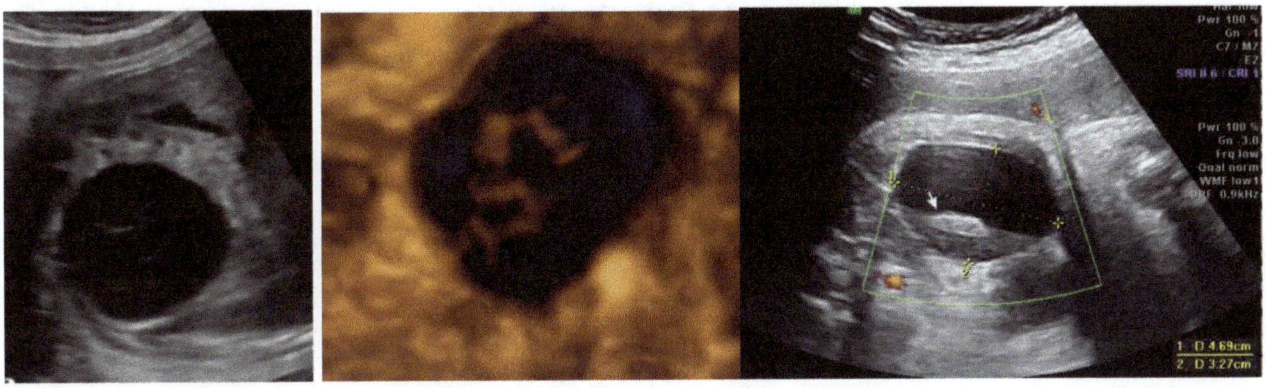

Figure 13. Fetal ovarian cyst: 2D and 3D surface rendering images. The evolution of the case led to the typical 'fluid–fluid' level aspect, due to the intracystic hemorrhage.

of ultrasound technology and due to the increase in the incidence of pregnancies that require hormonal treatment during the gestation period [2].

These ovarian tumors may be uni- or bilateral, sometimes multiple, and their appearance is as anechoic structures, thin-walled and having various sizes [5, 21–24]. Some authors described cases with solid tumors, teratomas or hemorrhagic cysts. To increase the accuracy of the diagnosis, MRI examination may be required (magnetic resonance imaging (MRI)) [22].

Fetal ovarian cysts have usually a good outcome; most of them progress to spontaneous resolution in the postnatal period. The most frequent complication of cysts is ovarian torsion. Other complications may be intracystic hemorrhage, rupture, dystocia during birth, etc. There are no guidelines for monitoring and treatment of this condition. The non-invasive monitoring by ultrasound seems to be the best approach in prenatal life [1, 5, 19–25] (**Figure 13**).

7.2. Hydrocolpos

Hydrocolpos is the accumulation of fluid in the vagina. When the fluid is observed on the vagina and the uterine body, the condition is called hydrometrocolpos. These diseases are caused by the persistence of the urogenital sinus or cloaca malformations [23]. The presence of a cystic mass in the presacral area, containing an anechoic fluid (suggesting urine) or sediment content, should guide the clinician to a diagnosis of urogenital sinus persistence [1, 2, 25].

8. Conclusions

The ultrasound diagnosis of renal and urinary tract abnormalities is generally based on the exclusion criteria, by comparison with the normal imaging one. In most cases, kidney or urinary tract abnormalities are diagnosed considering the appearance of amniotic fluid abnormalities, visualization of kidney size abnormalities or dilated appearance of the urinary tract. Congenital kidney abnormalities are often associated with the urinary tract malformation, and there is a wide range of anomalies resulting from disorders in the development process. It is important to differentiate abnormalities incompatible with life (as they require interruption of pregnancy) and asymptomatic/paucisymptomatic diseases in the postnatal life.

The genitalia anomalies must be treated by a multidisciplinary team that includes neonatologists, endocrinologists, urologists, perinatologists and medical geneticists with expertise in this field.

Author details

Sidonia Maria Sandulescu[1*], Ramona Mircea Vicol[2,3], Adela Serban[2,3], Andreea Veliscu Carp[2,4] and Vaduva Cristian[1,5]

*Address all correspondence to: ssidoniam@yahoo.com

1 University of Medicine and Pharmacy, Craiova, Romania

2 University of Medicine and Pharmacy, Bucharest, Romania

3 INSMC Alessandrescu-Rusescu, Bucharest, Romania

4 Clinical Hospital of Obstetrics and Gynecology Panait Sarbu, Bucharest, Romania

5 County Clinical Emergency Hospital of Craiova, Craiova, Romania

References

[1] Kurjak A, Chervenak FA, Vladareanu R. Donald School. Textbook of ultrasound in obstetrics and gynecology. Bucharest: Amaltea; 2012. ISBN 978-973-162-104-3. Pages 337-348

[2] CALLEN. Ultrasonography in Obstetrics and Gynecology. 6th ed. Dr Radu Vladareanu—Coordinator of the Romanian edition. Hypocrate; 2017. Pages 508-538

[3] Afroz R, Shakoor S, Salat MS, Munim S. Antenatal renal pelvic dilatation and foetal outcomes—A review of cases from a tertiary care center in Karachi, Pakistan. 2016. JPMA 66: 1597

[4] Stefan F. Nemec, Ursula Nemec, Peter C. Brugger, Dieter Bettelheim, Michael Weber, John M. Graham Jr., David L. Rimoin, Daniela Prayer. Male genital abnormalities in intrauterine growth restriction. Prenatal Diagnosis. 2012;**32**:427-431

[5] Palacios Loro ML, Segura Ramírez DK, Ordo˜nez Álvarez FA, Santos Rodríguez F. Congenital anomalies of the kidney and urinary tract. A vision for the paediatrician. Anales de Pediatría (Barcelona, Spain) 2015;**83**(6):442.e1-442442.e5

[6] Tudorache Ş, Cara M, Iliescu DG, Stoica A, Simionescu C, Novac LV, Cernea D. Fetal kidneys ultrasound appearance in the first trimester—Clinical significance and limits of counseling. Current Health Sciences Journal. 2016 January-March;**42**(1)

[7] Chou C-Y et al. Frequency of postnatal hydronephrosis in infants with a renal anterioreposterior pelvic diameter > 4 mm on midtrimester ultrasound. Taiwanese Journal of Obstetrics & Gynecology. 2015;**54**:554e558

[8] Chitayat D, Glanc P. Diagnostic approach in prenatally detected genital abnormalities. Ultrasound in Obstetrics & Gynecology. 2010;**35**:637-646

[9] Bernheim1 S*, Deschênes1,5 G, Schiff2,5 M, Cussenot3 I, Niel O. Antenatal nephromegaly and propionic acidemia: A case report. Bernheim et al. BMC Nephrology. 2017;**18**:110

[10] Maria Şorop-Florea, Ciurea RN, Ioana M, et al. The importance of perinatal autopsy. Review of the literature and series of cases. Romanian Journal of Morphology and Embryology 2017;**58**(2):323-337

[11] Capone VP, Morello W, Taroni F, Montini G. Genetics of congenital anomalies of the kidney and urinary tract: The current state of play. International Journal of Molecular Sciences. 2017;**18**:796. DOI: 10.3390/ijms18040796

[12] Tain Y-L MD Jr., Hsing L PhD, Lin C-Y MD, Hsu CN PhD. Incidence and risks of congenital anomalies of kidney and urinary tract in newborns—A population-based case–control study in Taiwan. Medicine February 2016;**95**(5)

[13] Reidy NUK. Developmental genetics and congenital. anomalies of the kidney and urinary tract. Journal of Pediatric Genetics. 2016;**5**:51-60

[14] Sirin Y, Susztak K. Notch in the kidney: Development and disease. The Journal of Pathology. 2012;**226**(2):394-403

[15] Vivante A, Kohl S, Hwang D, Dworschak G, Hildebrandt F. Single-gene causes of congential anomalies of the kidney and urinary tract (CAKUT) in humans. Pediatric Nephrology. 2014;**29**:695-704

[16] Ichikawa I, Kuwayama F, Pope J, Stephens F, Miyazaki Y. Paradigm shift from classic anatomic theories to contemporary cell biological views of CAKUT. Kidney International. 2002;**61**:889-898

[17] Sanna-Cherchi S, Ravani P, Corbani V, Parodi S, Haupt R, Piaggio G, Innocenti M, Somenzi D, Trivelli A, Caridi G, et al. Renal outcome in patients with congenital anomalies of the kidney and urinary tract. Kidney International. 2009;**76**:528-533

[18] Sanna-Cherchi S, Kiryluk K, Burgess KE, et al. Copy-number disorders are a common cause of congenital kidney malformations. American Journal of Human Genetics. 2012;**91**(6):987-997

[19] Muller F, Bernard MA, Benkirane A, Ngo S, Lortat-Jacob S, Oury JF, Fetal DM. Urine cystatin C as a predictor of postnatal renal function in bilateral uropathies. Clinical Chemistry. 1999;**45**:2292-2293

[20] Meizner I, Mashiach R, Shalev J, Efrat Z, Feldberg D. The 'tulip sign': A sonographic clue for in-utero diagnosis of severe hypospadias. Ultrasound in Obstetrics & Gynecology. 2002 Mar;**19**(3):250-253

[21] Ak›n MA, Ak›n* L, Ozbek** S, Tireli*** G, Kavuncuo.lu** S, Sander*** S, Akcakufl M, Gunefl T, Adnan Ozturk M, Kurto S. Fetal-neonatal ovarian cysts-their monitoring and management: Retrospective evaluation of 20 cases and review of the literature. Journal Of Clinical Research in Pediatric Endocrinology 2010;**2**(1):28-33

[22] Kwak DW, Sohn YS, Kim SK, In KK, Park YW, Kim YH. Clinical experiences of fetal ovarian cyst: Diagnosis and consequence. Journal of Korean Medical Science. 2006;**21**:690-694

[23] Hasiakos D, Papakonstantinou K, Bacanu AM, Argeitis J, Botsis D, Vitoratos N. Clinical experience of five fetal ovarian cysts: Diagnosis and follow-up. Archives of Gynecology and Obstetrics. 2008;**277**:575-578

[24] Katorza E, Pinhas-Hamiel O, Mazkereth R, Gilboa Y, Sex AR. Differentiation disorders (SDD) prenatal sonographic diagnosis, genetic and hormonal work-up. Pediatric Endocrinology Reviews. 2009;**7**:12-21

[25] Wang YC, Su HY, Liu JY, Chang FW, Chen CH. Maternal and female fetal virilization caused by pregnancy luteomas. Fertility and Sterility. 2005;**84**:509

4

Congenital Diaphragmatic Hernia

Adrian Claudiu Ratiu

Abstract

Over the past 20 years, prenatal detection of congenital diaphragmatic hernia (CDH) has improved worldwide, reaching up to 60% in Europe. Pulmonary hypoplasia and persistent pulmonary hypertension are the two main determinants of neonatal mortality and morbidity, so new tools have been focused on their evaluation. Fetal surgery for severe cases requires proper evaluation of the prognosis of fetuses with CDH. It is very important to identify reliable prenatal prognostic factors that can be used worldwide for several reasons: patient counseling is more accurate; the results of pre- and postnatal treatments will be comparable across different institutions; fetuses eligible for fetal surgery will be selected correctly; and a woman expecting a child with a very poor prognosis can prepare herself for the postnatal demise of her baby or, in some countries, opt for termination of pregnancy.

Keywords: congenital diaphragmatic hernia, thoracic anomalies, diaphragm anomalies

1. Introduction

Congenital diaphragmatic hernia (CDH) consists of a defect in variable size in the fetal diaphragm. It occurs more often on the left side and abdominal organs herniate into the thoracic cavity. Most if the time the diagnosis is made during the second trimester fetal morfology ultrasound examination. Diagnosis is based mainly on finding abdominal organs such as stomach, bowel, and liver in the chest cavity or in the presence of a chest mass which pushes the heart toward the lateral thoracic wall.

Although the surgical repair offers excellent results from the technical point of view, the problem with these patients are related to the impaired development of the lungs and their vasculature, therefore, the mortality and morbidity of these babies remain high even after surgery.

2. Spectrum of disease

2.1. Definition

Congenital diaphragmatic hernia (CDH) is defined by the presence of an orifice in the diaphragm that permits the herniation of abdominal contents into the thorax.

2.2. Epidemiology

CDH is a rare condition that occurs in <1–5:10,000 births [1]. The most common anatomic type encountered is the left-sided posterolateral hernia (Bochdalek hernia), including the vast majority of cases 85–90%, while the anterior hernia of Morgagni is rare. A bilateral defect accounts for 15–20% of cases; tissue defect involving most of the hemidiaphragm is called agenesis [2].

2.3. Causes

2.3.1. Environmental causes

No cases of CDH in humans have been unequivocally attributed to teratogenic or environmental exposures. Recently, a potential association with the immunosuppressive drug mycophenylate mofetil has been made, but the mechanism by which this drug could cause diaphragmatic defect is unknown [3].

2.3.2. Heritable causes

About 10% of all individuals with CDH have a chromosome abnormality. The most common abnormalities are trisomy 18 and isochromosome 12p (Pallister-Killian syndrome or PKS), although many additional abnormalities have been reported (**Table 1**). Some of the more common monogenic syndromes in which CDH occurs are listed in (**Tables 2** and **3**) [4].

2.4. Classification

There are six types of CHD (**Figure 1**):

1. Posterolateral defect (Bochdalek hernia) occurs most often on the left side and contains stomach, bowel, and spleen, and if right-sided, contains liver.

2. Parasternal defect (Morgagni hernia), located on anterior retrosternal or parasternal portion of the diaphragm, is rare and more often right-sided or bilateral and usually contains liver or bowel.

3. Other anterior hernias associated with Pentalogy of Cantrell are rare findings but are usually severe, probably derived from septum transversum. These cases are usually associated with Pentalogy of Cantrell (including defects in the midline abdominal wall supraumbilical, lower sternum, diaphragmatic pericardium, and heart).

Chromosome abnormality/locus	Frequency of congenital diaphragmatic hernia	
	Found in this disorder	**Attributed to this disorder**
Pallister-Killian syndrome/ (isochromosome or tetrasomy 12p)	~30%	? < 5%
Trisomy 13	Rare	Very rare
Trisomy 18	?1–2%	Rare among all CDH; most common chromosome abnormality in prenatally diagnosed CDH
Trisomy 21	Rare (Morgagni hernias > Bochdalek hernias)	Very rare
Del(4)(p16) (Wolf-Hirschhorn syndrome)	Rare	Very rare
+der (22) t(11;22)(q23;q11)	5–10%	Very rare
Del(15)(q26.2)	Unknown (?but possibly majority)	Unknown
Del(1)(q41-q42)	Unknown	Unknown
Del(8)(p23.1)	?30%	Unknown

Table 1. Common chromosome anomalies associated with CDH.

4. Central hernia is rare; the diaphragm defect involves the central tendinous (amuscular) part of the diaphragm. In these cases, the entire rim of diaphragmatic musculature is found to be present.
5. Hiatal hernia, extremely rare, occurs through a congenitally large esophageal orifice.
6. Diaphragmatic eventration is defined as an elevation or abnormal upward displacement of a part or entire normal diaphragm into the chest cavity. This rare type of CDH is caused by the existence of a thinner part of diaphragm which allows the upward displacement of abdominal organs.

For practical reasons regarding the imaging approach and counseling, it was proposed to classify CDH as intrapleural and mediastinal.

Intrapleural hernias occur through defects in the muscular diaphragm, which may result from deficient fusion of the pleuroperitoneal membranes and abdominal wall musculature or absence of the pleuroperitoneal membranes. Intrapleural hernia contents cause compressions on intrathoracic visceras, causing pulmonary hypoplasia and contralateral mediastinal shift. This category includes the traditionally classified Bochdalek hernias.

Mediastinal hernias can be classified into two types: retrosternal and central. Retrosternal hernias are categorized as Morgagni hernias, although a true Morgagni hernia is only a small anatomic located in the space between the sternal and costal heads of the diaphragm. True Morgagni hernia is considered to be a subtype of retrosternal mediastinal hernias, with larger

Syndrome	Frequency of CDH in this disorder	Mode of inheritance	Gene
Cornelia de Lange syndrome	?up to 5%	AD	*NIPBL*
			SMC3
	Unknown	XL	*SMC1A*
Craniofrontonasal syndrome	Rare	XL (but males less severely affected than females)	*EFNB1*
Denys-Drash syndrome	Rare	AD	*WT1*
Donnai-Barrow syndrome	~70%	AR	*LRP2*
Fryns syndrome	>80% (but ascertainment may be biased)	AR	Unknown (possible etiologic heterogeneity)
Matthew-Wood syndrome	~50%	AR	*STRA6*
Spondylocostal dysostosis (SCDO)	Rare	AR	*DLL3*
	Rare		*MESP2*
	Rare		*LFNG*
	Rare		*HES7*
Simpson-Golabi-Behmel syndrome	Rare	XL	*GPC3*

Table 2. Selected syndromes in which CDH is a feature.

ventral hernias which are defects in the central tendon stemming from septum transversum impaired development. Hiatal hernias, as their name shows, develop more through the esophageal hiatus and do not involve the central tendon. Differentiating ventral mediastinal hernias from intrapleural hernias is important because the intrapleural hernias, usually, do not lead to pulmonary hypoplasia, which is the major complication of CHD [5] (**Table 4**).

2.5. Embriology

The diaphragm starts to develop at approximately 4 weeks of gestation. It develops from several structures. The anterior central tendon develops from an infolding of the ventral body wall: the septum transversum. Another infolding on the posterolateral sides establishes the pleuroperitoneal membranes. Closure of the pleuroperitoneal canals occurs when the septum transversum fuses to the structures surrounding the esophagus, the esophageal mesentery, and connects to the pleuroperitoneal membranes. Closure of the pleuroperitoneal canals normally occurs around the eighth week of gestation in humans. The right side of the diaphragm closes before the left side [6].

The central portion and possibly anterior regions are thought to develop from the septum transversum, which is initially fused to the liver during development and becomes the unmuscularized central tendon of the diaphragm [7].

The posterolateral section, the place where Bochdalek hernia occurs, develops from the pleuroperitoneal folds (PPFs), which are triangular structures derived from mesoderm that form in

Syndrome	Gene (locus)
Apert syndrome	*FGFR2*
Beckwith-Wiedemann syndrome	Dysregulation of imprinted genes on 11p15.5
CHARGE syndrome	*CHD7*
C (trigonocephaly) syndrome	*CD96*
Coffin-Siris syndrome	Unknown
Czeizel-Losonci syndrome	Unknown
Gershoni-Baruch syndrome	Unknown
Goltz syndrome (focal dermal hypoplasia)	*PORCN*
Kabuki syndrome	Unknown
Marfan syndrome	*FBN1*
Mathieu syndrome	Unknown
Meacham syndrome	*WT1*
Microphthalmia with linear skin lesions syndrome	*HCCS*
PAGOD syndrome	Unknown
Pentalogy of Cantrell	Unknown
Poland anomaly	Unknown
Swyer syndrome	Unknown
Thoraco-abdominal schisis	Unknown

Table 3. Syndromes in which CDH is less frequently a feature.

the thorax in the early development of the diaphragm. These PPFs are part of the diaphragmatic connective tissue. The membranous diaphragm is later muscularized by migrating muscle precursor cells to the PPF from the cervical somites. This phenomenon happens before these cells proliferate, differentiate, and migrate onto the membranous diaphragm [8, 9]. The hypothesis is that a Bochdalek hernia occurs if the PPFs do not fuse with the septum transversum and the dorsal mesentery of the esophagus by the 10th week of gestation [4].

The lung originates as an outpouch of the ventral wall of the posterior end of the laryngotracheal tube and divides into two bronchial buds at 3–4 weeks of gestation [10]. As the two buds elongate, the primitive tubular foregut tube begins to pinch into two tubes, namely, the dorsal esophagus and the ventral trachea [11]. Further outgrowth of the lung-buds produces the secondary bronchi. In humans, the right lung has three lobes, whereas, the left lung is composed of two lobes. The branching of the primary bronchial buds are monopodial. Every secondary bronchus then undergoes progressive dichotomous branching as each branch bifurcates repeatedly. Reproducible branching in humans is completed at 16 generations in 16 weeks of gestation [12]. The last seven generations of airway are completed during the last part of gestation. Alveolization starts after 28–30 weeks in humans and is completed in postnatal period [13]. Reid [14] presented this process in her laws of development of the human lung:

1. The bronchial tree is completed by the 16th gestational weeks.
2. Alveoli, developed after birth, increase in number until 8 years of age and in size until the chest wall finishes growing.
3. Blood vessels are remodeled and increase, as new alveoli form, probably until the chest growth is complete.

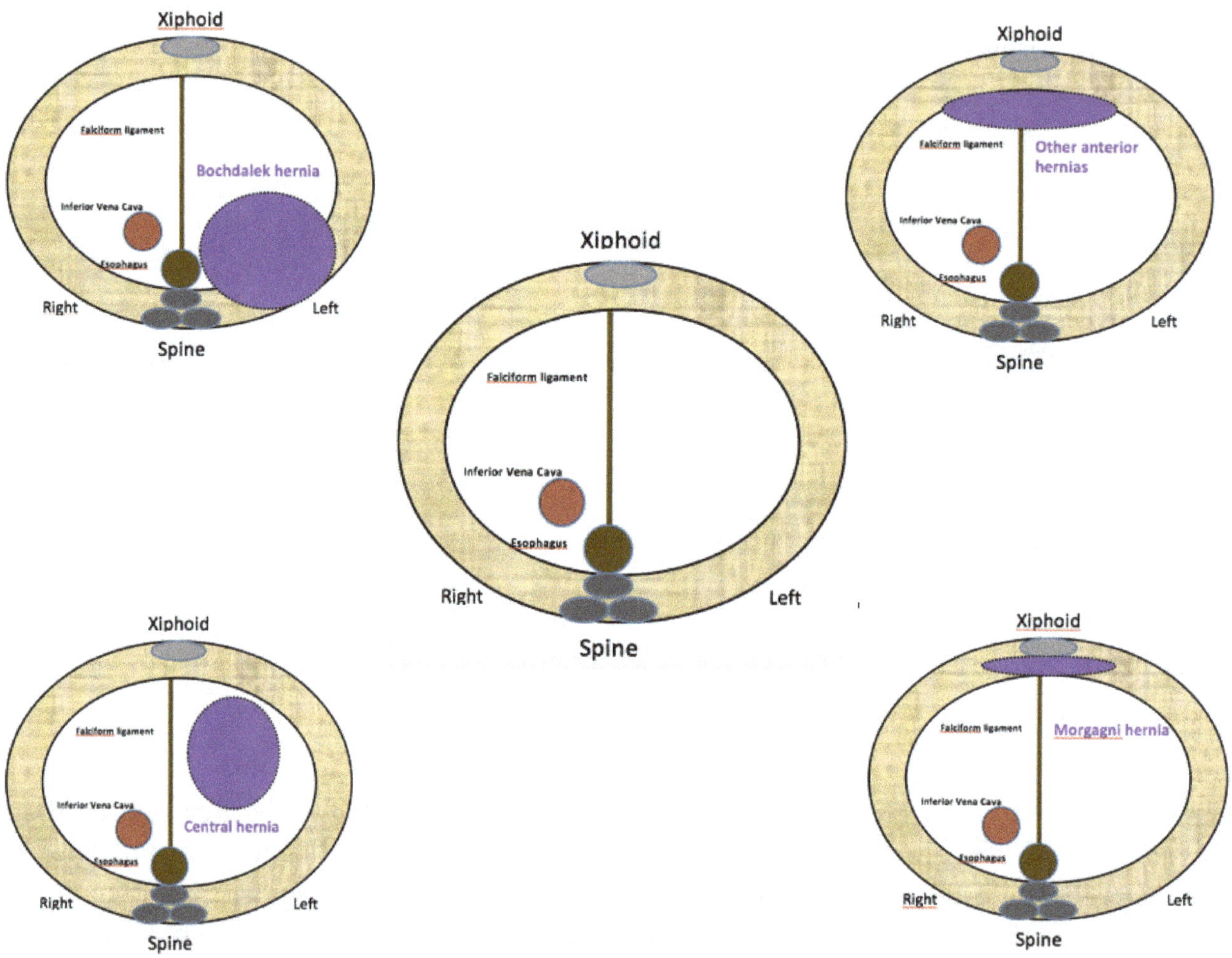

Figure 1. Types of congenital diaphragmatic hernia.

Hernia type	Location	Contents	Associated findings
Intrapleural	Lateral, usually left-sided	Stomach, bowel, spleen, variable-sized portions of the liver	Pulmonary hypoplasia
Mediastinal			
Ventral	Anterior and central	Liver, bowel	Pericardial effusion, pentalogy of Cantrell
Morgagni	Anteromedial, small, typically isolated	Liver, bowel	No pericardial communication
Hiatal	Posterior and central	Stomach, sometimes other organs	Congenital short esophagus

Table 4. Texas Children's Fetal Center classification of CDH.

2.6. Pathogenesis

The pathogenesis of CDH is poorly understood. The diaphragmatic defect is caused by delayed or impaired separation of the two compartments: thoracic and abdominal. This is due to closure of embryonic pleuroperitoneal canals influenced by the growth of the post-hepatic mesenchymal plate and of the pleuroperitoneal folds [15, 16]. In CDH, respiratory failure at birth is the result of pulmonary hypoplasia (PH), reduced airway branching, and surfactant deficiency. Extensive muscularization of the pulmonary vessels may result in persistent pulmonary hypertension (PPH) of the newborn. Historically, PH was believed to be the result of compression of the lungs by the herniating intrathoracic abdominal organs. However, our understanding of abnormal pulmonary development in relation to CDH has significantly improved and we know that pulmonary development is already affected prior to development of the diaphragmatic hernia, implicating that the lungs are primarily disturbed in their development before mechanical compression can happen [17, 18].

2.7. Associated anomalies

The most common associated anomalies are cardiovascular in 40–60% of live-born infants and in 95% of fetal demise; therefore, a detailed ultrasound examination must be performed in every case diagnosed with CDH [19] (**Table 5**).

2.8. Ultrasound diagnosis

Ultrasound evaluation of the thorax can be carried out easily until 25–26 weeks of gestation; after this period, the increased mineralization of the ribs limits the display of intrathoracic organs, especially for coronal or sagittal views. A number of thoracic anomalies evolve; they can appear only in the third trimester or they can regress before birth. Therefore, if an initial assessment of the thorax can be performed as early as at the 12th week of gestation, in order to follow up abnormal cases, late third-trimester scans may be needed.

Scanning planes: the most important view for the assessment of intrathoracic anatomy is the classic *four chamber view* of the fetal heart. In this plane, most thoracic viscera can be visualized, including the ribs, the sternum, and the cutaneous outline. The *midsagittal* and *parasagittal views* allow display of the diaphragm as a hypoechoic line below the lungs and the heart and above the liver and the stomach. The diaphragm shows a curved outline, convex toward the thorax.

Cardiovascular	VSD, ASD, tetralogy of fallot, hypoplastic left heart syndrome
Gastrointestinal abnormalities	Meckel diverticulum, anal atresia
Central nervous system	Neural tube defects, hydrocephalus, agenesis of corpus callosum
Limb abnormalities	Absence defects, polydactyly, syndactyly
Genitourinary abnormalities	Cryptorhydia, absent testes, ectopic kidney, horseshoe kidney
Eye abnormalities	Microphtalmia and anophtalmia

Table 5. Asociated anomalies.

Axial four-chamber view: the following structures should be checked: the two lungs appear as solid, homogeneous; weakly hyperechogenic that almost completely surrounds the heart, right larger than left lung; thoracic aorta behind the left atrium; the heart oriented toward the left; the ribs and overlaying cutaneous tissue; and posterior, the spine (**Figure 2**).

Three-vessel view: allows visualization of the thymus and its relationship with the great vessels and appears as a well-defined roundish solid structure interposed between the great vessels and the sternum. It is weakly hypoechogenic in comparison with the surrounding lungs. In front of the spine and behind the three vessels, the trachea, and, with some difficulty, the esophagus can be seen (**Figure 3**).

Midsagittal view: does not give significant information regarding the lungs because it is occupied mainly by the heart.

Right parasagittal view: the diaphragmatic hypoechogenic layer can be seen below the right lung.

Left parasagittal view: the diaphragmatic hypoechogenic layer can be seen below the left lung and the heart and allows to demonstrate that the stomach is located below the diaphragm.

The ultrasound diagnosis of CDH is, in general, indirect: the abnormal intrathoracic position of the stomach and/or the other migrated viscera and the displacement of the heart and the mediastinum is detected (**Figure 4**).

Left posterolateral CDH: in the *four-chamber view*, the stomach is in the left hemithorax or in the mediastinum (**Figure 5**).

Frequently, a few small bowel loops can be visualized near the stomach, while the heart and the mediastinum are pushed contralaterally. Much more rarely, the spleen and/or the left liver lobe may migrate as well. In few cases, only some ileal loops and/or the left hepatic

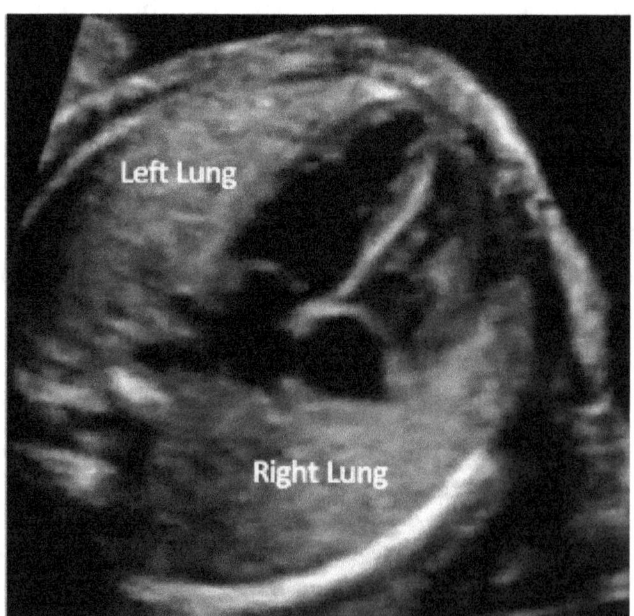

Figure 2. Four chamber view.

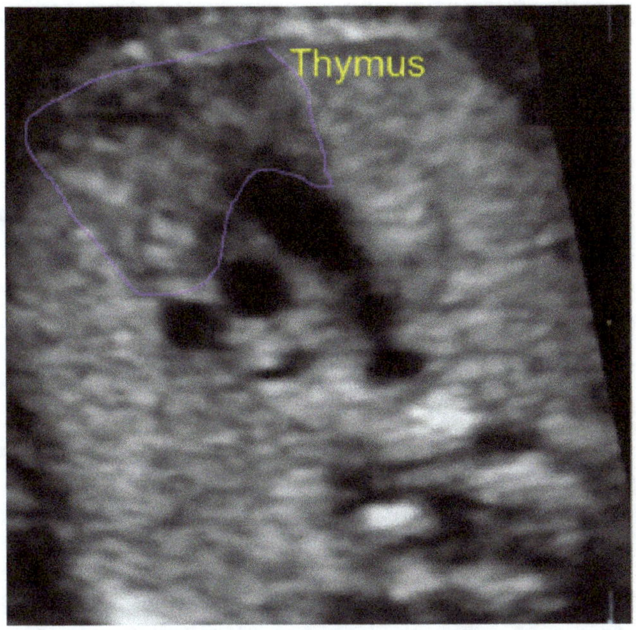

Figure 3. Three-vessel view. Note the thymus slightly hypoechogenic than lungs.

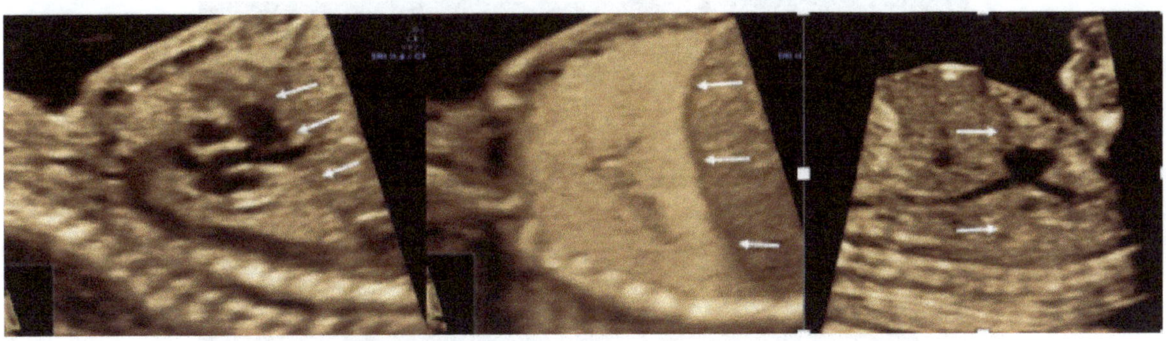

Figure 4. Sagittal view. Note the different echogenicity between lungs and abdominal viscera. Diaphragm appears as a hypoechogenic thin line.

lobe migrate into the thorax; therefore, the diagnosis is based only on dextrocardia and the unusual inhomogeneous appearance of the left hemithorax (**Figure 6**).

Kinking of the sinus venosus is a reliable sign in case of herniated left liver lobe; the bowing of the umbilical segment of the portal vein (portal sinuses) to the left of the midline and coursing of portal vessels to the lateral segment of the left hepatic lobe toward or above the diaphragm is considered the best predictor for liver herniation [20] (**Figure 7**).

It must be kept in mind that even though the diaphragmatic defect occurs in the first trimester, the visceral herniation is variable in time, from early second trimester to the first hour of life.

The sagittal views allow to detect some additional features that help confirm the diagnosis; the evidence of intrathoracic viscera on the four-chamber view is the basic requirement for a correct diagnosis of CDH.

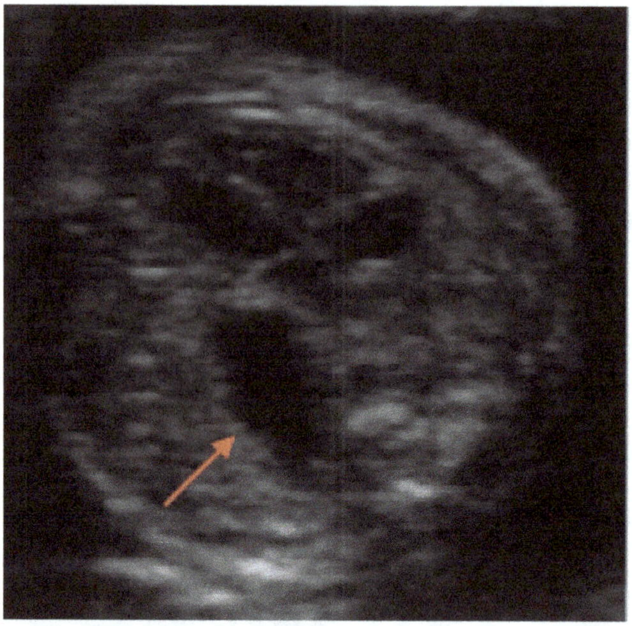

Figure 5. Left congenital diaphragmatic hernia. The stomach is in the left hemithorax and the heart is displaced to the right.

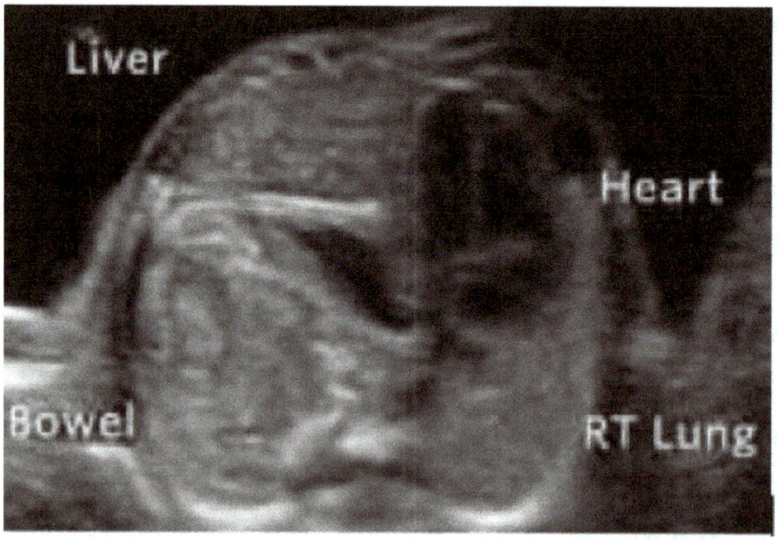

Figure 6. Left CDH. Herniation of left liver lobe and bowel loops. The heart is displaced to the right hemithorax.

Right-sided CDH: the diagnosis is difficult because the main feature, the intrathoracic displacement of the stomach, is absent because the defect is on the other side of the diaphragm. There are several indirect signs that lead to diagnosis. One is the leftward rotation of the heart with increase of the cardiac axis (**Figure 8**) and the upward displacement of the right hepatic lobe into the right hemithorax. This sign is best observed using color Doppler to identify the suprahepatic veins in the thorax because of the similar echogenicity of the lung and liver. Right-sided intrapleural hernias are less common, always contain liver, and may contain variable amounts of bowel and stomach. Rarely, intrapleural hernias may be bilateral; these tend to be associated with severe pulmonary hypoplasia. The midline position of the heart, the lack of

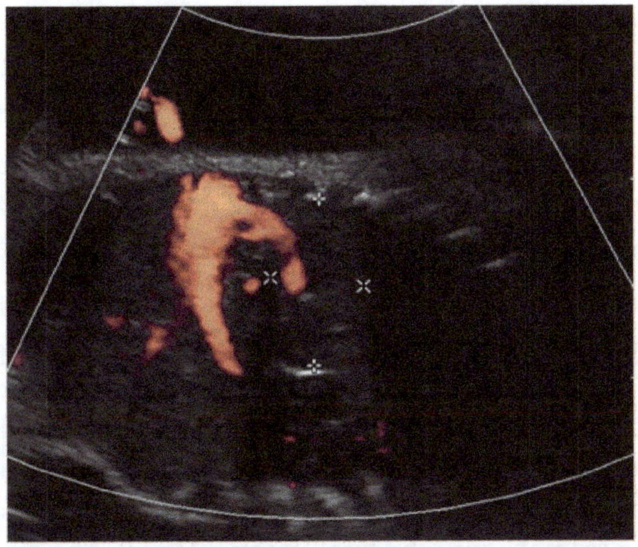

Figure 7. Portal vessels extending into the thorax. Left liver lobe (markers).

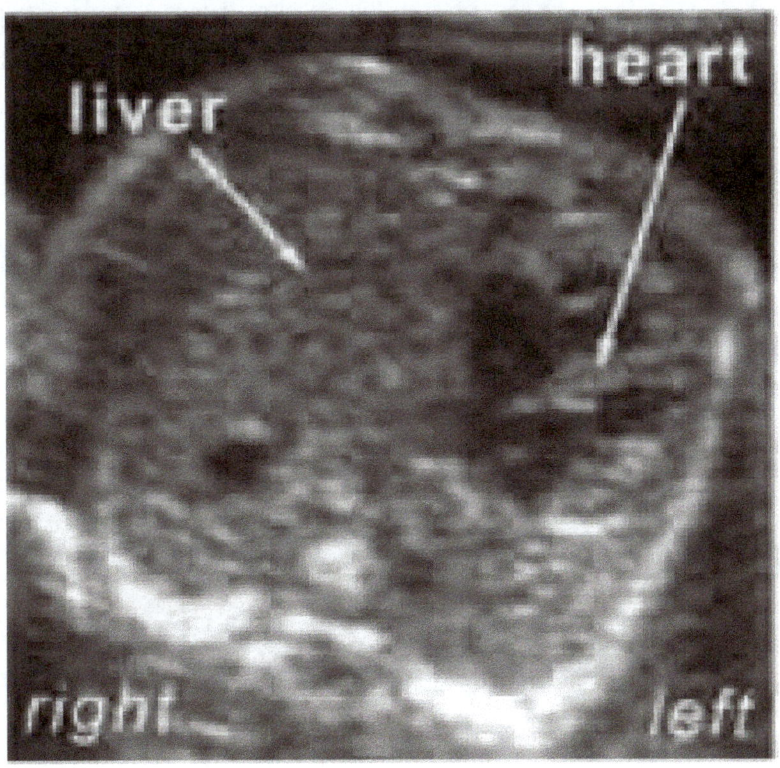

Figure 8. Leftward rotation of the heart with increase of the cardiac axis and upward displacement of the right hepatic lobe into the right hemithorax.

cardiomediastinal shift in cases of suspected intrapleural hernia should raise suspicion for the presence of bilateral intrapleural hernias.

Anterior and central CDH: the ventral type appears anteriorly because of the central tendons' defect. The central tendon of the diaphragm on his upper surface and the pericardium are communicating, if there is a defect at this site a pericardial effusion may develop. Ventral hernias may push the heart posteriorly but do not tend to cause pulmonary hypoplasia (**Figure 9**).

The smaller Morgagni hernia, usually is an isolated anterior defect and given its small size and location does not cause compression of thoracic organs. Morgagni hernias do not communicate with the pericardial space; therefore, this feature is a key element in differentiation from mediastinal hernias (**Table 6**).

Hiatal CDH: on ultrasound examination, it may appear as a hypoechogenic image behind the fetal heart in the posterior mediastinum, anterior to the vertebral body in continuity with a small fetal stomach located in the abdominal cavity just below the diaphragm in a median position. Parasagittal sonographic sections of the fetal thorax show an intact diaphragm on both sides. During the examination, stomach peristalsis may be visualized or the up and down movements of the stomach into the fetal thorax [21, 22]. The absence of liver in a hiatal hernia should help distinguish it from a right-sided intrapleural hernia.

The diagnosis of diaphragmatic hernia is rare during the first trimester. Early diagnosis has been associated with poor prognosis and the presence of additional defects [23, 24]. A diagnosis of CDH is suggestive if a displacement of the fetal heart in association with an intrathoracic mass having the appearance of the liver or stomach is detected.

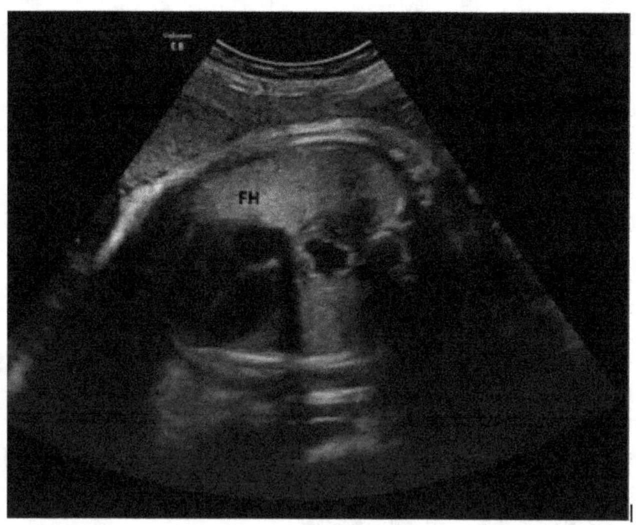

Figure 9. Transverse view of the fetal thorax with an anechogenic mass behind the heart; FH—fetal heart; Ao—aorta; S—stomach.

- Thoracic mass with mediastinal shift.
- Left-sided CHD: stomach is in thorax seen in *four-chamber view*, almost half of the cases have liver herniation.
- Right-sided CHD: almost always have liver herniation which is difficult to see; diagnosis is suspected in case of left mediastinal shift and Doppler reveals abnormal course of hepatic vessels.
- Polyhydramnios secondary to esophageal compression.

Table 6. Key sonographic features.

It was reported in a prospective study on 78,000 pregnancies at first trimester screening for chromosomal abnormalities by nuchal translucency thickness, 19 chromosomally normal fetuses with diagnosis of congenital diaphragmatic hernia. Only one of them was diagnosed in the first trimester; diagnosis was based on the visualization of the stomach in the thorax. In about one-third of the cases of diaphragmatic hernia, they found increased nuchal translucency. In the majority of the infants (83%) who died in the neonatal period due to pulmonary hypoplasia, nuchal translucency was increased, while the respective percentage for the survivors was 22%. The authors hypothesized that the accumulated nuchal fluid may be caused by venous congestion determined by intrathoracic compression due to early herniation of the abdominal organs [25].

The compression of herniated organs on esophagus or gastic outlet obstruction causes polyhydramnios which may became visible later in pregnancy. Another cause of polyhydramnios in cases with CDH is esophageal atresia with tracheoesophageal fistula, which may be very difficult to diagnose because the visualization of the proximal esophageal pouch is dependent on its being distended by swallowed amniotic fluid.

2.9. Differential diagnosis

Bronchogenic cysts (*foregut duplication*) contain several components of the bronchi, including respiratory epithelia, mucous glands, and cartilage and may occur anywhere along the length of the trachea or esophagus [26]. Most are diagnosed incidentally or if large enough, can compress the esophagus and/or trachea.

Congenital cystic adenomatoid malformation (CCAM): a developmental abnormality of the lung resulting from abnormal cell proliferation and decreased programmed cell death of lung tissue. Type I CCAM is most common and is distinguished by relatively large cysts and mucin production.

Cystic teratomas are benign tumors most often found in the anterior mediastinum. They consist of several differentiated cell types derived from endoderm, ectoderm, and/or mesoderm [27, 28].

Neurogenic tumors are the most common lesion found in the posterior mediastinum. They are likely to be of neural crest origin; the majority is benign: neurilemoma, neurofibroma, ganglioneuroma, pheochromocytoma, and neuroblastoma.

Pulmonary agenesis refers to partial or complete absence of lung tissue that is caused by failure of lung bud development.

Pulmonary sequestration results from primitive lung tissue that is not connected to the tracheobronchial tree. Sequestration may be intrapulmonary, occurring within the pleura of the normal lung or extrapulmonary, occurring outside the normal lung within its own pleural sac.

2.10. Prognostic indicators

The best validated measurement is contralateral lung area assessed by 2D ultrasound through the so-called lung area/head circumference ratio (LHR) [29]. Different methods for measuring were described but the most reproducible and accurate method involves tracing the lung contours.

Normal lung area develops four times more than the head circumference between week 12 and 32; therefore, the LHR needs to be adjusted according to gestational age. The effect of gestational age on LHR can be minimized by expressing the observed LHR as a ratio to the expected mean LHR for that gestational age.

2.10.1. *The lung area to head circumference ratio*

The lung-to-head circumference ratio (LHR) is a sonographic measure proposed to identify fetuses with congenital diaphragmatic hernia (CDH) that have a poor prognosis. The lung area contralateral to the CDH is measured at the level of *four-chamber view* by manual tracing of the lung which appears to be the most reproducible way of measuring the lung area [30]. The product is divided by the head circumference (HC) to obtain the LHR.

The lung area to head circumference ratio (LHR) = lung area/head circumference.

2.10.2. *Observed/expected lung-to-head ratio*

The observed LHR may be expressed as a percentage of the expected mean for gestational age as the observed/expected lung-to-head ratio O/E LHR [31, 32].

O/E LHR = (observed LHR/expected LHR) × 100

There has been proposed a four-step stratification of fetuses based on their observed/expected (O/E) LHR wherein it was also taken into account their liver position.

- Fetuses with an O/E LHR <15% have extreme pulmonary hypoplasia and there are no survivors reported.
- Fetuses with an O/E LHR between 15 and 25% have severe pulmonary hypoplasia and survival prediction is about 20%, those with the liver down having better prognosis than those with liver up in the thorax.
- Fetuses with an O/E LHR between 26 and 35% and those with an O/E LHR between 36 and 45% but with the liver up have moderate hypoplasia. They have an expected survival rate between 30 and 60%, which depends on the lung size.
- Fetuses with an O/E LHR between 36 and 45% with the liver down and those with an O/E LHR > 45% have mild hypoplasia and have better prognosis, >75% survival rate [33, 34] (**Table 7**).

• Prenatal prediction of postnatal outcome in CDH patients is based on ultrasound measurement of contralateral lung size and magnetic resonance total lung volumetry.
• The ratio of observed to predicted lung/head ratio is the most validated predictor for postnatal outcome; the liver position is also predictive.
• Fetal tracheal occlusion has been shown safe and feasible by minimally invasive means.

Table 7. Key points.

2.10.3. Fetal lung volumes

On fetal MR imaging there are several methods described for estimation of fetal pulmonary hypoplasia. All of these methods include the measuring of total fetal lung volume (TFLV). MR volumetry is considered the most accurate method for measuring ipsilateral lung and, therefore, for best estimation of fetal lung volumes, compared to three-dimensional ultrasound [35].

2.10.4. Fetal intervention

Because CDH is an anomaly with poor prognosis that can be identified in the prenatal period, it is justified to perform an intervention which improves lung function. Di Fiore and Wilson studied the concept of triggering lung growth by tracheal occlusion [36]. This was observed in an experiment of nature occurring in fetuses with congenital high airway obstruction syndrome (CHAOS), who display impressive lung growth. Through pregnancy, fetal lungs secrete fluid during their development, which creates a positive pressure under the glottis. Fluid secretion of the lung and a cyclical pressure change are essential for development and growth of the lung [37]. Fluid secretion increases the pressure in airways but during fetal breathing movements, the pressure gradient is normalized as glottis opens. This phenomenon creates cyclical periods of tissue stretch, which are important for an optimal balance between growth and differentiation [38]. Intrauterine tracheal occlusion acts like a closed glottis trapping the fluid causing subsequently increased tissue stretch, which triggers lung growth. The tracheal occlusion decreases the number of type II alveolocytes and lowers surfactant expression in occluded lungs [39–42]. This unwanted effect may be improved by either removing the tracheal occlusion before birth and/or by antenatal steroid administration [43, 44]. Experimentally, in-utero reversal of occlusion (clinically translated as a plug-unplug sequence) achieved morphologically better lung maturation [45].

3. Conclusions

As prenatal detection of fetal CDH improved in recent years, it is important to use standardized prognosis markers around the world. Currently, available markers are not 100% accurately predictive of outcome and their use is much less accurate in the presence of chromosomal anomalies or other malformations. This shows the fact that all fetuses diagnosed with CDH should undergo an ultrasound examination by a well-trained sonographer, as well as fetal echocardiography.

Author details

Adrian Claudiu Ratiu

Address all correspondence to: ratiu.adrian@umft.ro

University of Medicine and Pharmacy "Victor Babes", Timisoara, Romania

References

[1] Gallot D, Boda C, Ughetto S, Perthus I, Robert-Gnansia E, Francannet C, Laurichesse-Delmas H, Jani J, Coste K, Deprest J, et al. Prenatal detection and outcome of congenital diaphragmatic hernia: A French registry-based study. Ultrasound in Obstetrics & Gynecology. 2007;**29**:276-283

[2] Tudorache S, Chiuţu LC, Iliescu DG, Georgescu R, Stoica GA, Simionescu CE, Georgescu EF, Nemeş RN. Prenatal diagnosis and perinatal outcome in congenital diaphragmatic hernia. Single tertiary center report. Romanian Journal of Morphology and Embryology. 2014;**55**(3):823-833

[3] Parisi MA, Zayed H, Slavotinek AM, Rutledge JC. Congenital diaphragmatic hernia and microtia in a newborn with mycophenolate mofetil (MMF) exposure: Phenocopy for Fryns syndrome or broad spectrum of teratogenic effects? American Journal of Medical Genetics: Part A. 2009;**149A**:1237-1240

[4] Pober BR, Russell MK, Ackerman KG. Congenital diaphragmatic hernia overview. In: Pagon RA, Adam MP, Ardinger HH, et al., editors. Gene Reviews. Seattle (WA): University of Washington, Seattle; 1993-2017

[5] Mehollin-Ray AR, Cassady CI, Cass DL, Olutoye O. Fetal MR imaging of congenital diaphragmatic hernia. Radiographics. 2012;**32**:1067-1084

[6] Moore KL. The Developing Human: Clinically Oriented Embryology. 3rd ed. Philadelphia: WB Saunders; 1982

[7] Yuan W, Rao Y, Babiuk RP, Greer JJ, Wu JY, Ornitz DM. A genetic model for a central (septum transversum) congenital diaphragmatic hernia in mice lacking Slit3. Proceedings of the National Academy of Sciences of the United States of America. 2003;**100**:5217-5222

[8] Birchmeier C, Brohmann H. Genes that control the development of migrating muscle precursor cells. Current Opinion in Cell Biology. 2000;**12**:725-730

[9] Babiuk RP, Zhang W, Clugston R, Allan DW, Greer JJ. Embryological origins and development of the rat diaphragm. The Journal of Comparative Neurology. 2003;**455**:477-487

[10] Hopper AF, Hart NH. Foundations of Animal Development. Oxford: Oxford University Press; 1985

[11] Spooner BS, Wessels NK. Mammalian lung development: Interactions in primordium formation and bronchial morphogenesis. The Journal of Experimental Zoology. 1970;**175**:445-454

[12] Boyden EA. Development of the human lung. In: Brenneman J, editor. Practice of Pediatrics. Hagerstown, PA: Harper & Row; 1972

[13] Keijzer R, Puri P. Congenital diaphragmatic hernia. Seminars in Pediatric Surgery. 2010; **19**:180-185

[14] Reid L. The embryology of the lung. In: de Reuck AVS, Porter R, editors. Ciba Foundation Symposium. London: J. & A. Churchill Ltd; 1967. pp. 109-130

[15] Kluth D, Keijzer R, Hertl M, Tibboel D. Embryology of congenital diaphragmatic hernia. Seminars in Pediatric Surgery. 1996;**5**:224-233

[16] Greer JJ, Allan DW, Babiuk RP, Lemke RP. Recent advances in understanding the pathogenesis of nitrofen-induced congenital diaphragmatic hernia. Pediatric Pulmonology. 2000;**29**:394-399

[17] Jesudason EC, Connell MG, Fernig DG, et al. Early lung malformations in congenital diaphragmatic hernia. Journal of Pediatric Surgery. 2000;**35**:124-127, discussion: 128

[18] Keijzer R, Liu J, Deimling J, et al. Dual-hit hypothesis explains pulmonary hypoplasia in the nitrofen model of congenital diaphragmatic hernia. The American Journal of Pathology. 2000;**156**:1299-1306

[19] Puri P, Gorman F. Lethal nonpulmonary anomalies associated with congenital diaphragmatic hernia: Implications for early intrauterine surgery. Journal of Pediatric Surgery. 1984;**19**(1):29-32

[20] Bootstaylor BS, Filly RA, Harrison MR, Adzick NS. Prenatal sonographic predictors of liver herniation in congenital diaphragmatic hernia. Journal of Ultrasound in Medicine. 1995;**14**:515-552

[21] Ruano R, Benachi A, Aubry MC, Bernard JP, Hameury F, Nihoul-Fekete C, Dumez Y. Prenatal sonographic diagnosis of congenital hiatal hernia. Prenatal Diagnosis. 2004; **24**(1):26-30

[22] Di Francesco S, Matteo Lanna M, Napolitano M, et al. A case of ultrasound diagnosis of fetal hiatal hernia in late third trimester of pregnancy. Case Reports in Obstetrics and Gynecology. 2015;**2015**. Article ID 194090, 3 pages. DOI: 10.1155/2015/194090

[23] Garne E, Quataert P, de Vigan C. Congenital diaphragmatic hernia: A European population-based study of epidemiology, prenatal diagnosis and mortality. Prenatal and Neonatal Medicine. 1999;**4**:441-447

[24] Garne E, Haeusler M, Barisic I, Gjergja R, Stoll C, Clementi M, the Euroscan Study Group. Congenital diaphragmatic hernia: Evaluation of prenatal diagnosis in 20 European regions. Ultrasound in Obstetrics & Gynecology. 2002;**19**:329-333

[25] Sebire NJ, Snijders RJM, Davenport M, Greenough A, Nicolaides KH. Fetal nuchal translucency thickness at 10-14 weeks of gestation and congenital diaphragmatic hernia. Obstetrics and Gynecology. 1997;**90**:943-947

[26] Knudtson J, Grewal H. Thoracoscopic excision of a paraesophageal bronchogenic cyst in a child. JSLS. 2004;**8**:179-182

[27] Jaggers J, Balsara K. Mediastinal masses in children. Seminars in Thoracic and Cardiovascular Surgery. 2004;**16**:201-208

[28] Ionescu C, Haradja H, Gheorghiu D, Vladescu T, Pacu I, Dimitriu M. Prenatal ultrasound diagnosis of cervical teratoma. Gineco.ro. 2011;**7**(23):25-27

[29] Metkus AP, Filly RA, Stringer MD, Harrison MR, Adzick NS. Sonographic predictors of survival in fetal diaphragmatic hernia. Journal of Pediatric Surgery. 1996;**31**:148-151

[30] Peralta CFA, Cavoretto P, Csapo B, Vandecruys H, Nicolaides KH. Assessment of lung area in normal fetuses at 12-32 weeks. Ultrasound in Obstetrics & Gynecology. 2005; **26**:718-724

[31] Jani J, Nicolaides KH, Keller RL, Benachi A, Peralta CFA, Favre R, Moreno O, Tibboel D, Lipitz S, Eggink A, Vaast P, Allegaert K, Harrison M, Deprest J. Observed to expected lung area to head circumference ratio in the prediction of survival in fetuses with isolated diaphragmatic hernia. Ultrasound in Obstetrics & Gynecology. 2007;**30**:67-71

[32] Jani JC, Peralta CFA, Nicolaides KH. Lung-to-head ratio: A need to unify the technique. Ultrasound in Obstetrics & Gynecology. 2012;**39**:2-6

[33] Deprest JA, Flemmer AW, Gratacos E, Nicolaides K. Antenatal prediction of lung volume and in-utero treatment by fetal endoscopic tracheal occlusion in severe isolated congenital diaphragmatic hernia. Seminars in Fetal & Neonatal Medicine. 2009;**14**:8-13

[34] Ionescu C, Gheorghiu D, Pacu I, Sardescu G, Ionescu V. Prognosticul fetal în hernia diafragmatică congenitală stîngă. Obstetrica si Ginecologia. 2009;**LVII**(3):183

[35] Jani JC, Cannie M, Peralta CFA, Deprest JA, Nicolaides KH, Dymarkowski S. Lung volumes in fetuses with congenital diaphragmatic hernia: Comparison of 3D US and MR imaging assessments. Radiology. 2007;**244**(2):575-582

[36] DiFiore JW, Fauza DO, Slavin R, Peters CA, Fackler JC, Wilson JM. Experimental fetal tracheal ligation reverses the structural and physiological effects of pulmonary hypoplasia in congenital diaphragmatic hernia. Journal of Pediatric Surgery. 1994;**29**:248-256

[37] Moessinger AC, Harding R, Adamson TM, Singh M, Kiu GT. Role of lung fluid volume in growth and maturation of the fetal sheep lung. The Journal of Clinical Investigation. 1990;**86**:1270-1277

[38] Nelson SM, Hajivassiliou CA, Haddock G, et al. Rescue of the hypoplastic lung by prenatal cyclical strain. American Journal of Respiratory and Critical Care Medicine. 2005;**171**:1395-1402

[39] Probyn ME, Wallace MJ, Hooper SB. Effect of increased lung expansion on lung growth and development near midgestation in fetal sheep. Pediatric Research. 2000;**47**:806-812

[40] Luks FI, Roggin KK, Wild YK, et al. Effect of lung fluid composition on type II cellular activity after tracheal occlusion in the fetal lamb. Journal of Pediatric Surgery. 2001; **36**:196-201

[41] De Paepe ME, Papadakis K, Johnson BD, Luks FI. Fate of the type II pneumocyte following tracheal occlusion in utero: A time-course study in fetal sheep. Virchows Archiv. 1998;**432**:7-16

[42] O'Toole SJ, Sharma A, Karamanoukian HL, Holm B, Azizkhan RG, Glick PL. Tracheal ligation does not correct the surfactant deficiency associated with congenital diaphragmatic hernia. Journal of Pediatric Surgery. 1996;**31**:546-550

[43] Bratu I, Flageole H, Laberge JM, et al. Surfactant levels after reversible tracheal occlusion and prenatal steroids in experimental diaphragmatic hernia. Journal of Pediatric Surgery. 2001;**36**:122-127

[44] Davey MG, Danzer E, Schwarz U, Adzick NS, Flake AW, Hedrick HL. Prenatal glucocorticoids and exogenous surfactant therapy improve respiratory function in lambs with severe diaphragmatic hernia following fetal tracheal occlusion. Pediatric Research. 2006;**60**(2):131-135

[45] Flageole H, Evrard VA, Piedboeuf B, Laberge JM, Lerut TE, Deprest JA. The plug–unplug sequence: An important step to achieve type II pneumocyte maturation in the fetal lamb model. Journal of Pediatric Surgery. 1998;**33**:299-303

5

Prenatal Genetic Counseling in Congenital Anomalies

Mihaela Amelia Dobrescu, Florin Burada,
Mihai Gabriel Cucu, Anca Lelia Riza, Gratiela Chelu,
Razvan Mihail Plesea, Adela Cucu,
Alina Liliana Cimpoeru and Mihai Ioana

Abstract

The impact of genetic variability on embryogenesis and fetus development established medical genetics as essential for the prevention of congenital anomalies, early detection and appropriate management. Advances in ultrasonography equipment and technique allow early detection of many congenital malformations. In addition, genetic testing can be performed in a prenatal setting on a variety of biological samples obtained by invasive and noninvasive procedures: chorionic villus sampling, amniocentesis, cordocentesis, or maternal blood collection (i.e., cell free fetal DNA). In the past, only a small percentage of congenital anomalies had a readily identifiable etiology; genetic diagnostic procedures can provide at least some of the answers for the remaining unsolved cases. Undoubtedly, the need for appropriate case management and counseling justifies the importance of uncovering the underlying genetic cause of birth defects. In this chapter, we will focus on genetic counseling in congenital anomalies, including isolated congenital anomalies and preimplantation genetic diagnosis. Genetic counseling provides information and support, assisting parents in making informed decisions. Through this process, parents learn about the risk of having a newborn with a congenital malformation and the nature of the disorder and its natural history, are advised on available testing for that particular case, and discuss options for risk management and family planning.

Keywords: congenital anomalies, genetic counseling

1. Rationale for prenatal genetic counseling

Congenital anomalies are a major cause of stillbirths and neonatal mortality. Taking into consideration that in 2004 WHO estimated an incidence of about 7% in newborns, congenital anomalies are a major cause of morbidity and mortality worldwide.

Congenital anomalies can be caused by *chromosome abnormalities, single-gene defects, multifactorial inheritance,* or *epigenetic or nongenetic factors.* It is notable that in up to 50% of all cases no apparent identifiable cause can be found. Any microscopically detectable autosomal imbalance, such as trisomy, duplication, deletion, or monosomy, will result in severe structural and developmental abnormality, most of which are lethal conditions. Single-gene defects have been associated with congenital abnormalities that might involve one or more organs and systems with or without an obvious underlying embryological relationship. Multifactorial inheritance accounts for the majority of congenital abnormalities, including isolated malformations, in which genetic factors can clearly be involved.

It should be noted that although malformations are always thought to be congenital, not all congenital abnormalities are "literally" malformations. Anomalies due to an intrinsic, genetic (chromosomal aberration and gene mutation), or multifactorial factor represent approximately 45% of all congenital abnormalities. These are considered primary congenital malformations. Anomalies resulting from the action of an extrinsic factor—chemical, physical, biological agents, and possibly maternal condition—add up 5% of the congenital anomalies identified and are considered secondary congenital anomalies. For the remaining 50% of these abnormalities, the cause is unknown and therefore cannot be included in this classification [1].

The impact of genetic variability on embryogenesis and fetus development established medical genetics as essential for the prevention of congenital anomalies, early detection, and appropriate management. In the past, when dealing with congenital malformations, medical professionals had to face two major issues: a late detection of the anomaly and the lack of an identifiable cause. The act of disease prevention back then was virtually impossible.

Though, in the last decade of rapidly progressing genomic technologies, genetic diagnosis tools became widely accessible, playing an important role in both clinical practice and research. The completion of the Human Genome Project has contributed greatly to our understanding of the molecular basis of genetic disorders.

The importance of determining the genetic cause of birth defects lies in the need for appropriate case management and genetic counseling. Genetic counseling is meant to assist parents in making informed decisions. Through counseling, parents learn about the risk of having a newborn with a congenital malformation and the nature of the disorder and its natural history, are advised on available testing for that particular case, and discuss options for risk management and family planning.

All attempts must be made to arrive at as precise a diagnosis as possible by evaluating gestational history for environmental factors, family history for genetic factors, and patient anatomy for clues to embryologic etiopathogenic mechanisms. Evaluating family history for genetic factors, gestational history for environmental factors, and patient phenotype for information on embryologic mechanisms is mandatory to arrive at as precise a diagnosis as possible.

Genetic counseling may be hampered by the inaccurate recording of the above mentioned and the inherent uncertainty in interpreting them. Given the incompleteness of available data and the difficulty in interpretation, genetic counseling has a demanding and potentially difficult mission.

1.1. Prenatal genetic counseling—when and how

Genetic counseling is a complex medical act, which aims to help families, individuals, and couples to better understand the familial, medical, psychological, and reproductive consequences of the genetic contribution to specific health conditions. It can be offered both pre- and postnatally.

Fortunately, most babies are born healthy. However, in some pregnancies, a risk for birth defects or other genetic problems may be identified. Geneticists and genetic counselors provide prenatal genetic counseling services for individuals, couples, or families with a concern about the health of their unborn baby.

Prenatal counselling manages cases with risks by understanding prenatal screening and testing options. Increased chance of having a child with a birth defect or genetic condition makes the genetic consultations a necessity. The purpose of genetic counseling is to allow informed decision-making by communicating accurate and complete information and presenting objective diagnostic and therapeutic options [2]. To achieve its goal, information transfer must be made in a clear but neutral way, using simple language, respecting ethical and cultural values.

Pretest counseling. At this stage, the couple will be informed on the objectives of the counseling session regarding the suspicion of congenital anomaly for the pregnancy.

The genetic counselor/geneticist will lay down the alternatives the couple has for following up the pregnancy and explain the possibility and alternatives for testing for identifying the cause of the congenital anomalies identified. The geneticist must take into consideration that accepting to be tested may be influenced by psychosocial factors, such as ethnicity, sociodemographic status, and the presence of the partner during the counseling session [3].

If the couple expresses the desire for prenatal diagnosis, the counselor must present the objectives, benefits, risks, limitations, costs, and alternatives for each of the available screening and/or diagnosis techniques. The patient has the right to accept or refuse a given recommendation. At all times, it must be clear that testing is optional.

The counseling must go beyond making an informed choice for testing and what this step entails, but also preparing the couple for possible outcomes dictated by a positive or negative result.

Posttest counseling. Posttest counseling must explain thoroughly the significance of the result, the meaning of a positive or negative result, and go over the limitations of each test. It must also suggest other possible confirmatory or complementary tests or alternatives [2] and unconditionally support the patient's options, respecting the autonomy of his/her choice.

One of the most encumbering tasks of genetic counseling is presenting a family with the fact that their child has a genetic condition or birth defect. Most of the test results face the couple with a termination/no-termination decision.

As part of the informed decision-making process, the couple must be informed in detail on the clinical presentation and prognosis of the disorder identified. This is often problematic in chromosomal disorders: (1) genotypic variability—the phenotype will vary depending on the extent of the genetic defect and (2) phenotypic variability—the evolution of a case can vary greatly, even between carriers of the same type of anomaly.

1.2. "Why did it happen? Will it happen again? What can be done?"

These questions are perhaps among the most frequent during the counseling session and we will try to answer them briefly below. The probability reoccurrence is called "recurrence risk." Recurrence risk assessment and counseling is based on a combination of theoretic risk assessment and empiric data. Families and patients should be informed on the assumptions involved and the limitations of such estimates.

This chapter is focused on genetic counseling in congenital anomalies, caused by chromosomal, monogenic, or plurifactorial anomalies, as well as on preimplantation genetic diagnosis.

2. Genetic counseling in chromosomal congenital anomalies

Carrier and aneuploidy screening and diagnostic testing have expanded intensely over the past two decades [2], which is justifiable given the estimate of 5.3% of the neonates affected by a genetic disorder. Despite ultrasound and biochemistry reasons for recommending a prenatal diagnosis, genetic testing in pregnancy is optional. Decisions about undergoing testing should be expressed, consented, and based on individual patient's values and needs and guided by the geneticist during counseling sessions.

Congenital anomalies can be caused by chromosomal, monogenic, and multifactorial disorders [4]; out of which, chromosomal anomalies have a significant impact given their combined frequency of 1 in 153 pregnancies [5] and the reserved prognosis for many of them.

Aneuploidies are the most frequent chromosomal anomalies. Aneuploidies are numerical disorders (**Figure 1**)—the number of chromosomes differs to the normal state, called euploidy. Any of the chromosomes, autosomes, or heterosomes can be affected. Aneuploidies can be complete, involving the whole chromosome, or partial. From a single fertilized egg, more populations of cells of different genotypes can develop—this abnormal situation is called mosaicism. Due to their high incidence, three complete trisomies bear significance for the prenatal diagnosis: trisomy 21 (T21—Down syndrome), 18 (T18—Edwards syndrome), and 13 (T13—Patau syndrome).

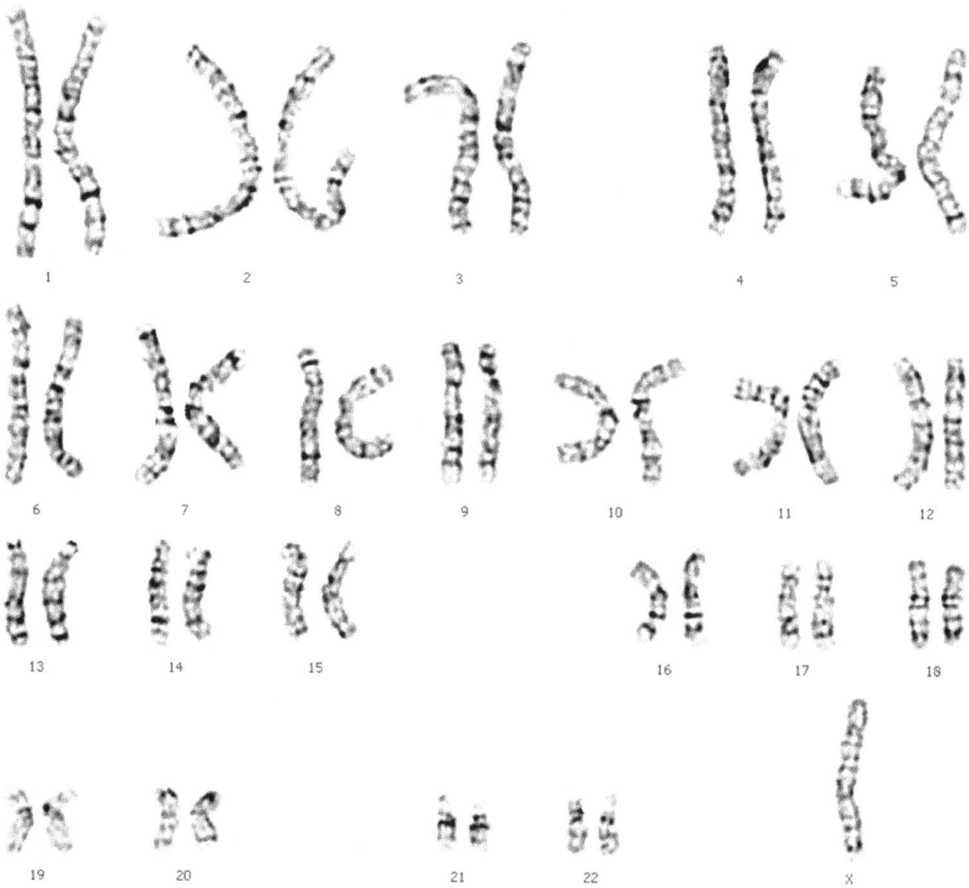

Figure 1. Karyotype 45,X—monosomy X.

Other chromosomal anomalies are structural, such as deletions, duplications, inversions, insertions, translocations, etc. (**Figures 2** and **3**). They are rare and require different diagnosis strategies, counseling, and management of the case.

Possible alternatives for screening ("Prenatal Biochemical and Ultrasound Markers in Chromosomal Anomalies") and diagnosis ("Genomic Testing for Prenatal Clinical Evaluation of Congenital Anomalies") are presented in detail in different chapters, due to their marked importance in genetic testing and counseling.

In the current section, we aim to cover several genetic counseling concepts in a few hypothetical situations of congenital anomaly with underlying chromosomal cause. Pre- and posttesting counseling are a prerequisite of all genetic counseling, but the genetic consult comprises also of a detailed assessment of medical history, psychosocial assessment, and family history, which we are not focusing on here [3, 6, 7].

The possible mechanism by which the chromosomal anomalies occur is usually due to errors in the cell division cycles: nondisjunction in the maternal meiotic division I, and, less frequently, paternal origin [8] or meiosis II [9].

The etiology is mostly unclear, but the probability of chromosomal anomalies increases with maternal age [4], and this is one of the most common etiological factors. Predisposition to

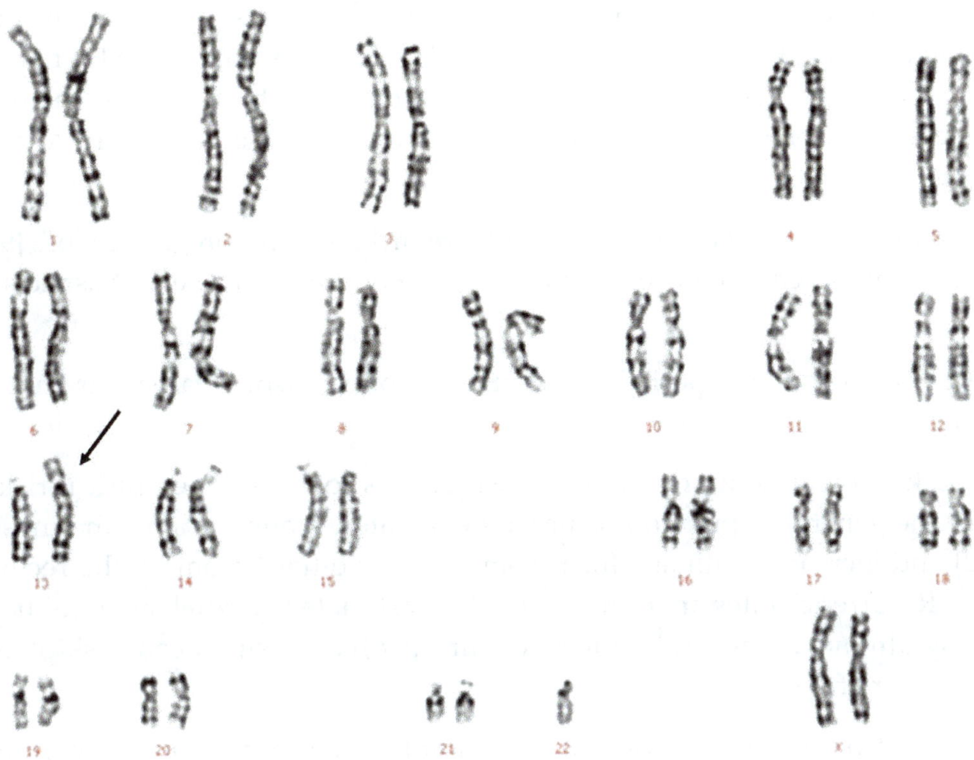

Figure 2. Karyotype 45,XX,rob(13;22)(q10;q10)—Robertsonian translocation.

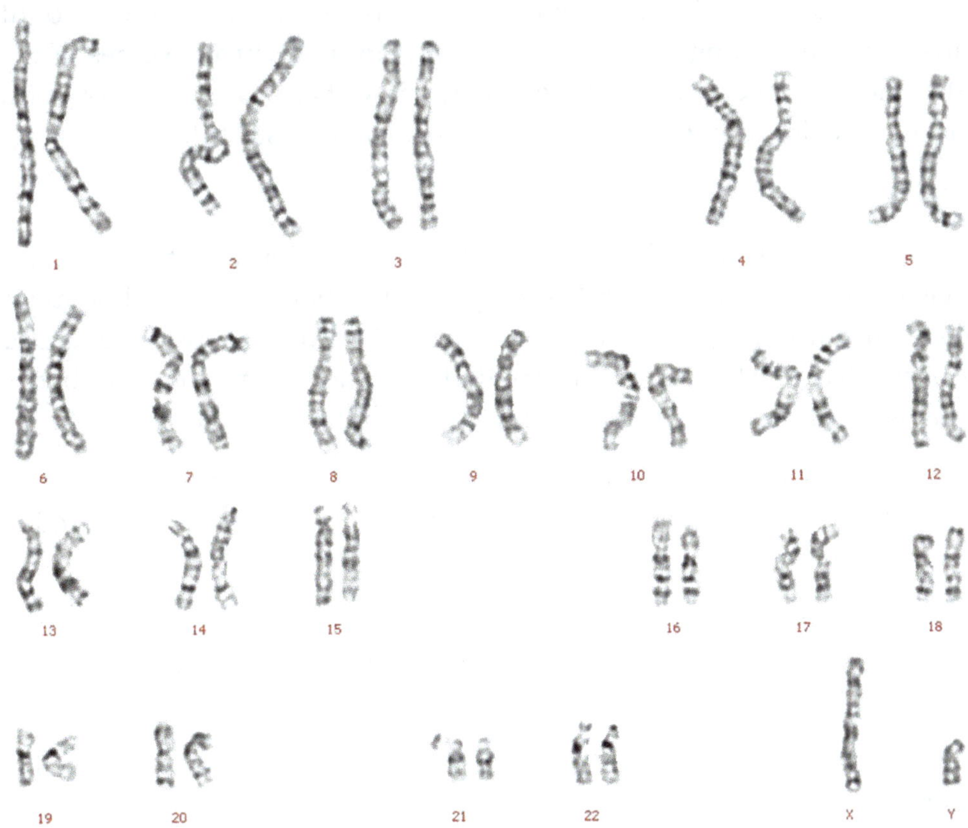

Figure 3. Karyotype 46,XY,t(1;15)(p36.3;q26.1)—reciprocal translocation.

oocyte aneuploidy is also seen in young women, gene expression alteration due to environmental factors and the influence of follicle-stimulating hormone (FSH) being possible culprits [10]. It is yet uncertain if the paternal age contributes to the risk of aneuploidy, if at all [11]. The contribution of different occupational or environmental factors is insufficiently documented.

Aneuploidies are most frequent causes of mental retardation and pregnancy loss [9]. It comes as no surprise that the chance of reoccurrence is one of the most relevant aspects of genetic counseling.

(a) Complete chromosomal, especially autosomal trisomies, when parents are not carriers of translocations

Recurrence risk in the absence of parent translocations follows the empirical risk—the risk measured in the general population, generally evaluated around 1% for the most common trisomy [12] and increases with age for trisomy 21. For other trisomies, the recurrence risk seems lower. Recurrence rates are rather difficult to estimate in sexual aneuploidies. Subjects with Down syndrome are generally infertile, but they have a significant risk of aneuploidy recurrence in their offspring [13].

(b) Chromosomal trisomies with one of the parents being a carrier of a chromosome 21 translocation

Down syndrome translocations are present in less than 4% of the cases. Translocations can occur de novo. For transmitted translocations, the recurrence risk depended on the affected parent: for instance, depending on the involved translocated chromosomes, if the mother is the balanced carrier, the risk is to that of the father, without any known reason for the discrepancy. A balanced translocation t(21,21) has 100% recurrence risk [14].

(c) Mosaicism

Generally, mosaicism cases have the lowest frequency contributions to the total of the trisomies. Mosaicism can occur de novo in the offspring, but parental germ line mosaicism contributes to the recurrence risk [15]. Reduced mosaic [16], meaning low percentage of modified cell lines, or partial trisomy [17], equivalent with duplication, generally has a better prognosis by comparison with a homogenous complete trisomy, but this is not a rule [18].

The couple must be informed that there is no prophylaxis or treatment to correct the aneuploidy, but genetic counseling can provide the support for medically informed decisions to guide the management of the case.

If the couple wishes to keep a pregnancy with chromosomal disorder, they must be informed on the obstetrical complications that may arise, the life expectancy, and the natural history of the disease neonatally and into adulthood.

A trisomy prenatal case, especially 13 or 18, may present with different obstetrical challenges: miscarriage and stillbirth are more frequent than compared to the general population. Structural anomalies of the fetuses lead to a negative prognosis after birth and low life expectancy [19].

Screening and diagnosis limitations for trisomy 13 lead to underdiagnosis of this aneuploidy. Genetic counseling should bring into discussion the viable fetuses in the second trimester (60% of the cases), when life expectancy is very hard to predict and there is no longer the alternative to terminate the pregnancy. It is crucial to inform the parents on the neonatal procedures for resuscitation, possibilities to correct certain defects so that the couple is prepared to face the trauma of having a child with lethal defect [20].

For trisomy 18, only 10% of the neonates survive longer than 1 year. Diagnosing this trisomy though genetic testing is essential for decision-making during the neonatal life, where critical emergency interventions and choosing invasive treatments are often required [21].

Trisomy 21 has a life expectancy of almost 60 years. Following up, the patient asks for collaborations with multiple medical specialties: cardiological, ENT, ophthalmology, endocrinology, to assess possible complications. During their pediatric life, other interventions are generally symptomatic and similar to their euploid peers [22]. The parents must be prepared though through genetic counseling for the possible difficulties due to motor and cognitive delay. Support in the patient's lifestyle can also come from nongovernmental associations and patient support groups, e.g., Down Syndrome International (https://ds-int.org/down-syndrome-your-country).

3. Congenital anomalies in monogenic diseases

Very often, genetic congenital anomalies are part of the clinical presentation of monogenic diseases; 7.5% of isolated or syndromic congenital anomalies are caused by monogenic disorders. Congenital anomalies can become obvious prenatally or at birth, and at times, they are noticeable only in later development, but in all cases, it happens between conception and birth.

The diagnosis of a monogenic disease is often established based on a conclusive family history, clinical examination, and pedigree pattern and confirmed through genetic testing.

With a known diagnosis, the risk of recurrence will be estimated according to the inheritance pattern of the disease. When definite diagnosis is not available, all attempts should be made to associate the clinical picture with a specific disease. If successful, precise genetic counseling can be offered. Situations when diagnosis cannot be demonstrated before birth are difficult to manage—the counselor will advise the couple when there is a lack of crucial medical information.

Should screening identify congenital anomalies during intrauterine life, couples will be faced with a pressing situation, as anomaly finding does not necessarily imply certain diagnosis. In this case, establishing the diagnosis should be aimed for whenever possible, as the first step in genetic counseling.

There are situations with a known diagnosis and known disease-causing mutation that allow prenatal diagnosis testing. Prenatal invasive diagnosis for monogenic disease running in the family, depending on its severity, should and will be recommended. If diagnosis can be readily established, then the recurrence risk can be calculated. Probability of inheritance based on Mendel's principles and conditional probability (also known as Bayesian analysis, based on Bayes' theorem on probability) are used to calculate genetic risk [1].

The risk of expressing a monogenic disease is dependent not only on the pattern of inheritance, but also on other factors such as the incidence of the disease, the presence of other affected members, the penetrance and variable expressivity, ethnicity, and the influence of environmental factors.

3.1. Autosomal dominant inheritance

An autosomal dominant disease is a condition expressed in both heterozygous, carrying one copy, and homozygous individuals, carrying two copies one from each parent. The disease is caused by a single gene defect located on an autosome. The affected individuals are usually heterozygous, and the homozygous genotype is associated with more severe features or can be lethal. Females and males exhibit the trait in approximately equal proportions and severity of clinical signs is similar between the two sexes. Both sexes are equally likely to transmit the mutation to their offspring. Mostly, the affected offsprings are descendants of an affected heterozygous and a normal parent. On average, half of the children will be heterozygous and express the disease and half will not. Rarely, homozygous are seen in autosomal dominant diseases. This status can be due to a higher frequency of a gene with mild effects, late onset (e.g. Huntington disease) or when both parents are affected (e.g. achondroplasia). Unusually, an affected homozygous parent will transmit the disease to all of his children. On the pedigree, a vertical transmission pattern is observed (**Figure 4**), and the disease phenotype is usually seen in one generation after another. The disease does not skip generations: if an individual has an autosomal disease, in most of the cases, one parent must also have it [1, 2].

Frequently, autosomal dominant disorders involve different organs and systems of the body; however, dominant conditions affecting one organ have been described (e.g., congenital cataract). The capacity of a single gene to affect unrelated organs is called *pleiotropy* (e.g., Marfan syndrome can affect the skeletal, ocular, and cardiovascular systems; some affected individuals have all features, whereas others may have almost none). In addition, the clinical features in autosomal dominant disorders can show remarkable variation between patients, even between the members of the same family. This difference between individuals is referred to as *variable expressivity* (e.g., in autosomal dominant polycystic kidney disease, some affected individuals develop renal failure in early adulthood, whereas others have just a few renal cysts that do not significantly influence renal function). Occasionally, the heterozygous and homozygous individuals express identical phenotype (complete dominance) [2, 23].

Sometimes, a dominant mutation is inherited, but the condition it determines is not expressed. In these cases, the gene has *reduced (incomplete)penetrance.* The term penetrance is used in monogenic inheritance to indicate the probability of a gene to influence the phenotype. A number of autosomal dominant diseases show an incomplete penetrance (e.g., polydactyly), meaning that a person has the mutation but shows no evidence of a disease. A gene is *completely penetrant* if each individual who inherited the mutation expresses clinical features (e.g., neurofibromatosis type I) [3].

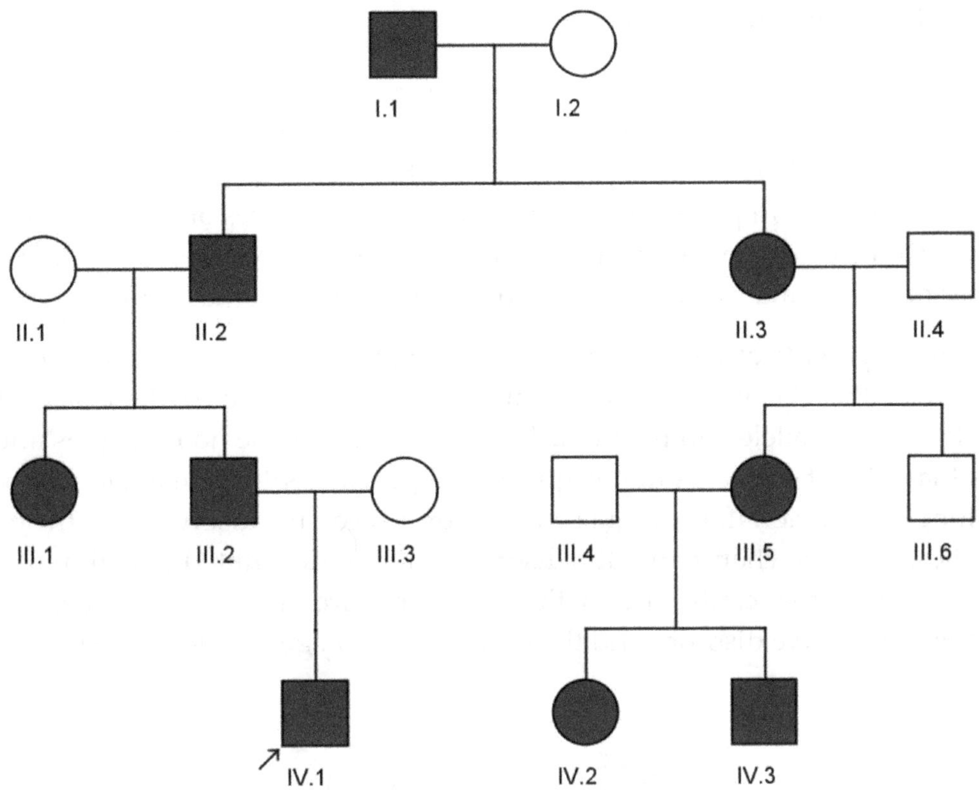

Figure 4. Autosomal dominant inheritance.

Often, known autosomal dominant conditions are seen in a person without an affected parent. The condition seems to be isolated and no clinical features are detected among other family members. In these cases, the disease can be attributed to a *"de novo" mutation* and the recurrence risk for siblings is very low. The mutation is found only in a gamete and the mutated gene is transmitted by one of the healthy parents. The percent of cases caused by de novo mutations is influenced by the severity of clinical features or the capability of reproduction. Osteogenesis imperfecta type II is exclusively caused by new mutations, the condition being perinatally lethal. Also, more than 80% of cases with achondroplasia are due to new mutations, and the proportion is significantly lower in polycystic kidney disease. In this case, it is important to know the family history to distinguish isolated cases and rule out incomplete penetrance or variation in expression. The detection of a specific mutation in a proband allows direct testing of the parents to exclude a disease with expression variability. Also, the detection of a specific mutation can help predict the severity of clinical features in some diseases [24].

Germline mosaicism is another mechanism documented in a number of autosomal dominant diseases such as tuberous sclerosis or osteogenesis imperfecta. Germline mosaicism, also known as gonadal mosaicism, is a condition in which the precursor (germ line) cells to egg and sperm cells are a mixture (mosaic) of two or more genetically different cell lines [1, 2]. The parents do not exhibit any clinical features because the somatic cells are not affected; only a proportion of eggs or sperm cells are carriers of the mutation. Two or more children are affected when there is no family history of disease. This condition is associated with increased recurrence risk for future offspring of a mosaic parent. Because mutation is a rare event, it is unlikely that this would be due to multiple mutations in the same family.

3.2. Autosomal recessive inheritance

An autosomal recessive disease is a condition expressed only in homozygous individuals with both mutant alleles. The parents of such homozygotes must be at least heterozygous for the disease allele and are usually referred to as carriers for that disorder (**Figure 5**). In most cases, the *loss-of-function* mutation is a process in which mutant allele reduces or removes the function of an enzyme. In the heterozygous state, the normal allele can compensate the mutant one, and in homozygotes or compound homozygotes with both mutant alleles, the disease occurs [1, 2, 4].

When two carrier parents of the mutant allele are matting, there is a 50% chance for each of them to transmit either the wild-type or the mutant allele. Thus, each of them has a 50% chance to transmit the mutant allele and further 25% of offspring may be homozygous affected. This also means that 50% of the cases the offspring will get one wild-type allele and one mutant allele, resulting in a carrier. If a parent is affected by a recessive disorder and the other is heterozygous there is a 50% chance that the disorder will be transmitted to children, depending on which allele the partner contributes with. All children are carriers when a parent is affected by an autosomal recessive disorder and the other is homozygous wild-type [1, 4].

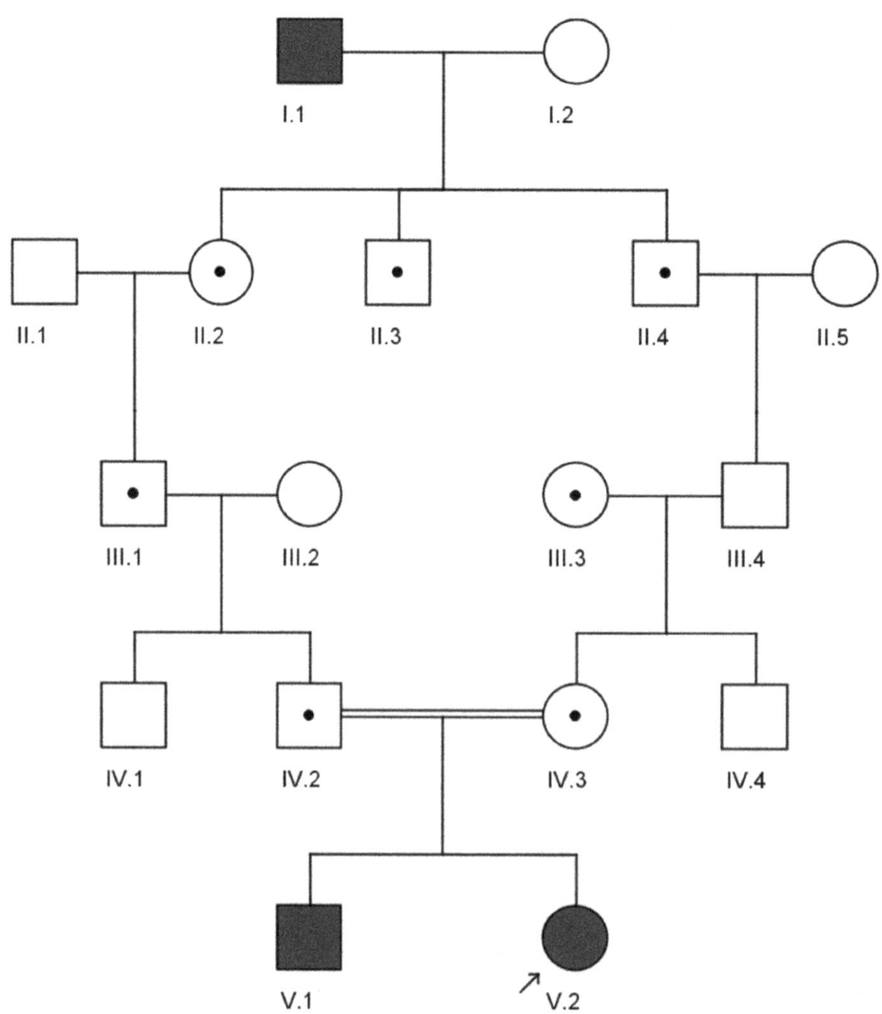

Figure 5. Autosomal recessive inheritance.

Consanguinity is referred to as a couple who have at least a common ancestor, meaning that they are relatives. Finding out that an individual with a genetic disorder is the result of a consanguineous couple is strong evidence for a recessive condition, although not certainty, because there is a greater chance that the parents would have inherited the mutant allele from their common ancestor and passed it down, than the possibility of finding a similar mutation in two unrelated individuals in the general population. In fact, this is true for very rare mutations (e.g., alkaptonuria or xeroderma pigmentosum). In contrast for common autosomal recessive disorders (e.g., cystic fibrosis), the incidence in general population is not significantly lower than in consanguineous marriages. Meaning that the rarer the mutation is in the general population, the more likely that the parents are related (consanguinity) [5].

There are specific recessive disorders for which it is not uncommon that two affected individuals will have children together. Such is the case for individuals with deafness or visual impairment who will benefit from the same social facilities or will be educated together. If the disorder is caused by the same mutation, then all their children would be affected; however, there are studies that show that normal children are born from these couples. The most common explanation is that the parents are homozygous for different genes, both causing deafness, and so the children are heterozygous for both mutations, also known as double heterozygote. This type of genetic heterogeneity is called *locus heterogeneity*. Heterogeneity can also be found in the same locus, as it would be the case of an affected individual who is heterozygote for both alleles, making him/her a *compound heterozygote*. Most affected individuals with recessive autosomal inherited disorders are compound heterozygotes, unless that specific mutation is rather common in the general population (as is the case with cystic fibrosis), or he/she is the result of a consanguinity marriage [1].

Another method of assessing recurrence risk is by calculating the genotype frequency, knowing the allele frequency. This is not as straightforward as it would seem because there is the matter of allele distribution in heterozygotes and homozygotes. This can be done by using the *Hardy-Weinberg Law*, but the population used on has to meet some criteria such as: (a) the population is large and the mattings are random; (b) there is no significant rate of new mutations; (c) there is no selection for any genotype; and (d) there is no significant migration disturbing the endogenous population allele frequency [6].

The presence of both homologous from a pair or chromosomal regions in an offspring coming from the same parent is called *uniparental disomy*. The uniparental disomy can be caused by an error in meiosis resulting in two different chromosomes coming from the same parent, which is called heterodisomy, or by an error in meiosis II, which will result in identical chromosomes transmitted from the same parent called isodisomy. This abnormality has been reported to be a rare cause for cystic fibrosis, in families where only one parent is heterozygote and the offspring takes both homologous chromosomes with the mutant allele from that parent [1, 4].

3.3. Sex-linked inheritance

This type of inheritance is linked to the genes found on the sex chromosomes. Inheritance patterns for the genes found on X chromosome relates to X-linked inheritance, while for the genes located on Y chromosomes, it is called holandric or Y-linked inheritance. The genes positioned on the X and Y chromosomes are unequally transmitted to males and females.

X-inactivation is a normal process, which appears in the early development of the embryo. The result is that most of the genes on one of the two X chromosomes in females are inactivated in each cell, ensuring the fact that, similar to males, females have only one functional X chromosome. One of the two chromosomes is randomly inactivated, meaning that approximately half of the cells in females have a functional X chromosome of maternal origin and the other half have the paternal one functional. This process interferes with both dominant and recessive X-linked inheritance as detailed below [5].

3.3.1. X-linked dominant inheritance

X-linked dominant inheritance is caused by a dominant mutant allele located on the X chromosome. Hemizygous males and both homozygous and heterozygous females are affected. Males are more likely to be severely affected given the fact that in females one of the X chromosomes will be inactivated (X-inactivation), unless the females are homozygous for that allele.

Affected heterozygote offsprings of both sexes have a 50% chance to inherit the mutant allele from an affected mother, which is similar in the autosomal dominant inheritance too (**Figure 6**). The difference between the autosomal and X-linked dominant inheritance refers to affected males. All daughters of an affected male will also be affected by inheriting the X chromosome with the mutant allele, whereas male offsprings will inherit the Y chromosome, thus avoiding the disorder. Affected females are twice more frequent than affected males, although females tend to have milder phenotypic manifestations. One example of an X-linked dominant inheritance disorder is the hypophosphatemic rickets [1, 2, 4].

In some cases, affected males with an X-linked dominant disorder are rarely seen, for example, Rett syndrome and incontinentia pigmenti. This is due to the fact that the presence of the mutant allele in male hemizygotes will result in an early embryonic development stop. In other cases, it seems that only females are affected because males are "speared." An example of a disorder that spares male hemizygotes is X-linked females—limited epilepsy and cognitive impairment. Females appear to be healthy at birth, yet they develop the affection from the second year of life, while males are unaffected their whole life. This disorder is caused by a loss of functional mechanism in the protocadherin gene 19, which is expressed in the neurons. The explanation for this particular case would be that random X-inactivation makes a mosaic expression of this gene in the cells of the central nervous system, which disrupts communications between neurons. In males, the brain is spared this miscommunication between neurons by seemingly a different protocadherin, which compensates the loss of the first [6].

3.3.2. X-linked recessive inheritance

X-linked recessive inheritance is caused by a recessive mutant gene located on the X chromosome. Almost all affected individuals are males (hemizygotes), while homozygotes affected females are rarely seen. The clinical features seen in females are mainly due to non-random X-inactivation [4].

All daughters of an affected male (hemizygous) will be carriers (heterozygotes) for a specific disorder, whereas the sons will inherit the Y chromosomes from the father and thus will be

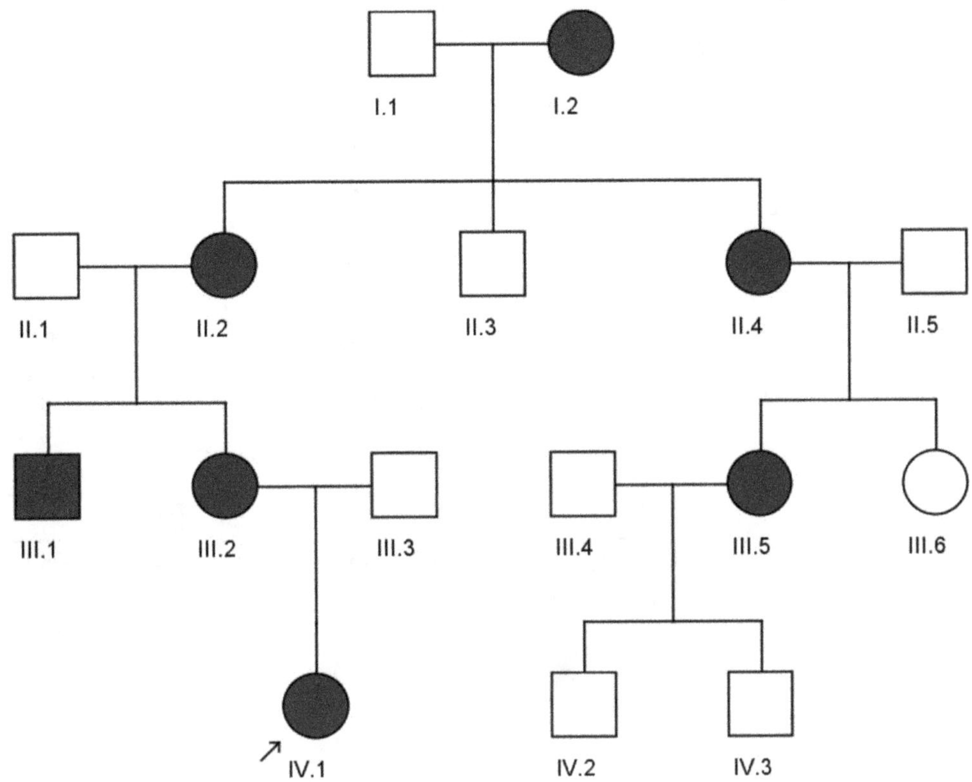

Figure 6. X-linked dominant inheritance.

unaffected by the disorder. For a female carrying the mutation, there is a 50% chance to transmit the mutant X chromosome to the offspring, as a result 50% of the daughters will be carriers and 50% of the sons will be affected (**Figure 7**). For a female to be affected means to inherit the mutant allele from each parent, which is very unlikely to happen, or another option is the presence of only one X chromosome (monosomy X) on which the mutation is present, making her a hemizygous for the allele, like in the case of males. A commonly known X-linked recessive disorder is hemophilia A caused by deficiency of factor VIII, a protein involved in clotting [1, 2, 6].

Sometimes, the females can express the phenotype. The most common situation is represented by a carrier female showing phenotypic features, phenomenon known as *manifesting heterozygote*. This manifestation is due to X-inactivation, which is not random anymore; rather, it has become unbalanced or skewed. The skewed X-inactivation can be both advantageous when the inactivated X chromosome in all or most cell lines and tissues is the one with the mutation and deleterious when inactivation occurs on the X chromosome containing the wild-type allele. This unbalance can be created through chance alone by selecting mostly one of the X chromosomes, rather than the other, or through different mechanisms like cytogenetic abnormalities (translocation) or removal of the cells containing the mutant allele [6].

The *germline mosaicism (gonadal mosaicism)* is an important mechanism in assessment of X-linked recessive inheritance risk and it was also seen in autosomal dominant inheritance. Because both male and female gametogenesis can be affected, it should be taken into account when the recurrence risk is assessed in apparently sporadically appeared X-linked disorders like Duchenne muscular dystrophy [1].

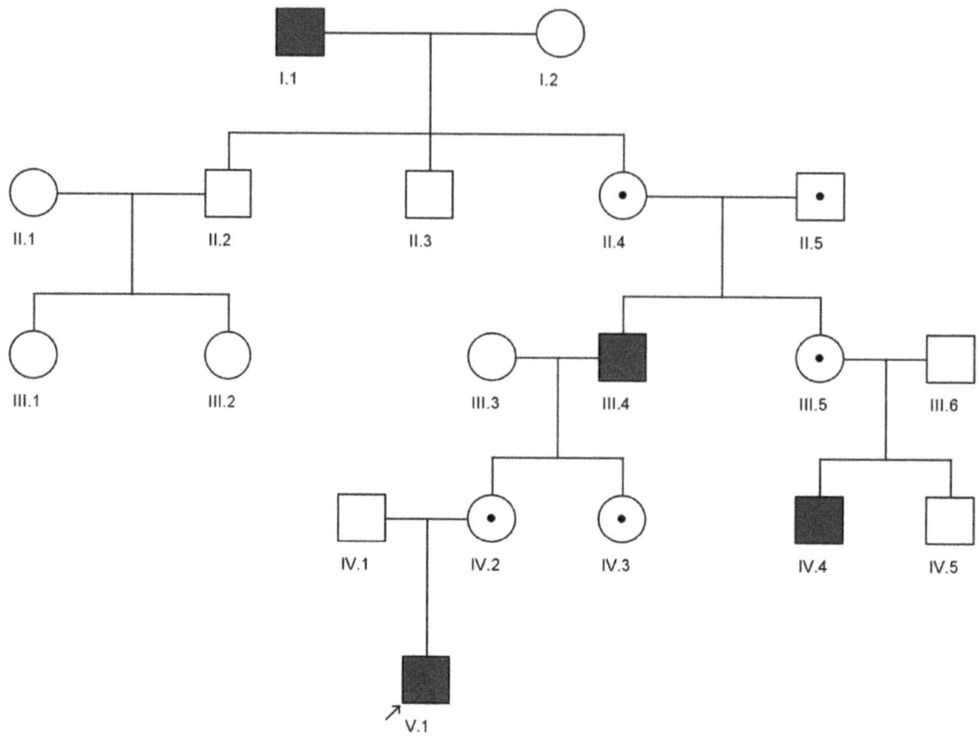

Figure 7. X-linked recessive inheritance.

3.3.3. Y-linked inheritance

Y-linked inheritance also known as holandric inheritance is caused by genes located on the Y chromosome. This is a rather straightforward type of inheritance as only males have Y chromosome, meaning that a male will transmit the mutant allele and thus the disorder to all his male descendants and none of his female ones.

4. Genetic counseling in multifactorial congenital anomalies

Multifactorial heredity describes a trait whose manifestations are determined by the activity of one or more genes in combination with environmental factors that can trigger, accelerate, or exacerbate the pathological process. Multifactorial diseases present a specific familial disposition, the incidence for close relatives of the affected individual being about 2–4%, unlike diseases determined by the mutations of a single gene (25–50%) [7].

These types of pathologies are classified into two main categories: (1) common diseases of adulthood (coronary disease, hypertension, diabetes, asthma, schizophrenia, etc.), having a prevalence of around 1–5%, and (2) isolated congenital abnormalities of the childhood (e.g. neural tube defects, cleft lip and anterior palate, congenital anomalies of the heart, varus equina), with an incidence of approximately 1–8% in newborns [25].

Congenital anomalies, also referred to as congenital abnormalities, congenital malformations, congenital disorders, or birth defects, are conditions of prenatal origin that describe developmental disorders of the embryo and fetus, potentially impacting its health and development [26]. There is a wide array of anomalies including structural and functional conditions that can fall under these headings [3].

Congenital anomalies are affecting 1–6% of pregnancies worldwide, making them a leading cause of morbidity and mortality in early life [8, 9, 27, 28]. In high-income countries, a quarter of the infant deaths is due to these anomalies [10, 29, 30]. Mortality in children under 5 years old escalates to 3.3 million [28].

These anomalies can occur in isolation (isolated congenital anomalies) or as a group of defects (multiple congenital anomalies). However, there is no generally accepted system of classification, or even an agreed definition of what constitutes a congenital anomaly [3].

Improvements in the sensitivity and availability of prenatal screening have helped decrease the number of children born with congenital anomalies [8, 31]. Even so, when the event arises, the diagnosis and the discussions around pregnancy termination create significant emotional distress [32]. Moreover, parents who have lost a child to a congenital anomaly or families with a pre-existing condition will be very concerned about the risk of recurrence in future pregnancies [11].

The role of genetic counseling is to provide guidance and support to the families being affected by these conditions [12, 24], yet the etiology of most congenital anomalies is multifactorial or unknown [33] and so an exact evaluation of the recurrence risk is hard to make for most anomaly groups and subtypes. There are a few population-based studies that offer some information concerning the recurrence risk [13, 14, 34]. All three studies conducted in the 1990s found that a congenital anomaly has twice the risk of occurrence in a future pregnancy if it has already been present, and the risk rises 5- to 12-fold if the same anomaly is present in the subsequent pregnancy [13, 14, 34]. These studies have also limitations, due to small sample size, lack or outdated classification, rendering them less useful. There is also more accurate data available in a recent article [3] that shows that for similar anomalies the recurrence risk for isolated congenital anomalies is 20-fold higher, while for dissimilar anomalies, the recurrence risk is 1.3-fold higher. Also, it was concluded in the article that the absolute recurrence risk varies between 1 in 20 and 1 in 30 [3].

General recurrence risk. Under these conditions, a number of general principles must be respected for genetic counseling. The empirical risk represents a medium risk for the respective disease in the population of which the proband (index case) is, and so it is possible that in the studied family the average risk is not the same as the real risk.

The overall empirical risk of recurrent fracture or progression for isolated congenital malformations with a frequency of 1–1000 newborns is about 2.5% for common diseases; at a frequency of 1–100, the risk is about 10%.

The risk of recurrence of the condition is influenced by a number of factors:

- The degree of kinship with the proband (index case). The risk of recurrence to first-degree relatives is much higher than for other people in the family; for example, the descendants and siblings of a proband with oral cleft have a risk of 3.15 and 2.79%, respectively, and the second- and third-degree relatives have much lower risks, 0.47 and 0.27%, respectively.

- The presence of a more severe condition in the proband. If the proband has a unilateral oral cleft, the risk to siblings is 1.9%, and if the proband has bilateral oral cleft, the risk rises to 6.6%.
- The presence in the family of several affected individuals. In the case of labia, if two siblings are affected, the risk for the next birth is 10%; if a parent and child are affected, then the risk for another affected child is 14%.
- Sex of the proband. The risk increases if in the family there are sick individuals of a certain sex at which the illness is normally less frequent (i.e., developmental dysplasia of the hip in boys and pyloric stenosis in girls).
- Consanguinity increases the risk of recurrence because the risk genes are inherited from both sides.

If for certain isolated congenital anomalies there is no information on the empirical risk in a given population, the risks may be recalculated based on the population frequency and the severity of the condition, as well as the number of affected individuals.

Recurrence risks per pathology. Regarding *congenital anomalies of the heart*, the recurrence risk is greater on the horizontal line (brotherhood) than on the vertical line for first-degree relatives and it revolves around 2–4%, whereas for second-degree relatives, the risk is reduced, becoming similar to that of the general population [35]. On the other hand, though, if the affected parent is the mother, the recurrence risk is significantly higher than the one for which the father would have been the carrier of the anomaly.

Cleft lip when associated or not with anterior palate represents the most common facial congenital anomaly, being present in over 20% of the cases and also having a positive family history.

At birth, the fact that the child has an affected mother and that she has another affected child increases the prevalence. The recurrence risk for patients that have first-degree relatives with this disease is 32 times greater than in the general population for cleft lip and anterior palate and 56 times greater for anterior palate alone, even though patients with cleft lip have a high familial recurrence of almost 4%.

In regard to *neural tube defects*, recent studies have pointed that if the proband would be the first affected child in the family then the recurrence risk for the following children would be 3.15%, whereas for the second affected sibling, the risk for recurrence would be around 10–11.76%. Some studies also showed that the risk is higher for female children and for the first and last siblings of a mother.

Congenital hip dislocation has a 5% recurrence risk if an affected sibling is already present. An increased risk of male probing according to sex ratio (8 males per 1 affected female) is encountered in people affected by this congenital anomaly.

Varus equina seems to be twice as frequent in girls as in boys, while in families that have one child with this condition, the occurrence risk for the following children is 30 times higher than that of the general population being approximately 7.3%.

The indirect setting, based on family history, of an increased individual risk of the disease will allow for the direct determination by molecular tests of genetic risk factors, possibly specific medical actions of early diagnosis.

To summarize, genetic counseling in isolated congenital anomalies relies on information gathered from population-based studies, on new and future discoveries related to the etiology of these disorders, and other factors such as the degree of kinship with the proband, presence of a more severe condition, more than one individual affected in the same family, or consanguinity for calculating the recurrence risk for the respective condition.

Genetic counseling is about guidance and support for the patient and the patient's family, so a great deal of attention must also be directed toward careful wording when explaining the risk and decisions that need to be made.

5. Preimplantation genetic diagnosis (PGD)

Preimplantation genetic diagnosis is a multistep procedure that analyzes the genetic material from a single or several cells, with the purpose to avoid a pregnancy affected by a specific disease. The biological samples were obtained during assisted reproductive treatment (ART) by the biopsy of oocyte polar bodies or embryos. PGD requires a multidisciplinary and highly experienced team in ART and genomic evaluation at single-cell level [15, 16].

Indications for PGD. Usually, PGD is provided to couples at risk of conceiving abnormal offspring with monogenic or chromosomal disorders. Thus, PGD is suitable for couples where one member is affected by a dominant disorder or both are known carriers of mutant alleles for a recessive disease, or one of them carries a balanced chromosome rearrangement that predisposes him/her to transmit and unbalanced chromosomal abnormality, often deletion or duplication [16, 17]. The presence of a gene mutation or chromosomal abnormality in a member or members of a family must be identified before PGD to allow the detection of a particular genetic abnormality before implantation and further the transmission of a specific disorder to children. Only normal embryos are transferred to the uterus to initiate the pregnancy knowing that the embryo is not a carrier for a specific abnormality, thus decreasing the risk of having an offspring affected by a specific genetic disorder. Many of these diseases are associated with an early death or severe mental and congenital abnormalities. The monogenic diseases diagnosed through PGD include autosomal recessive conditions (e.g., β-thalassemia, cystic fibrosis, spinal muscular atrophy, and sickle cell disease), autosomal dominant conditions (Huntington's disease, myotonic dystrophy, and Charcot-Marie-Tooth disease), or X-linked recessive conditions (fragile X syndrome, Duchenne muscular dystrophy, and hemophilia) [18].

PGD is also available to help parents in creating embryos that are human leucocyte antigen (HLA) compatible with a child affected by a severe blood disease, thus the selected sibling serving as a donor. PGD is an appropriate choice for carrier couples who also have infertility problems and plan to use assisted reproductive treatment anyway or for couples with an ethical or religious objection to pregnancy termination. PGD can also be used for the detection of a variety of cancer predispositions (e.g., familial breast cancer) [19, 20].

Biopsy procedures and genetic analysis technique. Genetic testing can be performed using biological samples obtained by one of the following: polar body, cleavage-stage embryo, or blastocyst biopsy [15, 16].

Polar body biopsy. First and second polar bodies are haploid cells produced in the first and, respectively, second meiotic division of oogenesis. The genetic evaluation of both polar bodies is required to precisely establish the genetic status of the oocyte. Because polar bodies are not a part of the zygote, this technique is mainly performed in some countries where embryo biopsy is unauthorized by law. Polar body analysis only provides data about mutations or aneuploidies of maternal origins. The chromosome abnormalities occurring postmeiotically (e.g., mosaicism and polyploidy), limited amount of genetic material, and doubling the number of samples for analysis have made the need to perform this type of biopsy questionable [36, 21].

Cleavage-stage embryo biopsy. Cleavage-stage biopsy is usually performed on day 3 when early embryo consists of approximately 6–10 cells. At this stage, the cells are still totipotent and are not yet adhering to one another, allowing the extraction of a single blastomere for genetic testing. Limited amount of genetic material and high rates of mosaicism observed in early embryos can lead to misdiagnosis at this stage. The biopsy of two blastomeres was associated with deleterious effects on embryo development and is recommended to be avoided [22, 37].

Blastocyst biopsy. The embryo reaches the blastocyst stage on day 5 or 6 after fertilization. The blastocyst contains about 100 cells and comprises the outer trophectoderm and inner cell mass. During blastocyst biopsy, 5–10 trophectoderm cells are retrieved; thus, more material for genetic diagnosis is available. The ethical and safety considerations related to early embryo biopsy are overcome somewhat because the trophectoderm cells will differentiate into trophoblast cells and further go on to form placenta and other extraembryonic tissues, and not participate to form the embryo [15, 23]. Recent studies showed that this type of biopsy has no effect on reproductive capacity of a blastocyst [16, 24]. However, only about 40–50% of preimplantation embryos will reach this stage in vitro. Because the time to obtain a genetic diagnosis is very limited to perform a fresh embryo transfer, mostly frozen embryo transfer is performed after vitrification [15, 16, 36].

Genetic analysis techniques. After the biological material is available for biopsy, the genetic analysis can be performed. The evaluation is based on only a single cell or very limited genetic material. For fresh embryo transfer, the genetic diagnosis must be done within 24–36 h. The single-gene mutations are detected using molecular genetic methods (PCR, PCR-multiplex, RTqPCR, whole genome amplification, or even next-generation sequencing) and chromosomal abnormalities (e.g., translocation and aneuploidies) by cytogenetic techniques (FISH, array CGH, and SNP array) [16, 25].

The embryo testing using genetic methods with the aim to detect *de novo* chromosomal aneuploidies is known as preimplantation genetic screening (PGS) [26]. PGS analyzes whether a single cell or a small number of cells biopsied from a preimplantation embryo is euploid before transferring it to the uterus. PGS is not PGD, being mainly offered to couples with advanced maternal age, recurrent implantation failure or recurrent miscarriages, and other conditions associated with high risk for aneuploid embryos in order to increase the success rate of IVF (~30%). PGS can be performed using FISH, multiplex quantitative PCR, or chromosomal microarrays [16, 27, 28].

Genetic counseling. A clinical genetic consultation provided by a geneticist with practice in ART is required to the couples before starting PGD treatment. Its purpose is to confirm the genetic diagnosis, to evaluate the reproductive status of the couple, and to provide information about the disease, mode of inheritance, recurrence risk, genetic testing, and reproductive options, including PGD [38].

Genetic counseling by a qualified geneticist or a certified genetic counselor is recommended to the couples to receive support and appropriate information in a nondirective manner and with no pressure, allowing them to make the best choice. Family history, reason for PGD, what is PGD, alternative reproductive options and side effects of treatment, the limitations of testing, success rates (about 30%), and possible outcome options should be discussed, including an unsuccessful cycle [29, 30].

Also, a multiple birth should be considered when ART is used. Thus, the couple should understand and consider the physical, psychological, and financial impact of treatment [31].

An important part of genetic counseling is to establish the reason for choosing PGD. In most cases, the couples choose PGD to avoid termination of pregnancy due to a genetic disease or to know earliest that the pregnancy is unaffected by a specific genetic abnormality [17]. Other reasons for PGD include a previously affected child or a loss of a child, recurrent abortions, or infertility. When parents are carriers for a recessive disorder, more embryos may be carriers for a mutant allele. The couple must be informed about the genetic status of the embryos and in the absence of a clinical feature in carriers, these can be considered for transfer to increase the number of available embryos. The issue of genetic testing of children for carrier status should be discussed prior to offering prenatal diagnosis to confirm the PGD result.

Sex selection is not allowed by law in many countries, while in others, it is allowed. Except some recessive X-linked disorders where females may have a mild phenotype, in these cases, the female embryos should be excluded for transfer, and the parents should be able to choose not to know the sex of their embryos.

After implantation, a new contact with a geneticist is required. Occasionally, when PGD is used, a misdiagnosis can occur; therefore, prenatal diagnosis should be offered. Prenatal diagnosis requires an invasive testing (chorionic villus sampling and amniocentesis) associated with the risk of losing the pregnancy, and many of them may refuse the confirmatory test [29].

The postnatal confirmatory diagnosis from blood is in contrast to recommendations for testing in childhood, which specify that unless there are clinical benefits to testing minors, testing for carrier or late disease conditions should be delayed until the child is old enough to understand the implications and be part of the decision making. In most cases, a successful PGD cycle will result in an ongoing pregnancy and a healthy live born infant. However, a follow-up after birth is recommended.

6. Ethical considerations

Biomedical ethics is based on applying various principles in order to create a framework of moral analysis that allows the practitioner to make an optimal decision in agreement with the patients' wishes/needs and their point of view.

Medical genetics is one of the medical fields in which, from the very beginning, sensitive ethical issues have been raised; their importance subsequently became more and more undeniable due to technological advances and discoveries in the field (see Human Genome Project, Next Generation Sequence, and Whole Genome/Exome Sequencing).

Of all the areas of genetics, prenatal diagnosis raises the most fervent debates and, consequently, ethical dilemmas. It is one of the chapters that are hard to fit in an accurate guide for the clinician, sufficient enough to use and make sure he has done or said what is needed to ensure that the health of the patient and family is protected.

The particularity of this field is derived from the existence of two entities whose rights must be taken into account: on one hand, the "patient," the unborn fetus at different stages of development at the time of the diagnosis request, and on the other hand, the mother/couple requesting the diagnosis. Although the phrase"on one hand and … on the other side" might seem inappropriate, it still reflects reality, because not always the rights of the patient are on the same side as those of the parents. And here lies the first dilemma: autonomy vs. benefit.

6.1. Ethical principles and prenatal counseling

In order to improve medical practice in medical genetics and implicitly in prenatal genetic diagnosis, a set of essential ethical principles was developed to support a clinical decision [32, 35]:

1. Respecting the autonomy of a person referring to the right of a patient to make his/her own decision without any constraint but at the same time informed by a genetic counseling in a nonlinear and impartial manner, without prejudices.
2. The "do not harm" obligation and the "doing good" duty reflect on the degree of necessity of the two desires. Obviously, it is desirable to do well (benefit), but in this process, it is much more important to avoid mistakes before getting the right benefit (e.g., presymptomatic testing for early-onset diseases) [33].
3. Confidentiality protects the patient's genetic data from various other parts. The data could be provided only with the patient's consent and only if the doctor considers them relevant. However, the doctor may not respect confidentiality if the genetic data are relevant for the relatives and the patient is not able to properly inform them about familial medical conditions.
4. Equal access to patients for care and treatment: this concept is the most difficult to apply due to the insufficient resources.

Prenatal diagnosis (PD), and here we will only refer to invasive PD, involves a genetic test that allows the diagnosis of a fetus with a serious genetic disorder (and there is an issue of what "serious" means in the opinion of specialists), followed by communication of the data to parents. The purpose of prenatal genetic testing is exclusively medical and testing criteria should be clearly established [34].

When PD is recommended, the couple will be informed, regardless of their perspective on abortion because sometimes it can be useful for psychological and medical training for the birth of a child with a congenital anomaly [34]. However, PD is a voluntary decision of the couple who will decide if the suspected condition requires diagnosis testing or termination of the pregnancy.

The distinctiveness of PD consists in this one-sided decision of the pregnant woman whose sentence affects both herself and the unborn child; if a woman is able to make an independent and well-considered decision, she must have the necessary knowledge to act in the context that PD does not only give information about a potential termination of a pregnancy but also it provides information that will prepare the parents for the birth of an affected child.

For this purpose, pretesting counseling is vital, and it will determine not only the risk of the fetus being affected, but also the chances of it being normal, it will inform about the conditions that can be diagnosed and their consequences not only on the fetus but also on the care/treatment options. Furthermore, it will also provide counseling regarding the limits of the test, the possibility of an irrelevant or unexpected result, and the couple's options after testing.

If a PD is established, the physician should discuss with the pregnant woman about all the possible aspects of the clinical features, including the heterogeneity of the clinical manifestations. The informed choice of the pregnant woman/couple in the diagnosis of a fetus with congenital malformations will be respected and protected without prejudice, giving importance and priority to the family and sociocultural background in which the couple and the future malformed child will spend their lives.

In the case of PD without medical indication, when the testing is only based on pregnancy/couple's anxiety, it will be done but with a low priority in allocating resources compared to PD associated with medical reasons. The practice of PD testing with the intention of selecting the child's sex (except for X-linked diseases) is not permitted, as well as the testing of paternity (excepting the pregnancy after an incest or rape) [34].

Particularly, the evolution of technology with the implementation of NGS in PD complicates the ethical aspects because, although genetic diagnosis has been improved, the method has some limitations, some of them common with those of the usual methods of PD [35]:

1. Diagnosing a disease for which there is no treatment.
2. Neither the severity of the clinical manifestations nor the progression of the disease can always be predicted only by conducting a genetic test.
3. There are not yet genetic tests established for all genetic diseases.
4. The results require a complex interpretation because the test provides a lot of data.
5. No test is 100% safe; the safety is dependent on the disease and the used method.
6. Laboratory errors sometimes do occur.
7. Not all pathogenic variants could be detected and interpreted.
8. The cost of the method is very expensive and not all the patients have financial resources.

In conclusion, ethical aspects surrounding PD are multiple and demanding for both the physician and parents, but using the qualified knowledge of a professional, exposed with much tact and patience, the couple will correctly understand the implications of the problem and their possible solutions/the lack of solutions and will take the best decision based on these aspects and according to their own convictions.

Author details

Mihaela Amelia Dobrescu*, Florin Burada*, Mihai Gabriel Cucu, Anca Lelia Riza, Gratiela Chelu, Razvan Mihail Plesea, Adela Cucu, Alina Liliana Cimpoeru and Mihai Ioana

*Address all correspondence to: amelia_dobrescu@yahoo.com and florinburada2000@yahoo.com

Medical Genetics Regional Center (CRGM), Dolj, Human Genomics Laboratory, University of Medicine and Pharmacy of Craiova, Craiova, Romania

References

[1] Covic Mircea SD, Ionel S. Genetica Medicala. 2 ed. Romania, Iasi: Polirom; 2011. pp. 515-523

[2] Fonda Allen J, Stoll K, Bernhardt BA. Pre- and post-test genetic counseling for chromosomal and Mendelian disorders. Seminars in Perinatology. 2016 Feb;**40**(1):44-55

[3] Handbook of Genetic Counseling/Trisomy 18—Wikibooks, open books for an open world

[4] Wieacker P, Steinhard J. The Prenatal Diagnosis of Genetic Diseases. Deutsches Ärzteblatt International. 2010;**107**(48):857-62

[5] Verma IC, Puri RD. Global burden of genetic disease and the role of genetic screening. Seminars in Fetal & Neonatal Medicine. 2015 Oct;**20**(5):354-363

[6] Handbook of Genetic Counseling/Trisomy 13—Advanced Maternal Age—Occupational Exposures—Wikibooks, open books for an open world

[7] Handbook of Genetic Counseling/Down Syndrome—Trisomy 21-1—Wikibooks, open books for an open world

[8] Ioannou D, Tempest HG. Meiotic nondisjunction: Insights into the origin and significance of aneuploidy in human spermatozoa. Advances in Experimental Medicine and Biology. 2015;**868**:1-21

[9] Griffin DK. The incidence, origin, and etiology of aneuploidy. In: Jeon KW, editor. International Review of Cytology. Academic Press; 1996. pp. 263-296

[10] Vialard F, Boitrelle F, Molina-Gomes D, Selva J. Predisposition to aneuploidy in the oocyte. Cytogenetic and Genome Research [Article]. Switzerland; 2011;**133**(2-4):127-135

[11] Fonseka KGL, Griffin DK. Is there a paternal age effect for aneuploidy? Cytogenetic and Genome Research. [Article]. 2011;**133**(2-4):280-291

[12] Cereda A, Carey JC. The trisomy 18 syndrome. Orphanet Journal of Rare Diseases. 2012 Oct;**7**:81

[13] Bijanzadeh M. The recurrence risk of genetic complex diseases. Journal of Research in Medical Sciences. 2017;**22**:32

[14] Selikowitz M. Down Syndrome. Oxford: OUP; 2008

[15] Uehara S, Yaegashi N, Maeda T, Hoshi N, Fujimoto S, Fujimori K, et al. Risk of recurrence of fetal chromosomal aberrations: Analysis of trisomy 21, trisomy 18, trisomy 13, and 45,X in 1,076 Japanese mothers. Journal of Obstetrics and Gynaecology Research. 1999;**25**(6):373-379

[16] Chen CP, Wang LK, Chern SR, Chen YN, Chen SW, Wu PS, et al. Mosaic trisomy 17 at amniocentesis: Prenatal diagnosis, molecular genetic analysis, and literature review. Taiwanese journal of Obstetrics & Gynecology. 2016 Oct;**55**(5):712-717

[17] Bregand-White J, Saller DN, Clemens M, Surti U, Yatsenko SA, Rajkovic A. Genotype-phenotype correlation and pregnancy outcomes of partial trisomy 14q: A systematic review. American Journal of Medical Genetics Part A. 2016 Sep;**170**(9):2365-2371

[18] Baty BJ, Blackburn BL, Carey JC. Natural history of trisomy 18 and trisomy 13: I. Growth, physical assessment, medical histories, survival, and recurrence risk. American Journal of Medical Genetics. 1994;**49**(2):175-188

[19] Dotters-Katz SK, Kuller JA, Grace MR, Laifer SA, Strauss RA. Management considerations for ongoing pregnancies complicated by trisomy 13 and 18. Obstetrical & Gynecological Survey. 2016 May;**71**(5):295-300

[20] Pawelec M, Dzugalik M, Pietras J, Belza L, Latkowski L. Medical and ethical considerations related to viable fetuses with trisomy 13 in the 36th week of pregnancy—A review of the literature. Advances in Clinical and Experimental Medicine. 2015 Sep-Oct;**24**(5):911-921

[21] Rosa RF, Rosa RC, Zen PR, Graziadio C, Paskulin GA. Trisomy 18: Review of the clinical, etiologic, prognostic, and ethical aspects. Revista Paulista de Pediatria. 2013 Jan-Mar;**31**(1):111-120

[22] Ranweiler R. Assessment and care of the newborn with down syndrome. Advances in Neonatal Care. 2009 Feb;**9**(1):17-24; Quiz 5-6

[23] Bradley S, James T. Medical Genetics: An Integrated Approach. 1st ed. McGraw-Hill Education/Medical; 2014

[24] Harper PS. Practical Genetic Counselling. 7th ed. UK: CRC Press; 2010

[25] Covic Mircea SD, Ionel S. Genetica Medicala. 2 ed. Romania, Iasi: Polirom; 2011. pp. 677-680

[26] DeSilva M, Munoz FM, Mcmillan M, Kawai AT, Marshall H, Macartney KK, et al. Congenital anomalies: Case definition and guidelines for data collection, analysis, and presentation of immunization safety data. Vaccine. Netherlands; 2016;**34**(49):6015-6026

[27] CfDC, Prevention. Update on overall prevalence of major birth defects—Atlanta, Georgia, 1978-2005. Morbidity and Mortality Weekly Report. 2008 Jan;**57**(1):1-5

[28] Christianson A, Howson CP, Modell B. March of Dimes: Global report on birth defects, the hidden toll of dying and disabled children. 2005

[29] Oakley L, Maconochie N, Doyle P, Dattani N, Moser K. Multivariate analysis of infant death in England and Wales in 2005-06, with focus on socio-economic status and deprivation. Health Statistics Quarterly. London, England: the Stationery Office; c1999-2009;**42**(1):22-39

[30] World Health Organization. Birth defects. Sixty-Third World Health Assembly Provisional Agenda Item. 2010;**11**:32-33

[31] Boyd PA, Devigan C, Khoshnood B, Loane M, Garne E, Dolk H, et al. Survey of prenatal screening policies in Europe for structural malformations and chromosome anomalies, and their impact on detection and termination rates for neural tube defects and Down's syndrome. BJOG : An International Journal of Obstetrics and Gynaecology. 2008 May;**115**(6):689-696

[32] Asplin N, Wessel H, Marions L, Georgsson Öhman S. Pregnancy termination due to fetal anomaly: Women's reactions, satisfaction and experiences of care. Midwifery. 2014 Jun;**30**(6):620-627

[33] World Health Organization, Prevention CfDCa. Birth Defects Surveillance Training: Facilitator's Guide. 2015

[34] Basso O, Olsen J, Christensen K. Recurrence risk of congenital anomalies—The impact of paternal, social, and environmental factors: A population-based study in Denmark. American Journal of Epidemiology. Oxford University Press for the Johns Hopkins Bloomberg School of Public Health; 1999 Sep;**150**(6):598-604

[35] Covic M, Stefanescu D, Sandovici I, Gorduza VE. Genetica Medicala. III ed. Polirom; 2017. pp. 636-655

[36] Xu K, Montag M. New perspectives on embryo biopsy: Not how, but when and why? Seminars in Reproductive Medicine. United States; 2012 Aug;**30**(4):259-266

[37] Goossens V, De Rycke M, De Vos A, Staessen C, Michiels A, Verpoest W, et al. Diagnostic efficiency, embryonic development and clinical outcome after the biopsy of one or two blastomeres for preimplantation genetic diagnosis. Human Reproduction. 2008 Mar;**23**(3):481-492

[38] Technology PCotSfAR, Medicine PCotASfR. Preimplantation genetic testing: A practice committee opinion. Fertility and Sterility. 2007 Dec;**88**(6):1497-1504

6

Congenital Abnormalities of the Fetal Heart

Dominic Gabriel Iliescu, Ştefania Tudorache,
Dragos Nemescu, Monica Mihaela Cirstoiu,
Simona Vlădăreanu, Claudiu Marginean,
Iuliana Ceausu, Daniel Muresan,
Marius Calomfirescu Vicea, Mona Elena Zvanca,
Cezara Muresan, Laura Monica Cara,
Ciprian Laurentiu Patru,
Roxana Cristina Drăguşin and Maria Sorop-Florea

Abstract

Congenital heart defects (CHDs) are the most frequent congenital malformations, the costliest hospital admissions for structural defects and the leading cause of infant general and malformations related mortality. Fetal echocardiography represents a skilled ultrasound examination, because of the complexity, physiological and structural particularities of the fetal heart. The efficiency of the cardiac scan is reported with great variation, depending on the scanning protocol, examiner experience and equipment quality but CHDs remains among the most frequently missed congenital abnormalities.

Keywords: heart defects, congenital, ultrasonography, echocardiography

1. Epidemiology. Incidence and risk factors for cardiac abnormalities

Congenital heart defects (CHD) are the most frequent congenital malformations (5–12 per 1000 live births), the costliest hospital admissions for structural defects and represent the leading cause of infant general and malformations related mortality (42%) [1, 2]. Prenatal CHD detection allows proper counseling, provides the options of pregnancy termination [3], in utero treatments (antiarrhythmics, valvuloplasties, etc.) [4–7] and allows for delivery planning in a referral center [8–11].

CHD etiology includes many genetic, environmental and teratogenic factors [12–16], but 90% of heart malformations have no identified cause. Conversely, the risk may be reduced with periconceptionally folic acid intake [17].

2. Indications and settings for fetal echocardiography (FECG)

A detailed sonographic examination, used to characterize fetal cardiac anatomy has traditionally been reserved for high-risk populations [18–22]: advanced maternal age, more than 35 years old, family history of CHD or disorders that involves potential CHD, infectious, autoimmune or metabolic diseases, exposure to drugs and teratogens. FECG was also proposed in certain pregnancy findings: structural defects, non-immune hydrops, arrhythmia, suspected chromosomal abnormalities, enlarged nuchal translucency, monochorionic multiple gestation. Nowadays, professional guidelines recommend a screening heart evaluation to all pregnancies, as most of the CHD cases are not associated with known risk factors [38–45].

Guidelines and training requirements have been developed [18, 19]. An accurate visualization of heat features is commonly achieved at 18–22 gestational weeks. FECG is a relatively brief but skilled ultrasound examination, because of the complexity and prenatal physiological and structural particularities of the fetal heart. Consequently, FECG has not been widely implemented, and the prenatal diagnosis of even severe CHD varies considerably, with less than half prenatally detected.

3. Fetal heart evaluation. The cardiac sweep and longitudinal views

Optimal views of the fetal heart are obtained when the cardiac apex is orientated toward the anterior maternal wall. Heart anatomy is evaluated using a sequential segmental analysis, starting from the venous plane (atria with veins connections), following the blood flow to ventricles and great arteries [23]. The information regarding fetal heart anatomy is achieved by examining five axial and three longitudinal scanning planes [18, 19, 24], described below, with examples of cardiac abnormalities. In general practice, only the axial sectional planes are evaluated during the cardiac sweep [25] (**Figure 1**).

1. **Upper abdominal view** facilitates the evaluation of normal abdominal situs by identifying the stomach, descending aorta and inferior vena cava position (**Figure 1(1)**).
2. **Four-chamber view (4CV)** is visualized in the lower half of the fetal chest, where the heart, with crux cordis occupying its central portion and a complete rib are present (**Figure 1(2)**). The evaluation parameters include:
    - *Situs*—the heart is normally left-sided, namely levocardia, or situs solitus. Rarely, a complete situs inversus is present. In the presence of an abnormal heart situs CHD but also congenital diaphragmatic hernia should be considered (**Figure 2**), as the presence of significant ectopic abdominal content in the chest displaces the heart.

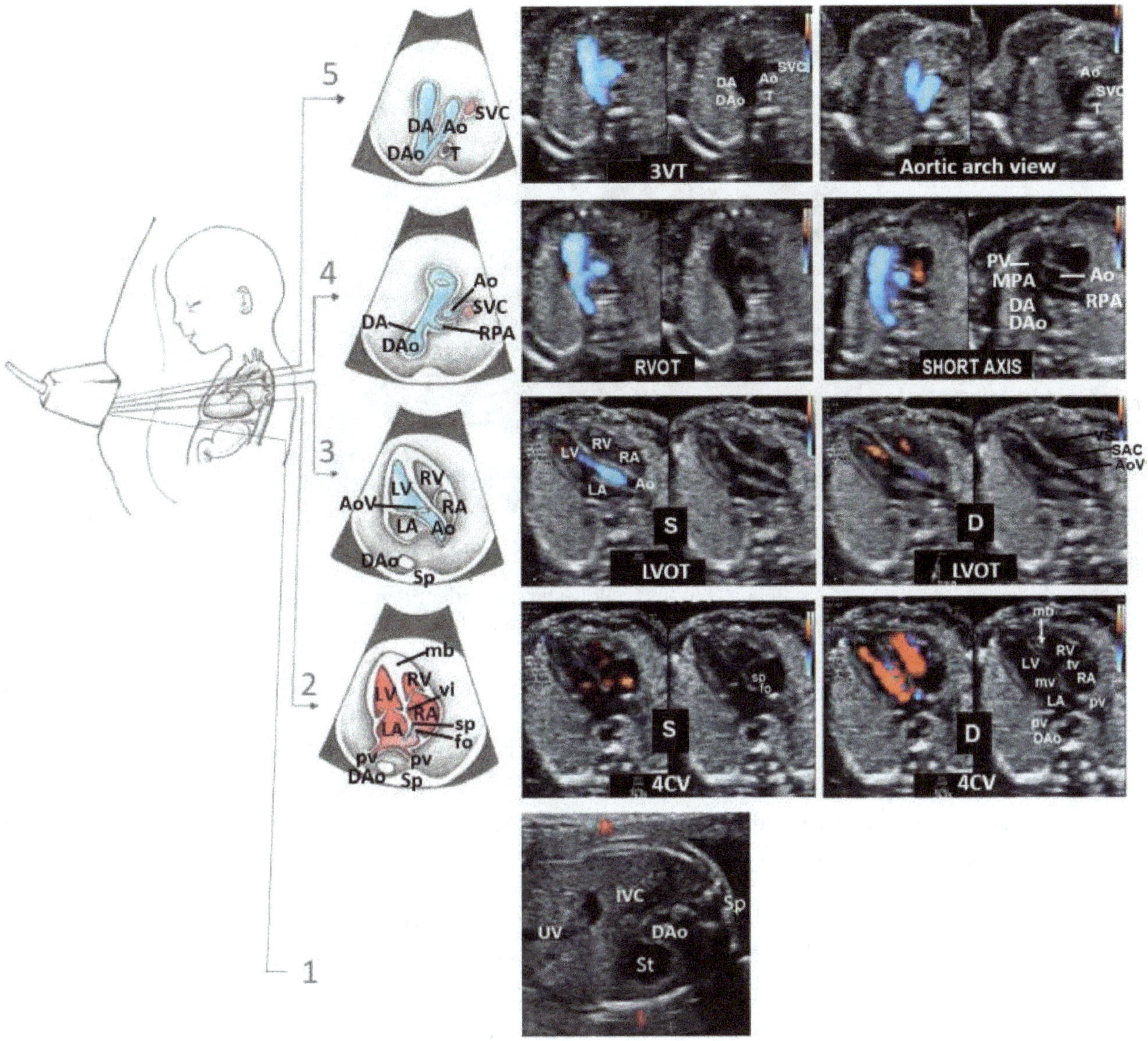

Figure 1. Normal heart visualized during fetal cardiac sweep. Visualization of the cardiac transverse planes, by sweeping the transducer from the four-chamber plane toward the fetal neck as shown in the left of the image. Schematic presentation of the cardiac planes in duplex mode (gray-scale and color Doppler) that become apparent: (1) upper abdominal view, and abdominal situs; (2) four-chamber view (4CV). The atrioventricular Doppler flow is red because of the direction toward the direction during diastole. When the atrioventricular are closed, during systole, the atrioventricular flow is absent; (3) left ventricular outflow tract (LVOT). Note the continuity of the ventricular septum (VS) with the aortic wall. When the aortic valve (AoV) is closed, during diastole, the aortic flow is absent; (4) right ventricular outflow tract (RVOT) and (5) three-vessel and trachea (3VTV) and aortic arch views. L, left; R, right; St, stomach; D, diastole; and S, systole; UV, umbilical vein; DAo, descending aorta; IVC, inferior vena cava; SVC, superior vena cava; LV, left ventricle; RV, right ventricle; LA, left atrium; RA, right atrium; mb, moderator band; mv, mitral valve; tv, tricuspid valve; vi, valve insertion; pv, pulmonary veins; sp., septum primum; fo, foramen ovale, DAo, descendent aorta; MPA, main pulmonary artery; DA, ductus arteriosus; RPA, right pulmonary artery; PV, pulmonary valve Sp, spine; T, trachea. Modified with permission [26].

- *Heart axis*—normally, the apex points toward the left side at 45 ± 15–20° (**Figure 1(2)**). Some studies on CHDs suggested that an abnormal cardiac axis is present in more than two-thirds of the cases [27] (**Figure 15C**).
- *Area of the heart,* is abnormally increased if higher than 1/3 of the thorax area, or cardio-thoracic circumference ratio is above two standard deviations [28] (**Figure 3**). It can arise

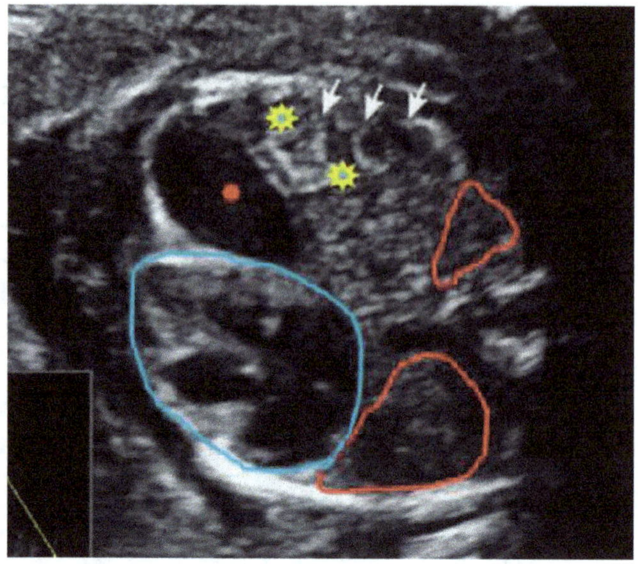

Figure 2. Two-dimensional US images in the cross-sectional plane of the thorax at the level of the four-chamber view of the heart. Stomach (red star) and small bowel loops (yellow stars) are identified intrathoracic and displaces fetal heart (figured by the blue tracing line) to the right; the lungs areas are highlighted by red tracing lines. With permission, Tudorache et al. [34].

from a number of situations which include CHD, particularly tricuspid atresia or dysplasia, including Ebstein's anomaly, twin to twin transfusion syndrome, fetal dilated cardiomyopathies, hydrops fetalis, or may be due to abnormal shunting from arteriovenous malformations, as the vein of Galen malformation or placental chorioangioma (**Figure 3**).

- *The atria* present similar size. The pulmonary veins enter the posterior left atrium and both vena cava enter the anterior right atrium (**Figure 1(2)**). Various condition may alter this spatial relation, as fetal isomerism and the normal atrial dimensions, where Ebstein's anomaly is the most representative condition (**Figure 4**).
- *The ventricles* should be visualized with similar width and contractility. The right ventricle is anterior, with more coarse lining and trabeculation. Abnormal shape of the ventricular wall lining may be an indicator for cardiac tumors, as tuberous sclerosis (**Figure 5**) or rhabdomyoma (**Figure 6**). Normally, the left ventricle forms the apex of the heart, the right ventricular apex contains the moderator band and septal insertion of the tricuspid valve is more apical than the mitral valve (**Figure 1(2)**). In later gestation, the right ventricle becomes slightly larger, but 2D or M-mode nomograms correlated with the gestational age or fetal biometry and Z-scores for fetal heart area and axis and cardiothoracic ratio, atrioventricular valve annuli, ventricular lengths and walls thickness, but also for emerging vessels, are available [29, 30].

  A diminutive ventricle may be associated with significant CHD, as the hypoplastic left/right heart syndrome (**Figure 7**). Also, an abnormally small left ventricle may be an indirect sign of aortic coarctation (**Figure 19A**). However, less significant cardiac abnormalities may associate a larger right heart, as the persistence of left superior vena cava (**Figure 8**).
- *Ventricular septum integrity* is better evaluated from a lateral incidence, with the ultrasound beam perpendicular to the septum. A dropout of echoes or an opening of the

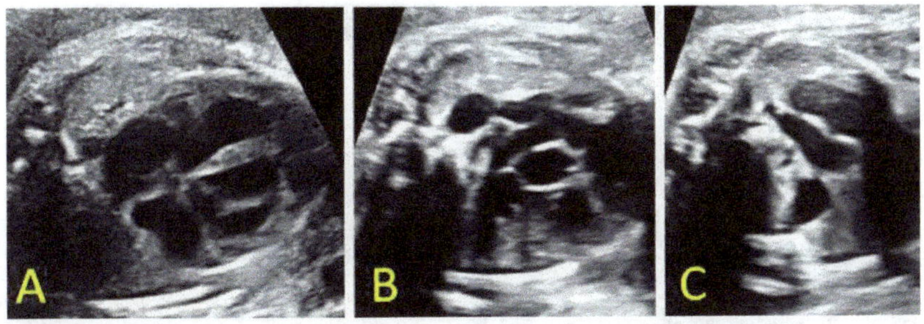

Figure 3. Cardiomegaly. (A) Increased area of the heart, occupying half of the thorax area. (B and C):Outflow tract appears dilated in relation to the fetal thorax.

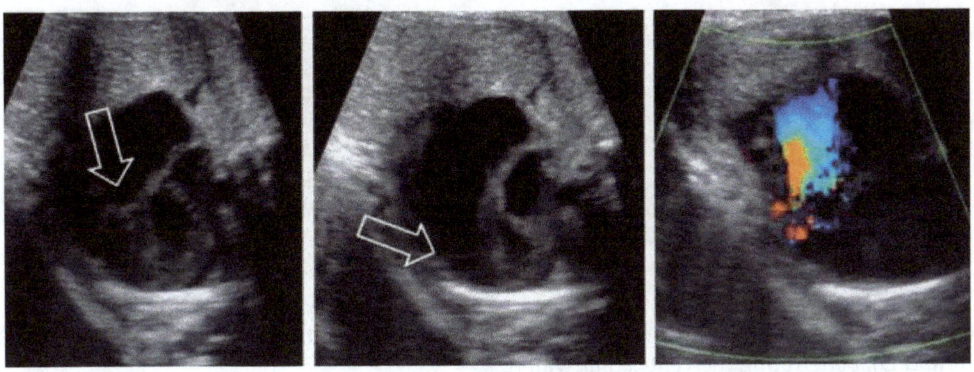

Figure 4. Ebstein's anomaly. The arrow indicates the dysplastic tricuspid valve with septal and posterior leaflets of the tricuspid valve displaced toward the apex of the right ventricle. Color Doppler investigation shows significant valvular regurgitation.

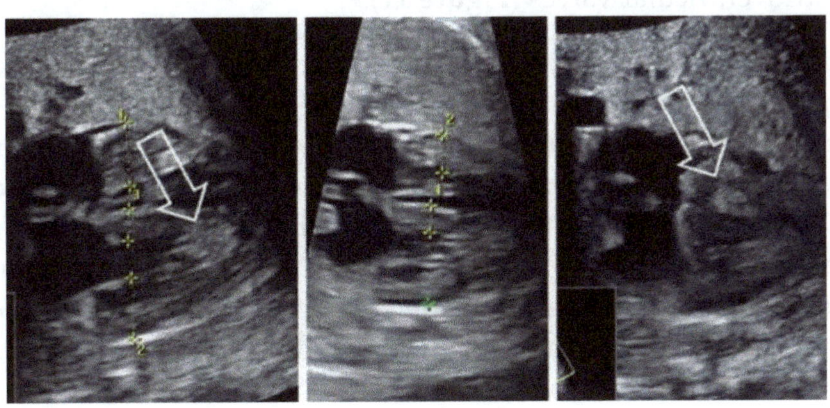

Figure 5. Tuberous sclerosis. Increased thickness of ventricular walls and presence of solid tumors in ventricular cavities, highlighted with open arrows.

ventricular septum, causing communication between the two ventricles suggests the diagnosis. The entire septum must be swept (**Figure 9**) for a more confident diagnosis, and Doppler investigation enhances the diagnosis, especially for small defects (**Figure 10**). Ventricular septal defects are the most common cardiac abnormality and accounts for almost one third of all cardiac defects.

- *Atrial septum primum* presence, at the crux of the heart, along the *atrioventricular valves* insertion which is more apical for tricuspid valve. Atrioventricular septal defects, known

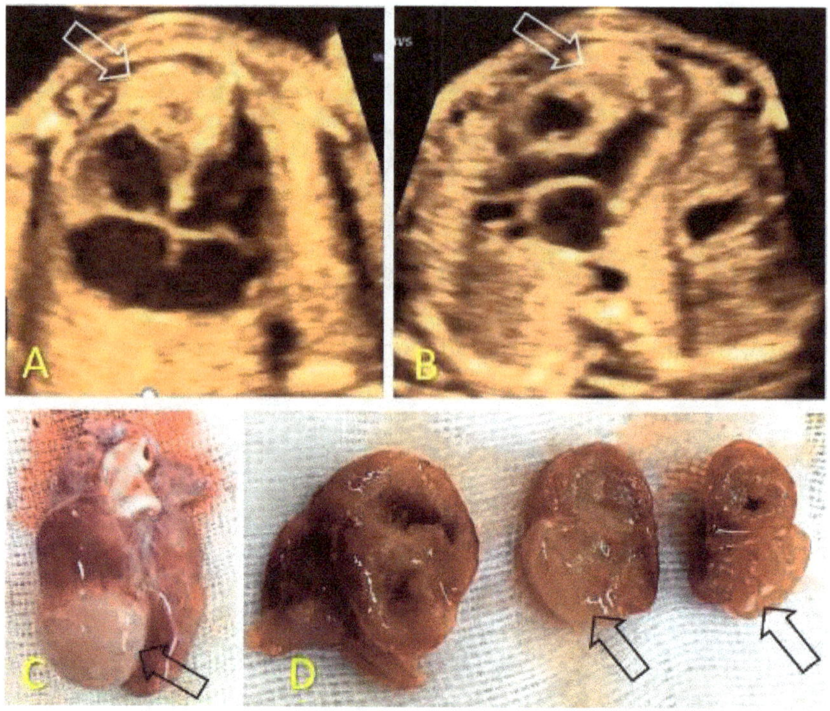

Figure 6. Rhabdomyoma of the right ventricle, visible in 4CV (A) and left ventricle outflow tract view (B), and confirmed postabortum (C and D), penetrating the ventricular wall (C).

as endocardial cushion defects are situated in the central core of the heart. It involves the association of septum primum and ventricular septal defect and a variable degree of abnormal atrioventricular valves (**Figure 11**).

- *Foramen ovale* represents about one third of the atrial septum and the flap bulges in the left atrium. A restrictive foramen ovale, because of a narrow foramen ovale orifice, or premature adhesion of the foramen ovale valve to the atrial septum, has repeatedly been discussed as a cause of fetal hemodynamic compromise [31]. Foramen ovale aneurysm is defined as dilatation of the atrial septum with bulging of the septum at least half the distance to the left atrial wall (**Figure 12**), is primarily a defect of septum primum which results in: septum primum bulging, loss of the normal biphasic motion of foramen ovale and arrhythmia. Associated abnormalities include: atrial septal defect, tricuspid atresia, hypoplastic right heart, aortic stenosis, transposition of the great vessels, Ebstein anomaly, atrioventricular valve and pulmonary venous obstruction.

- *Pericardial effusion* should be absent, or less than 2–4 mm. Greater effusions usually occur as a component of hydrops, as one of the earliest findings, and are also associated with cardiac structural abnormality, arrhythmia and an increased incidence of chromosomal anomalies (**Figure 12**) [32, 33].

- *Heart rate and the regularity* of the rhythm is assessed based on the cardiac cycle length measured using M-mode or pulsed Doppler interrogation. Most common arrhythmias are transient and without clinical relevance, as brief episodes, less than 1–2 minutes of a bradycardic, tachycardic or irregular heart rhythm.

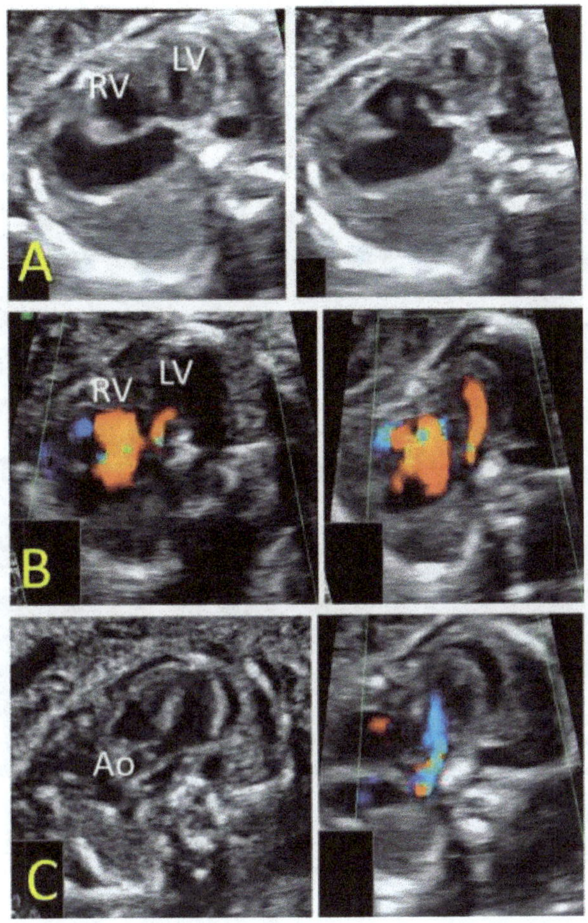

Figure 7. Hypoplastic left heart syndrome (HLHS), with discordance of the heart chambers, ventricular cardiomyopathy and hypertrophic left ventricle (A), markedly reduced filling at Doppler evaluation (B), fibroelastosis, and reduced aortic caliber and flow (C).

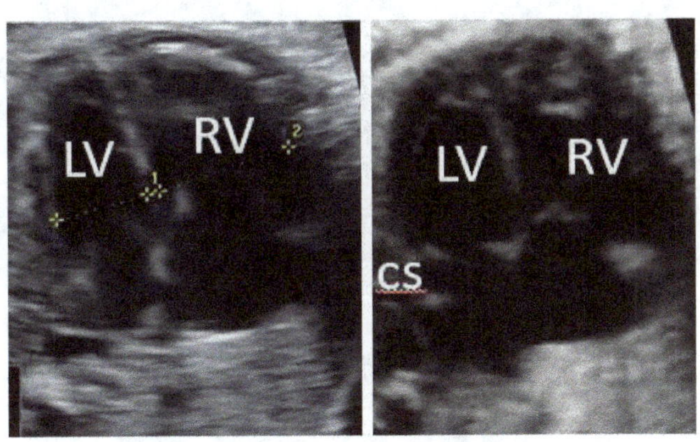

Figure 8. Discordance of the cardiac ventricles, with enlarged right ventricle and dilated coronary sinus (CS), in the presence of persistent left superior vena cava.

Irregular cardiac rhythm represents the most common rhythm anomaly and is almost always associated with isolated premature atrial contractions (PACs). Frequently blocked PACs will result in bradyarrhythmia that can mimic bradycardia (**Figure 13**). In rare cases, irregular rhythm may progress to supraventricular tachycardia.

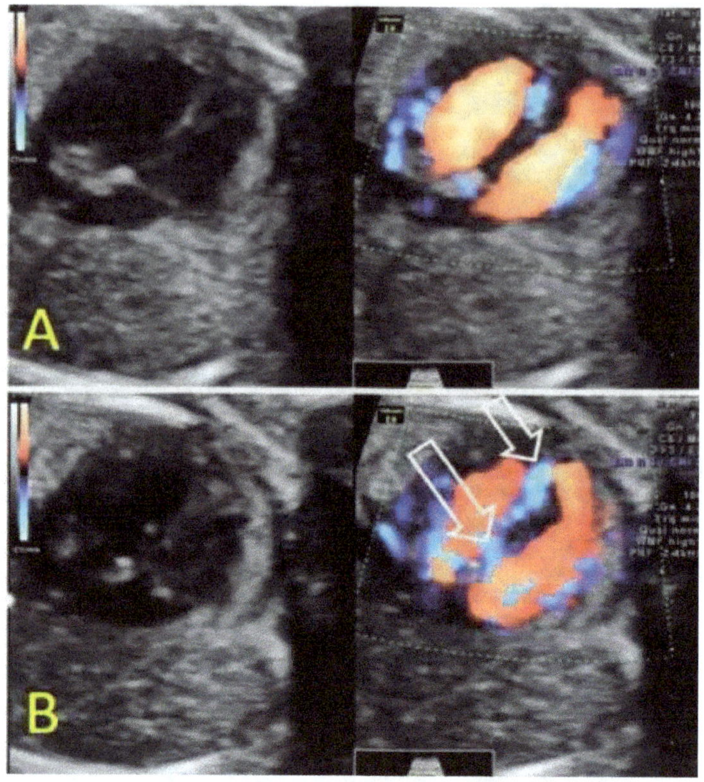

Figure 9. Multiple VSDs, apical and membranous, unapparent in certain 4CV incidence at gray-scale and color Doppler evaluation (A), but present in nearby planes, as the cardiac sweep is conducted (B). The entire interventricular septum must be carefully swept.

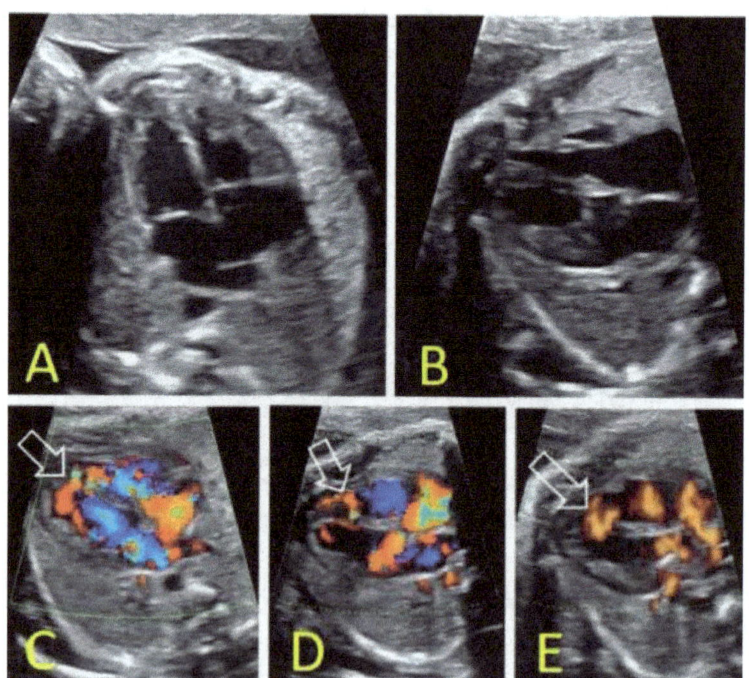

Figure 10. Multiple VSDs, apical and muscular, inapparent in gray-scale evaluation. (A): Apparently normal ventricular septum in apical and (B): lateral four-chamber view. (C–E): Muscular VSDs diagnosed using color Doppler in lateral four-chamber view—open arrows.

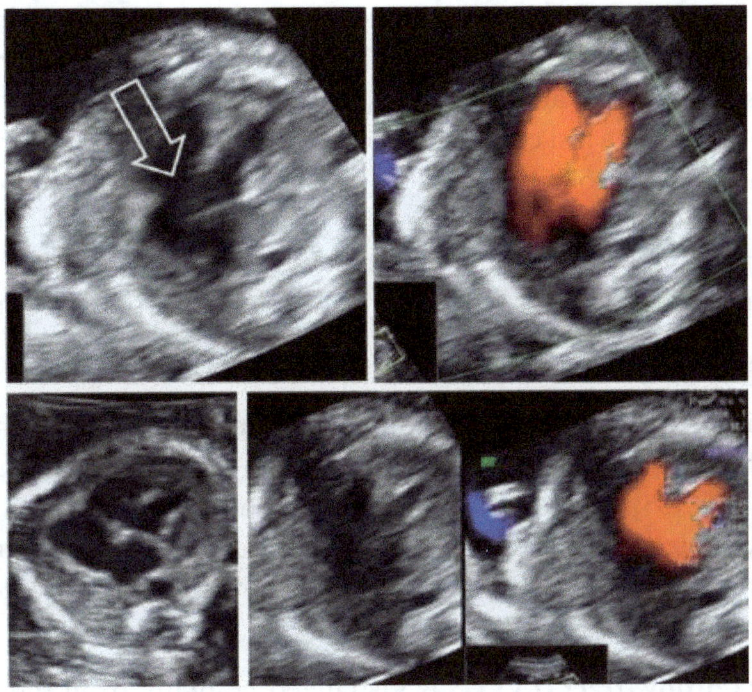

Figure 11. Atrioventricular septal defect. A large defect (open arrow) is present in the area where normally crux cordis is identified.

Fetal bradycardia represents a persistently slower heart rate, of less than 100–120 beats/min. More concerning is the observation of sustained bradycardia induced by sinus bradycardia, atrial bigeminy and complete heart block. Heart block is frequently associated with maternal anti-Ro autoantibodies and CHD and the most common condition is an unbalanced atrioventricular septal defect associated with left isomerism.

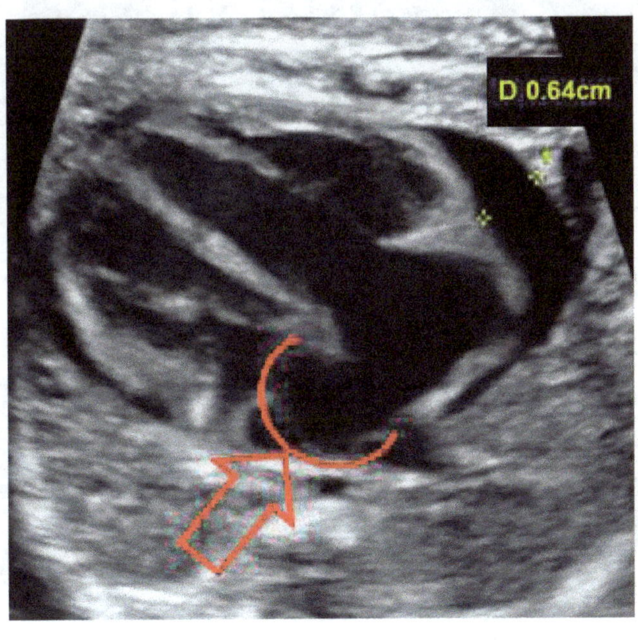

Figure 12. Foramen ovale aneurysm (red arrow) in a case where pericarditis is associated.

Fetal tachycardia implies atrial and ventricular rates above 180 bpm. Fetal anemia, hypoxia, infections, and maternal thyrotoxicosis may induce this condition. The main causes of fetal tachycardia are supraventricular tachycardia (**Figure 14**), the most common cause, with atrioventricular re-entry due to a fast conducting accessory pathway), sinus tachycardia, and atrial flutter (with atrial rate 300–500 bpm and only every second or third atrial beat conducted across the atrioventricular node, resulting in ventricular rates of 150–250 bpm). The use of echocardiography is important to differentiate these conditions and their hemodynamic impact, because the severe conditions may lead to low cardiac output, hydrops and fetal demise.

- *Coronary sinus*, may be demonstrated by fine sweeping caudally from the 4CV (**Figure 8**).

Given all these information, the 4CV is much more than a simple count of cardiac chambers, but certain abnormalities, especially involving great vessels, cannot be detected at the 4CV level alone [35]. Recent revised and updated guidelines and recommendations from several professional bodies [18, 36, 37] plead for the routinely screening evaluation of the outflow tract views along the 4CV, based on strong medical evidence regarding the prenatal detection of CHD [38–40].

3. **Left ventricular outflow tract (LVOT)** is visualized cranially from the 4CV plane and directed toward the fetal right shoulder. In this five-chamber view, the ascending aorta appears arising from the left ventricle (**Figure 1(3)**), with no proximal *transversal branching*, allowing for its differentiation from the main pulmonary artery.

- *Septoaortic continuity*, should be visualized as a continuous line between ventricular septum and aortic wall. The discontinuity of this structure is seen in the presence of a

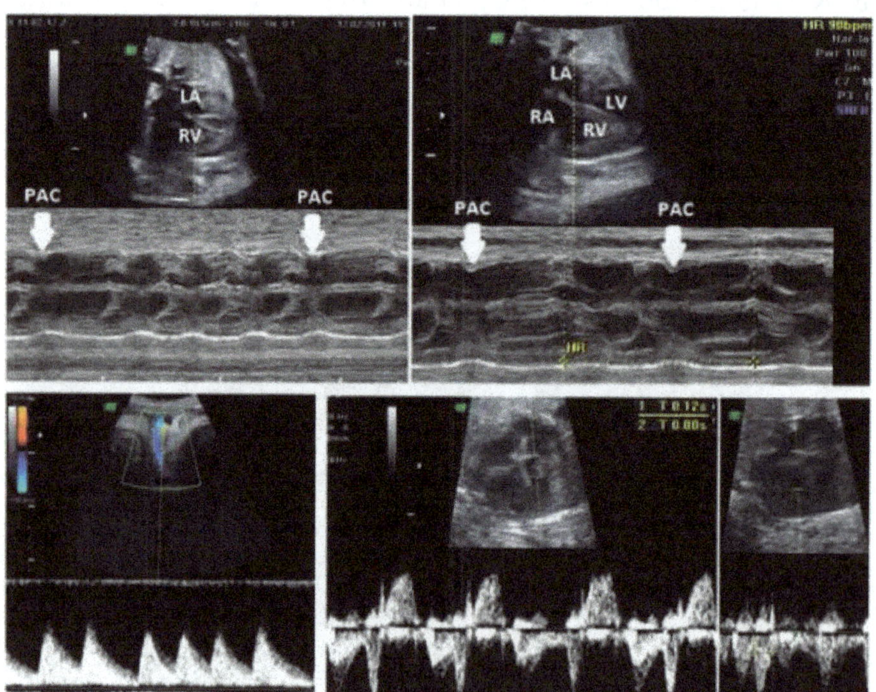

Figure 13. Fetal bradyarrhythmia, M-mode and pulsed Doppler evaluation. Premature atrial contractions (PACs, highlighted with arrows) are blocked, resulting in bradycardic irregular cardiac rhythm. Normal values for the mechanical PR interval by pulsed Doppler interrogation at the mitral-aortic region in prediction of heart block risk.

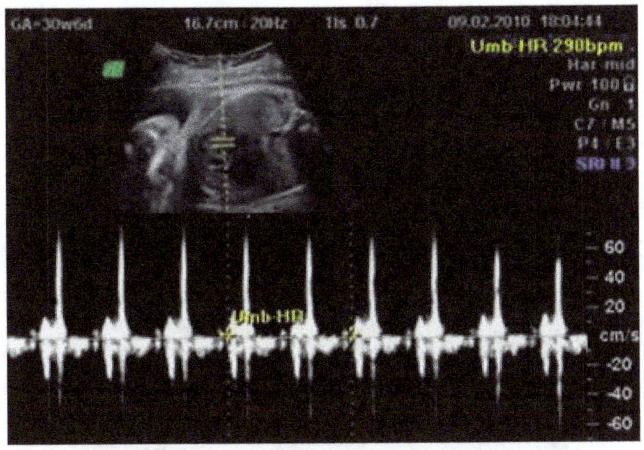

Figure 14. Tachyarrhythmia and measurement of cardiac rhythm using pulsed Doppler.

sub-aortic septal defect that is frequently associated with overriding. A good example of this condition is present in tetralogy of Fallot cases (**Figure 15**).

- The *aortic valve* cusps should open freely, disappearing in systole and not thickened. Aortic dysplastic and stenotic valves do not fully open this will decrease the blood flow into the aorta. Aortic stenosis impairs the left ventricular development, leading to hypoplastic left heart syndrome (**Figure 16**).

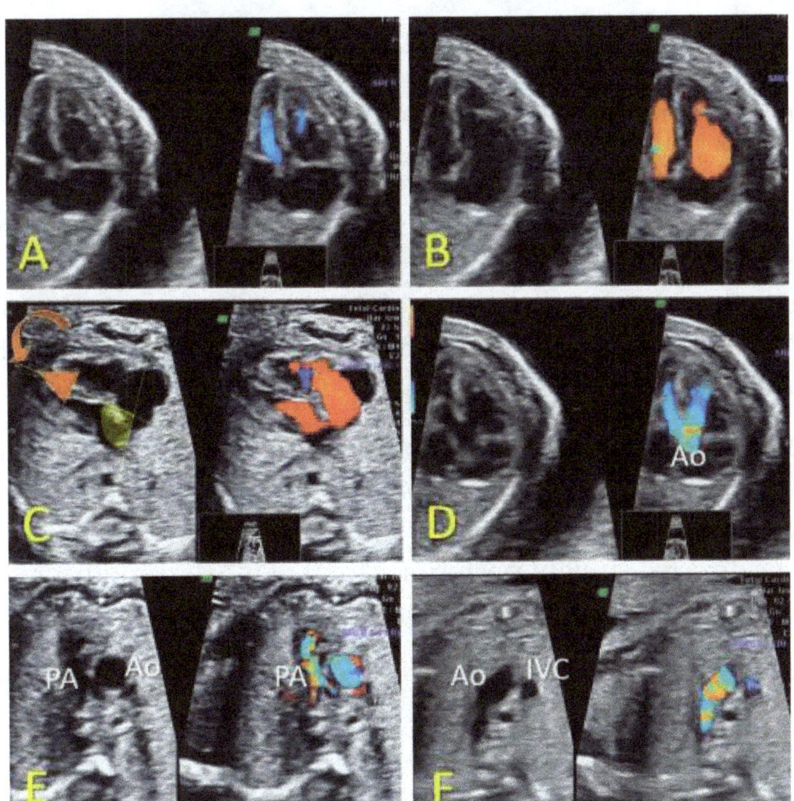

Figure 15. Tetralogy of Fallot. Inapparent four-chamber view (A and B) with increased cardiac axis (C). Septal defect with septoaortic discontinuity and aortic root overriding at the level of mixing flows form ventricles (D). Diminutive stenotic pulmonary artery is identified in right outflow tract view (E) and three-vessel and trachea view (F).

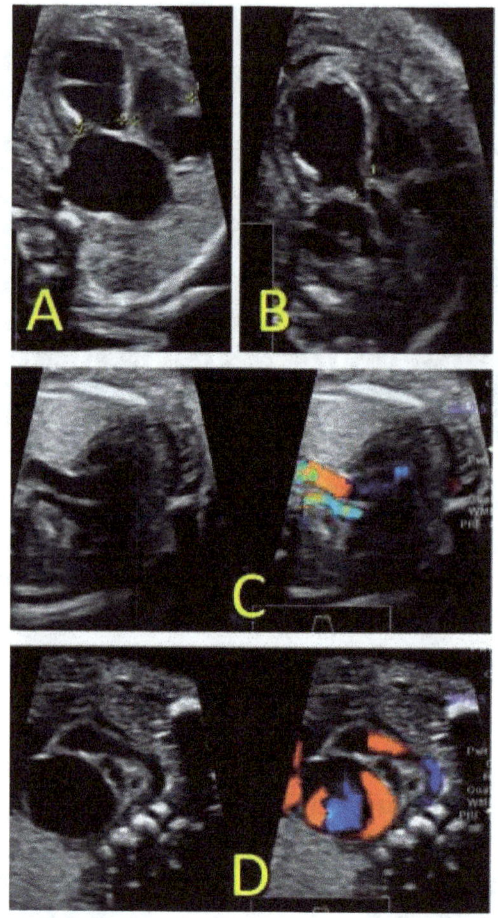

Figure 16. Aortic stenosis. Abnormal left ventricle with atretic inlet and fibroelastosis (A), stenotic aortic root (B) and aortic arch in axial (C) and longitudinal (D) views.

- *The width* of the aorta should be approximately equal with the pulmonary artery. Unbalanced blood flows through the outflow tracts as in Fallot Tetralogy, determine a larger aorta, because the aortic root receives blood from both ventricles due to overriding (**Figure 15D** and **E**). Valvular dysplasia and aortic arch stenosis/coarctation (**Figure 16**) determine a smaller aortic caliber.

4. **Right ventricular outflow tract (RVOT)** and short axis view are visualized cranially from the LVOT plane (**Figure 1(4)**), where the main pulmonary artery root arises from the anterior right ventricle with a short and straight course and soon *branching* into a large vessel, the ductus arteriosus directed straight posteriorly toward the descending aorta as an extension of the main artery, and the smaller pulmonary arteries directed laterally.

   - The pulmonary *valve cusps* should have a similar aspect as described for the aortic valves. The dysplastic stenotic valves may appear thickened and with incomplete opening during systole (doming) (**Figure 17A**) and determine pulmonary stenosis.

   - The approximately equal *width* of the two outflow tracts should be noted. Pulmonary stenosis may be associated with valvular stenosis, total anomalous pulmonary venous drainage, septal defects, supravalvular aortic stenosis, Noonan syndrome and tetralogy of Fallot. On color and pulsed Doppler investigation, pulmonary stenosis cases display turbulent or retrograde flow in and increased velocities distal to the valve (**Figure 17B**

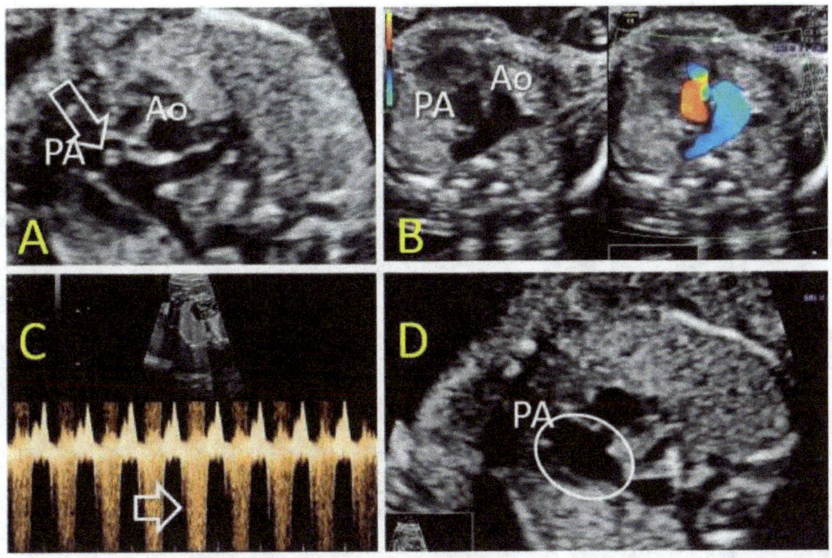

Figure 17. Pulmonary stenosis. (A): Dysplastic pulmonary valves, with incomplete opening and doming; (B): reversed and turbulent flow in the RVOT; (C): post-stenotic increased velocities in pulmonary artery course; (D): post-stenotic dilatation.

and **C**), with PSV higher than the aortic flow. A post-stenotic dilatation of the proximal pulmonary artery may be seen (**Figure 17D**). A variable degree of hypoplastic right ventricle with hypertrophic wall, dilatation of the right atrium, and tricuspid insufficiency may be present, while congestive heart failure and hydrops may occur in severe stenosis.

- *Spatial relationship* evaluation should note crossing of aorta at a right angle and characteristic early transversal branching of the pulmonary artery (**Figure 1(4)**). In the absence of these ultrasound features, transposition of the great arteries should be suspected (**Figure 18**).

5. **Three-vessel and trachea view (3VTV)** is obtained sliding cranially in the upper thorax during cardiac sweep (**Figure 1(5)**). Superior vena cava (SVC) on the right side, the aortic arch and ductal arch, anterior and to the left of the aorta, are visualized. The approximately equal arterial arches form a *"V"-shaped confluence* toward the descending aorta, in the left of the spine. This plane is also used for thymus evaluation [41].

   This view may be altered with regard to several features. Their width may be discrepant, as due to aortic coarctation, where the aortic isthmus is significantly smaller than the arterial duct (**Figure 19**). However, this diagnosis is challenging and affected by high rates of false-positive diagnoses. Thus, to improve detection, a multiple-criteria prediction model is adopted, as a combination of isthmic/duct and ventricular diameters ratios and Z-scores, visualization of CoA shelf and isthmic flow disturbance [42, 43].

   Another abnormality of 3VTV plane is represented by the impossibility to identify all the three vessels. One of the arterial arches may not be seen, as in the presence of an interrupted aortic arch (**Figure 20**), or more than three vessels may be present, as in persistent left superior vena cava (**Figure 21**).

   The superior vena cava may be identified contralateral, on the left side, as in the persistent of left superior vena cava (**Figure 8**).

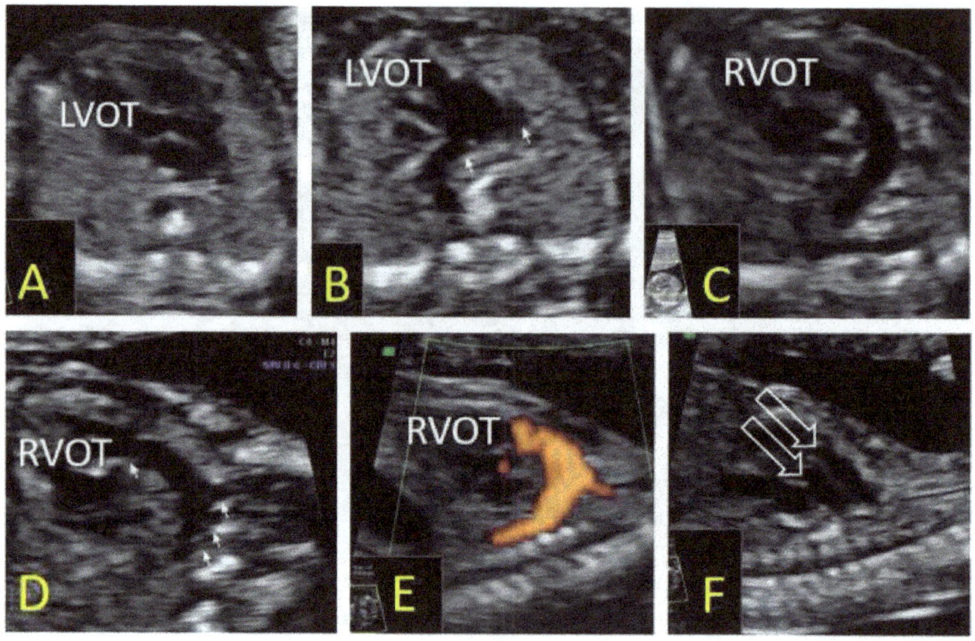

Figure 18. Transposition of the great arteries. (A): Emergence of the vessel arising from the left ventricle, showing early branching (B) that suggest pulmonary outflow tract. (C): Emergence of the vessel arising from the right ventricle with no evident branching in the transversal plane. (D): Sagittal view of the thorax showing branching characteristic to aortic arch of the vessel arising from the anterior ventricle in gray scale and after power Doppler is applied (E). (F): Parallel course of the great vessels.

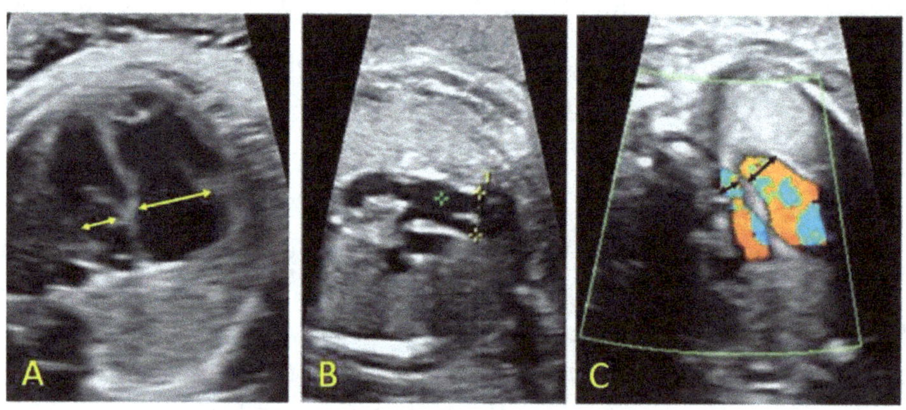

Figure 19. Discrepancy between the large right ventricle, pulmonary root and arterial duct and the diminutive left ventricle, aortic arch and isthmus in aortic coarctation. Calculations for mitral and tricuspid valves (A), arterial arches (B), isthmus and ductus (C).

Absence of a normal "V"-sign confluence of the arterial arches can be used to detect aortic arch abnormalities: right aortic arch, double aortic arch (**Figure 22**) and interrupted aortic arch (**Figure 20**).

6. Aortic and ductal arches views

- *The aortic* and *ductal arches* are visualized in longitudinal planes aligned with the respective ventricular outflow tracts. Aorta origins from the middle of the heart, with a typical "hook" shape, with the neck vessels arising longitudinally (**Figure 23A**).

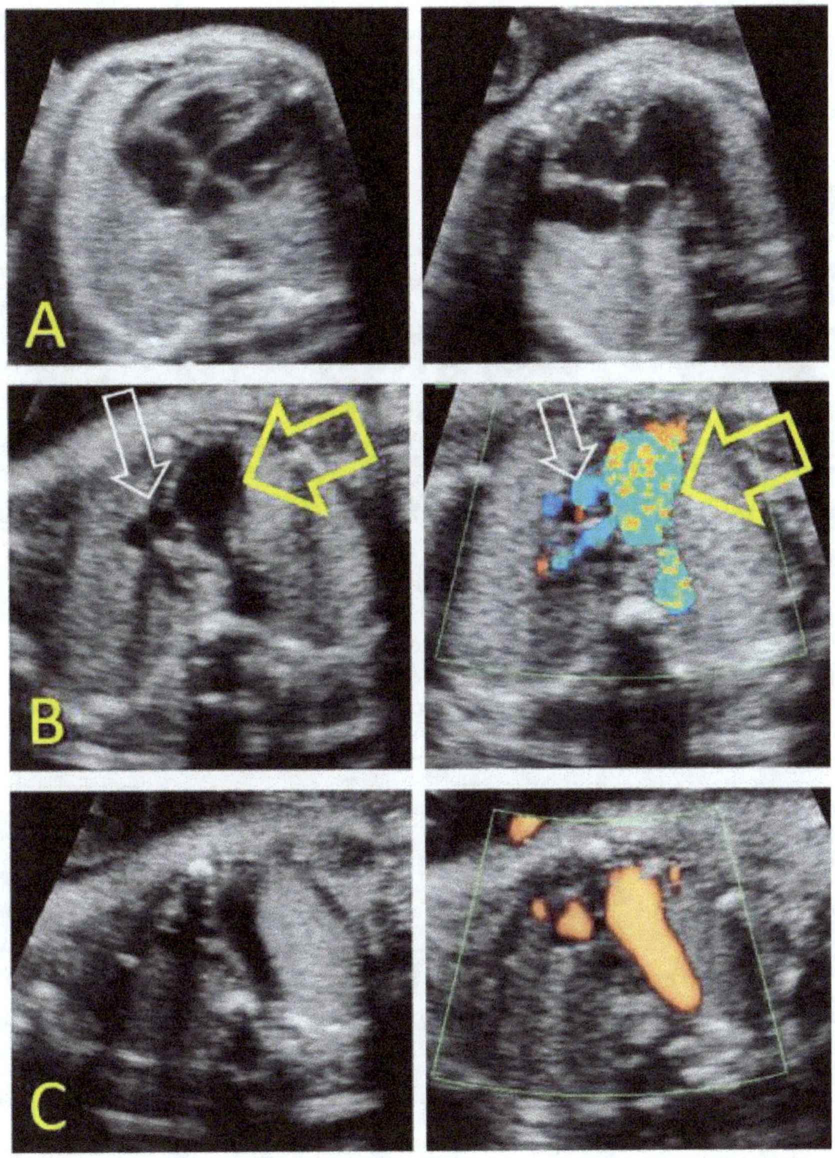

Figure 20. Interrupted aortic arch. (A): The ventricular discordance is not present, because of the septal defect, not evident in four-chamber views, but sub-aortic, when the entire septum is swept. (B): Enlarged pulmonary trunk (yellow arrow), and thin aorta (white arrow) in 3VT view. (C): Discontinuity of aortic arch in upper mediastinum axial planes.

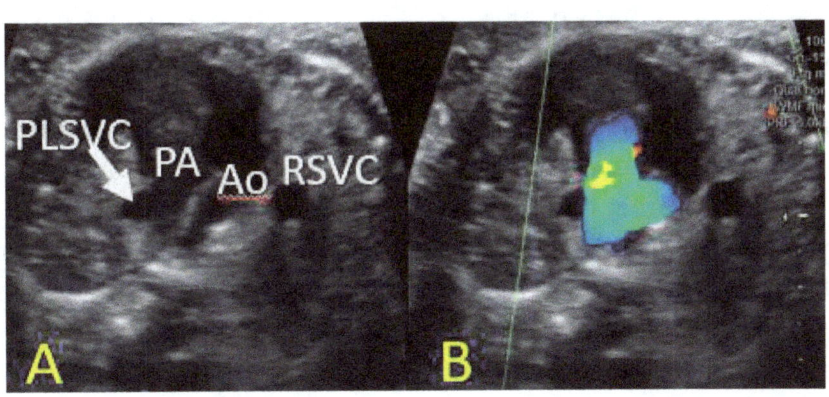

Figure 21. Persistent left superior vena cava (PLSCV), indicated with arrow in duplex gray-scale (A) and color Doppler (B) evaluation.

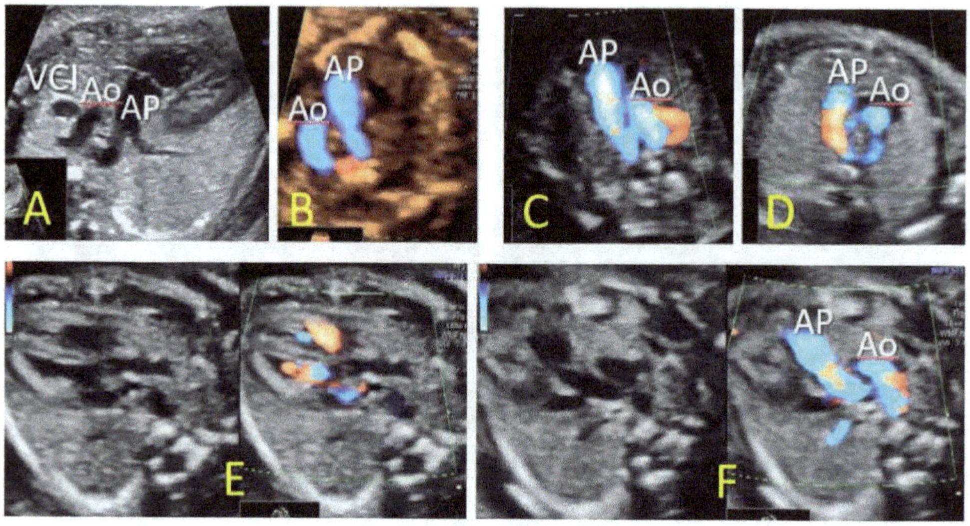

Figure 22. Right aortic arch (RAA) types. RAA and left ductus, forming a "U" shape of the arterial arches confluence as an almost complete vascular ring (A and B). Note the aorta coursing to the right of the spine, on the same side with superior vena cava (A), and a visible vascular incomplete ring behind the trachea. Double aortic arch, color Doppler evaluation (C and D) with complete vascular ring between the aortic branches. RAA with right ductus (E and F), described before with normal heart [44], duplex mode evaluation. Both arterial arches are directed to the right of the spine, resulting a "V"-shaped confluence on the right of the spine.

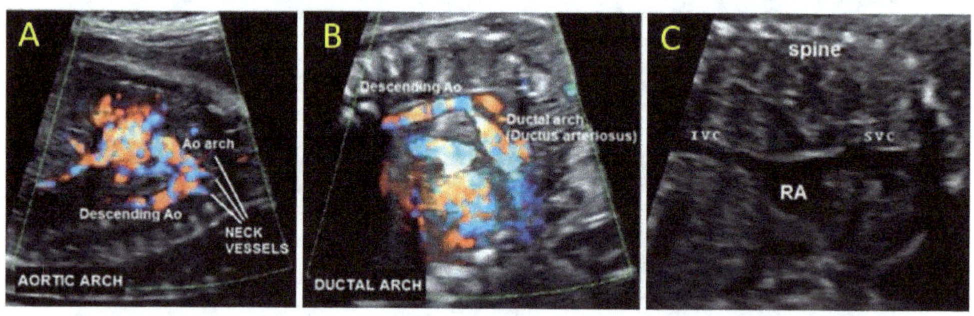

Figure 23. Aortic (A) and ductal (B) arches in longitudinal view. Note the differences mentioned in the text, regarding the origin, curvature and branching. (C): Bicaval view. IVC, inferior vena cava; SVC, superior vena cava; RA, right atrium.

A diminutive caliber accompanied by an altered shape may be present in aortic arch coarctation (**Figure 24A**) or stenosis (**Figure 16D**). Also, the course of the arch may be misshaped and interrupted, with lack of communication with the descending aorta, as in interrupted aortic arch (**Figure 24C**).

The vessel may appear irregular and thin, as in pulmonary stenosis (**Figure 24B**), or heavily dilated, as in aortic arch stenosis or interruption (**Figure 24D**). The ductus may be absent, as is usually in the most frequent variant of absent pulmonary valve syndrome-associated with tetralogy of Fallot. Another type of the syndrome—accompanied by tricuspid atresia, is characterized by a normal or narrowed ductus arteriosus, along the dysplastic right ventricle. Contrarily, the isolated type of absent pulmonary valve syndrome, with intact ventricular septum, associates a severe right ventricular hypertrophy with pulmonary artery and ductus arteriosus dilatation.

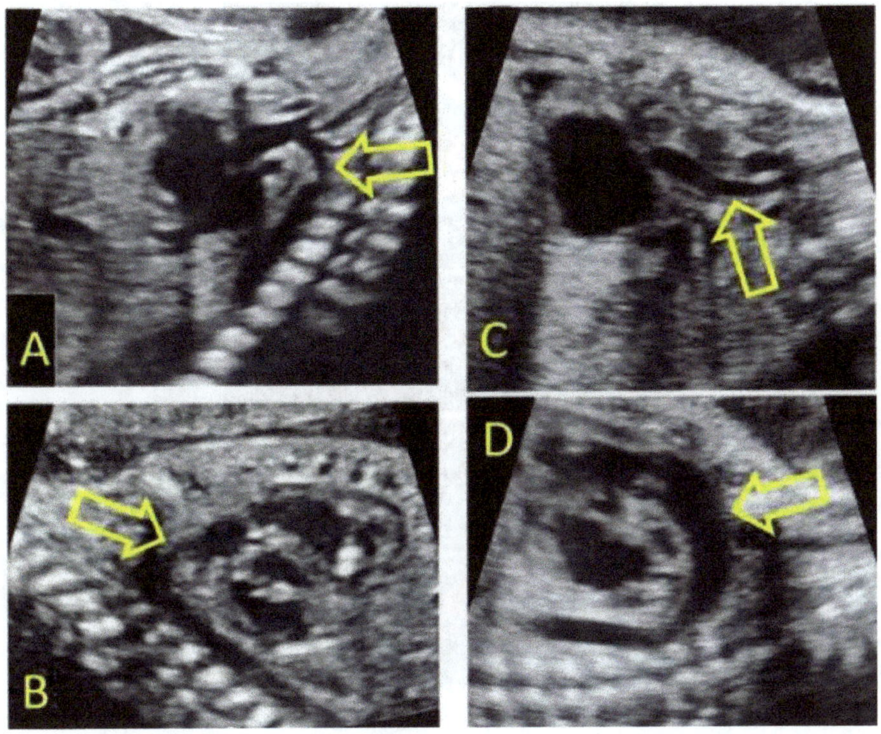

Figure 24. Pathologic aortic and ductal arches in longitudinal view. (A): Aortic coarctation with stenotic isthmus (arrow); (B): pulmonary valvular stenosis, with irregular course and stenotic ductal areas; (C and D): interrupted aortic arch, with ascending aorta that fails to curve, but courses straight cranially (C), and heavily enlarged ductal arch (D).

- *Superior and inferior vena cava views*/caval long-axis view/bicaval view is found longitudinally on the right of the spine, in line with the superior and inferior vena cava confluence with the right atrium (**Figure 23C**). The normal aspect is altered in fetal isomerism, interrupted inferior vena cava or persistent left superior vena cava.

4. Doppler imaging

Color Doppler and *high definition directional power flow* sonography allows for a better understanding of the cardio-vascular anatomy and function [18, 45, 46], particularly in detecting regurgitation, small septal defects and first trimester anatomic and physiological features of heart, as presented below. The ductus venosus appearance, flow and connections depend on the Doppler identification and interrogation of this small vascular structure. Agenesis of ductus venosus was associated with a high incidence of cardio-vascular and genetic abnormalities (**Figures 25** and **26**).

Pulsed Doppler sonography is an adjunct to evaluate the cardiac rhythm, but also the blood flows at the level of various arteria or venous vascular sites and valves.

B-flow and classic power Doppler display in some cases greater sensitivity in imaging cardio-vascular blood flow, but they are not routinely used.

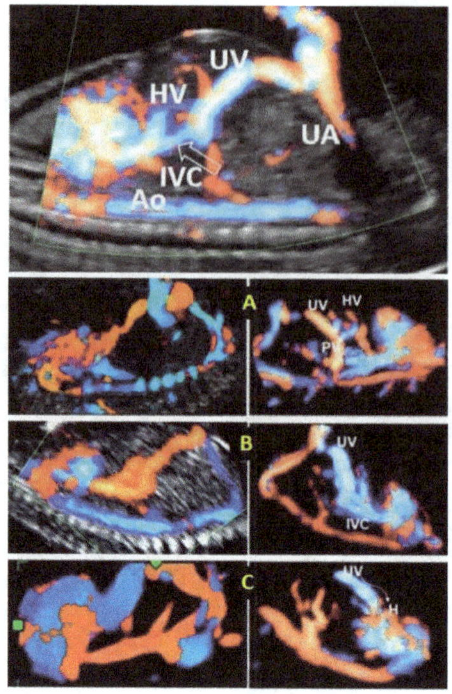

Figure 25. The upper image presents the normal appearance of ductus venosus in 2D color Doppler imaging. (A–C): Agenesis of ductus venosus: with hepatic (A), caval (B) and cardiac (C) drainage. UV, umbilical vein; IVC, inferior vena cava; H, heart; HV, hepatic veins; UA, umbilical artery; PV, portal vein; Ao, aorta.

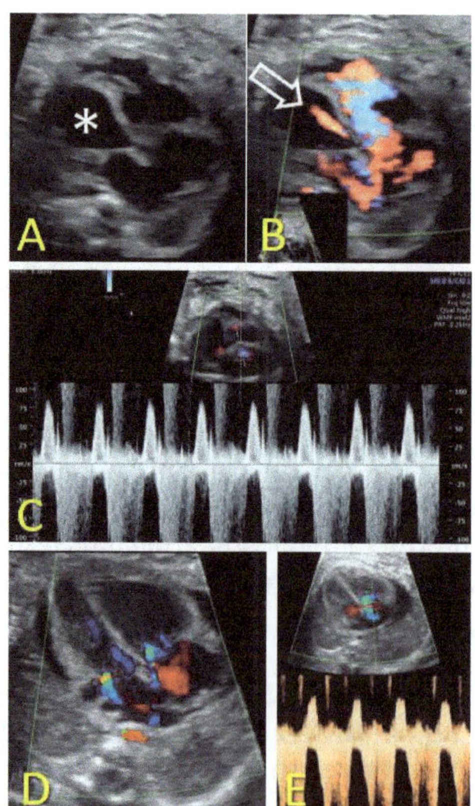

Figure 26. Applications of color and spectral Doppler. (A): Critical aortic stenosis with dysplastic left ventricle (*), atretic valve and aortic regurgitation (arrow, (B)). (C): Same case, tricuspid regurgitation, pulsed Doppler evaluation. (D): Atrioventricular valves regurgitation associated with cardiomegaly. (E): Same case, spectral Doppler evaluation of atrioventricular flow.

5. 4D spatiotemporal image correlation (STIC)

Volume datasets obtained with 4D STIC ultrasonography allow the evaluation of virtual planes not available for direct visualization with 2D technique, and facilitates the reconstruction of the spatial relationships between the cardio-vascular structures (**Figure 27**). This technology has the potential to increase the CHD detection rate by decreasing the dependency on sonographer skills and experience. However, due to the expensive costs and lack of specialists for training and interpretations, the technique is not routinely used.

In selected cases, it may offer important information as the comprehensive assessment of complex CHD cases [47–50] and the evaluation of cardiac function and quantification of fetal hemodynamic parameters, such as cardiac output [51].

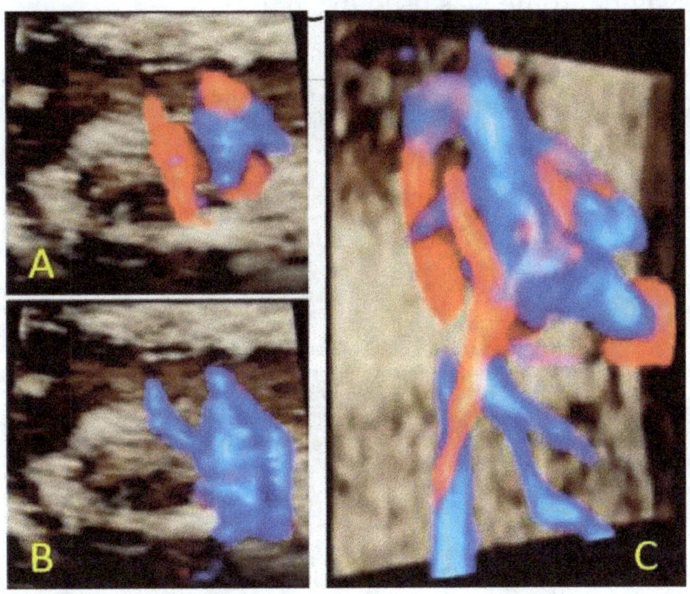

Figure 27. Double outlet right ventricle in 4D STIC. Axial planes show the origin of the great vessels (A) and the communication of the pulmonary artery with the left ventricle, due to a septal defect (B). Oblique longitudinal plane with the anterior origin of the two outflow tracts (C).

6. Cardiac function

It should be considered for suspected structural or functional cardiac anomalies [18, 19]. Some *qualitative* markers are identified during standard scanning: cardiomegaly, atrioventricular valve regurgitation, and hydrops. The *quantitative* assessment of heart function includes the study of myocardial movement such as tissue Doppler, myocardial/ventricular strain, strain rate imaging, fractional shortening and the myocardial performance index [52–54].

7. Efficiency of the fetal cardiac scan

Although the most frequent congenital malformations, CHDs are among the most frequently missed [18, 55]. The efficiency of the cardiac scan is reported with great variation, depending on the scanning protocol, examiner experience, equipment quality and scanning conditions [18, 56–58]. It appears that the use of 4CV alone detects up to 77% of CHD, while adding OTV increases prenatal detection to 83–92% of major abnormalities.

8. Early evaluation of the fetal heart, at the first trimester (FT) morphogenetic scan

Congenital heart defects appear during the first 8 weeks of the fetus development, thus cardiac sonography at the genetic scan, during 11–13 gestational weeks (GW) is feasible (**Figure 28**) and identifies numerous abnormalities (**Figures 29–35**) [59–61]. The rate of complete cardiac evaluation increases with gestational age, from 20% at 11GW, to more than 92% at 13–15 GW, especially when transvaginal route was used [62, 63].

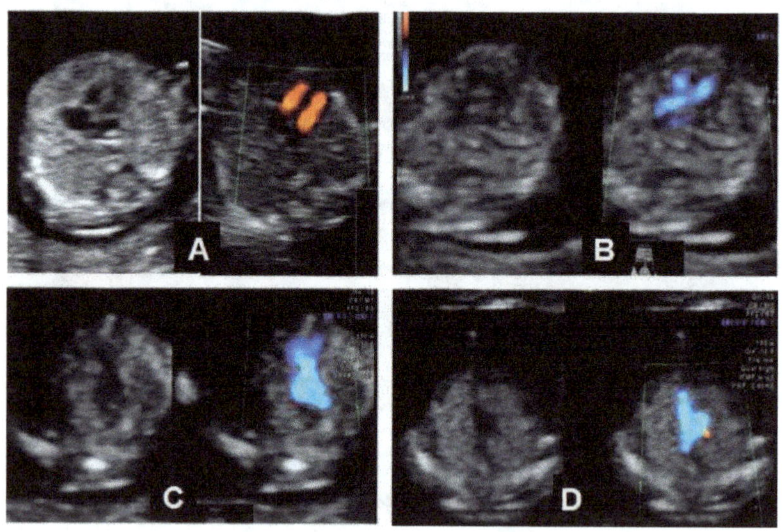

Figure 28. FT cardiac sweep of a normal heart, duplex mode. (A): 4CV plane: gray-scale imaging shows, crux cordis and pulmonary veins entering left atrium; color Doppler imaging shows equal atrioventricular flow and no flow between ventricles. (B): LVOT plane with the aortic emergence, septoaortic continuity and aortic flow. (C): Crossing of the great vessels. (D): 3VT plane – the confluence of arterial arches on left of spine with normal direction and equal flow.

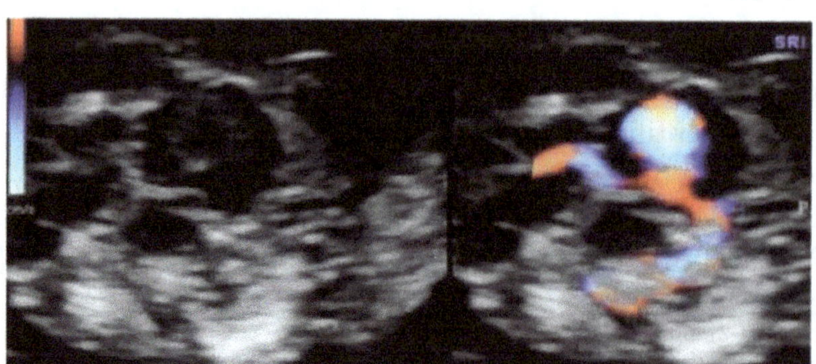

Figure 29. Monoventricular heart.

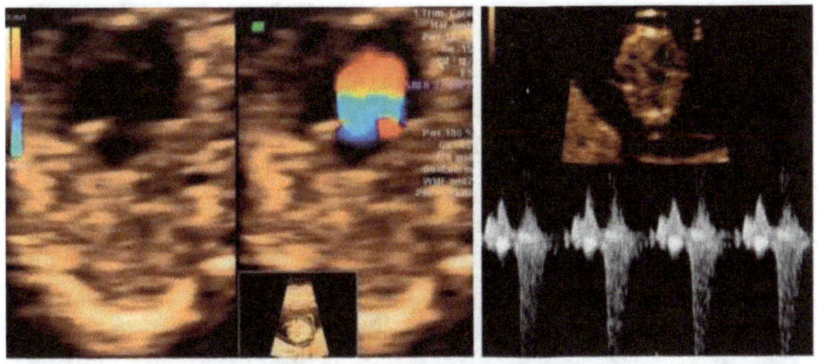

Figure 30. Atrioventricular septal defect. Thickened common valve, large communication between the cardiac chambers, absence of crux cordis and regurgitation.

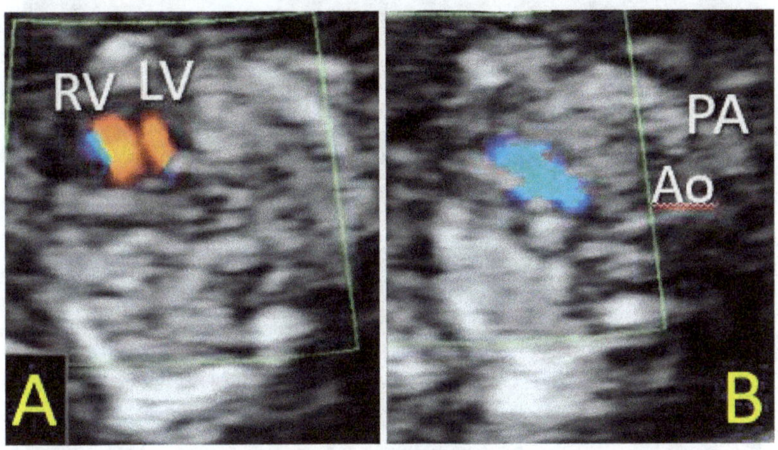

Figure 31. Hypoplastic left heart. A diminutive left ventricle (A) and aorta (B) are identified with the aid of color Doppler. RV, left ventricle; LV, left ventricle; PA, pulmonary artery; Ao, aorta.

Regarding the *imaging technique*, gray scale is the basis of a reliable fetal cardiac scan in the ST, but much less informative in the FT [64].

For safety reasons, routine use of pulsed color Doppler is advised against in the FT [65], although tricuspid and ductus venosus flows are commonly used [66–72] and color Doppler improves early visualization of cardio-vascular features, due to the low discrimination of the heart structures in gray-scale mode [73–75], while respecting the ALARA principle (As Low As Reasonably Achievable) [76].

At a lesser extent, the FT *examination protocol* is similar to the second trimester cardiac scan [77, 78], as presented in **Figure 28**. 4D-STIC is feasible in the FT and likely to improve CHD detection in expert hands.

The *efficiency* of FT cardiac scan varies widely (detection rate 5.6–90%), depending on the protocol used, population risk and scanning route (TV, TA or both). High detection rates for major CHD were reported even in unselected or low risk population 80–90%, when using an extended standardized protocol [74, 75]. A systematic review of the literature [79] reported a pooled sensitivity and specificity of 85% (95% CI, 78–90%) and 99% (95% CI, 98–100%),

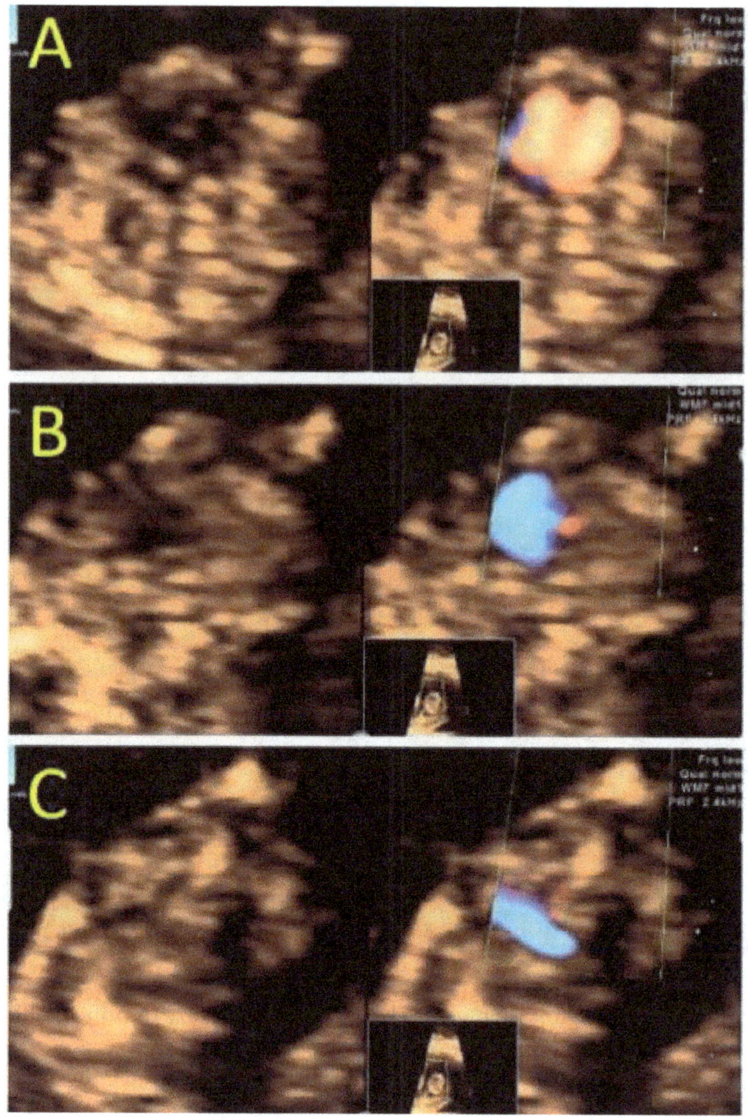

Figure 32. Transposition of great arteries. Inapparent four-chamber view (A), with parallel course of the arterial arches (B) and the impression of only one arterial arch at the level of 3VT view (C).

respectively. Thus, FT cardiac scan has a high accuracy in major CHD detection and a reasonable accuracy to diagnose normal heart. We should underline during parents counseling that normal fetal cardiac features examinations at any time of pregnancy do not exclude CHD, as some diseases evolve in utero and become apparent later during pregnancy: coarctation of aorta, pulmonary stenosis, tetralogy of Fallot, hypoplastic left heart syndrome, cardiomyopathy or cardiac tumors [80–83]. Ventricular septal defects are the earliest missed lesions because of the small size of the lesion and low flow velocities in the FT. A normal cardiac scan in the FT should not be considered a replacement for the second trimester echocardiography.

Markers for cardiac abnormalities (**Figure 36**) may also be useful in early pregnancy, as increased nuchal translucency (NT) and abnormal ductus venosus and tricuspid flows. Increased *NT* was associated with cardiac dysfunction and abnormalities, even in chromosomally normal fetuses, but not obviously related to any particular type of cardiac anomaly [84–86]. The prevalence of CHD when NT is the 95th percentile is up to 20% [87] and about six times higher

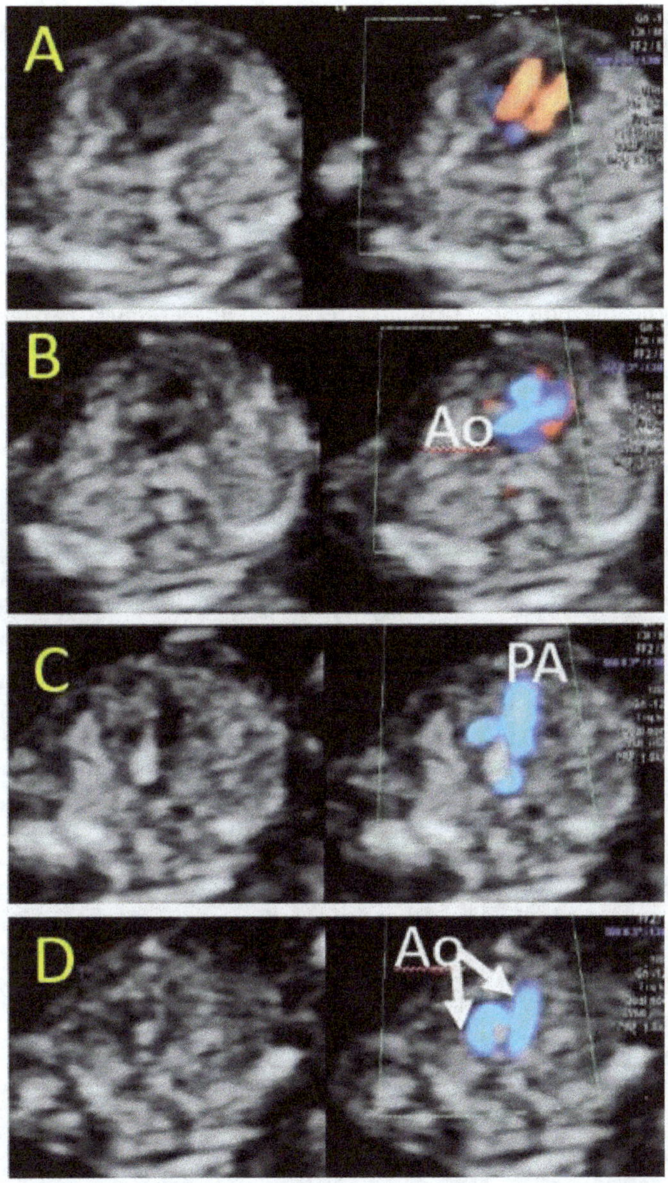

Figure 33. Double aortic arch. Four-chamber view with normal appearance (A), normal emergence of the aorta (B) and pulmonary artery (C), with the aorta coursing to the right of the spine and dividing in two branches that form a vascular ring around the trachea (D).

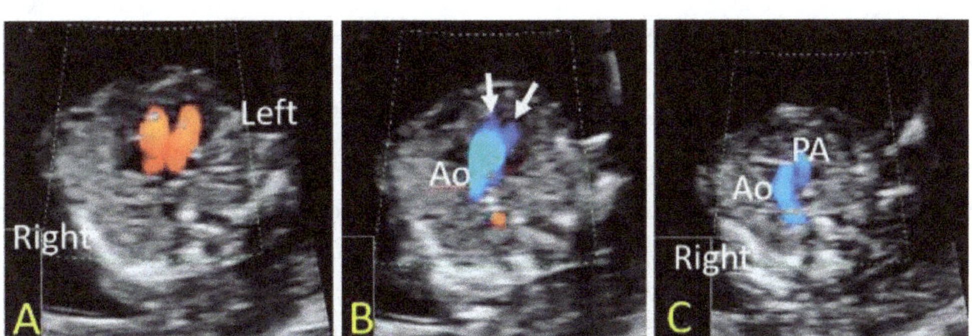

Figure 34. Tetralogy of Fallot with right aortic arch. (A): Normal appearance of atrioventricular flows; (B): overriding aorta; (C): aorta coursing to the right of the spine along the diminutive pulmonary artery.

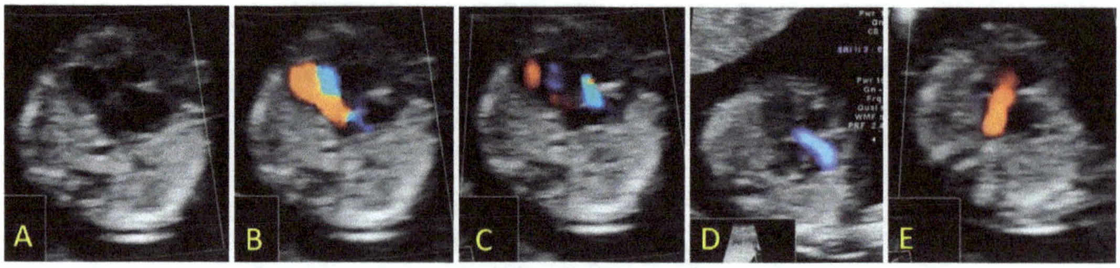

Figure 35. Hypoplastic right heart syndrome. Tricuspid atresia with intact septum. (A): Dysplastic thickened tricuspid valve in 4CV assessment, with lack of antegrade blood flow (B) and regurgitation (C). Normal aortic flow is visualized (D), and reversed ductal flow (E), by using color Doppler.

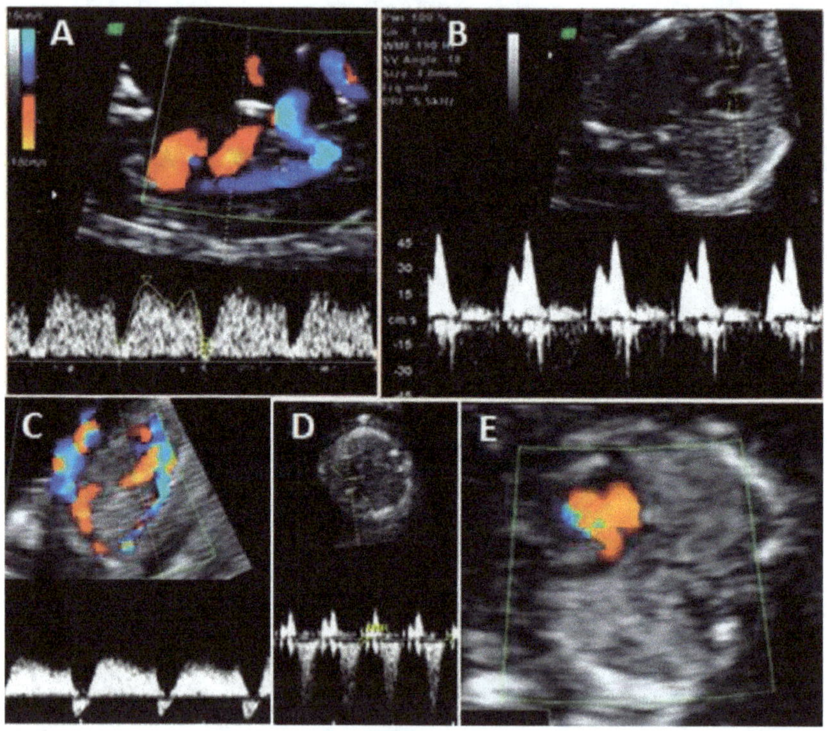

Figure 36. Normal flows at the pulsed Doppler interrogation of ductus venosus (A) and tricuspid valve (B). Ductus venosus with reversed a-wave (C) and tricuspid regurgitation (D) in fetus with atrioventricular septal defect (E).

than unselected population for NT ≥99th percentile [88]. Still, NT measurement is not a reliable screening test for CHD during FT, because of the overall low detection rates for CHD (around 15%) in unselected or low-risk populations [89, 90].

The performance of early screening for CHD achieved by measurement of fetal NT is improved by the assessment of ductus venosus and tricuspid valve flow pattern. In fetuses with enlarged NT (above 95 centile) and *absent or reversed a-wave in DV flow* the risk for major CHD is tripled [91]. The finding of reversed a-wave in chromosomally normal fetuses increases by almost 10 times the risk of CHD, with a predominance of right-heart anomalies regardless of the measurement of NT [86]. Also, chromosomally normal fetuses with *tricuspid valve regurgitation* have an 8-fold increased risk for CHD [92, 93].

Author details

Dominic Gabriel Iliescu[1], Ştefania Tudorache[1], Dragos Nemescu[2*], Monica Mihaela Cirstoiu[3], Simona Vlădăreanu[4], Claudiu Marginean[5], Iuliana Ceausu[3], Daniel Muresan[6], Marius Calomfirescu Vicea[7], Mona Elena Zvanca[3], Cezara Muresan[8], Laura Monica Cara[9], Ciprian Laurentiu Patru[1], Roxana Cristina Drăguşin[1] and Maria Sorop-Florea[1]

*Address all correspondence to: dnemescu@yahoo.com

1 Department of Obstetrics and Gynaecology, University of Medicine and Pharmacy, Craiova, Romania

2 Department of Obstetrics and Gynaecology, University of Medicine and Pharmacy, "Gr.T.Popa", Iasi, Romania

3 Department of Obstetrics-Gynecology, University of Medicine and Pharmacy, Bucharest, Romania

4 Department of Neonatology, University of Medicine and Pharmacy, "Carol Davila", Bucharest, Romania

5 Department of Obstetrics and Gynaecology, University of Medicine and Pharmacy, Targu-Mures, Romania

6 Department of Obstetrics and Gynaecology, University of Medicine and Pharmacy, "Iuliu Hatieganu", Cluj-Napoca, Romania

7 Secretary, Romanian Society of Ultrasound in Obstetrics and Gynecology, Bucharest, Romania

8 Department of Obstetrics and Gynaecology, University of Medicine and Pharmacy, "Victor Babes", Timisoara, Romania

9 Department of Public Health, University of Medicine and Pharmacy, Craiova, Romania

References

[1] Rosano A, Botto LD, Botting B. Infant mortality and congenital anomalies from 1950 to 1994: An international perspective. Journal of Epidemiology and Community Health. 2000;**54**:660-666

[2] Donofrio MT, Moon-Grady AJ, Hornberger LK, et al. Diagnosis and treatment of fetal cardiac disease a scientific statement from the American Heart Association. Circulation. 2014;**129**:2183-2242

[3] Chenni N, Lacroze V, Pouet C, Fraisse A, Kreitmann B, Gamerre M, Boubli L, D'Ercole C. Fetal heart disease and interruption of pregnancy: Factors influencing the parental decision-making process. Prenatal Diagnosis. 2012 Feb;**32**(2):168-172. DOI: 10.1002/pd.2923

[4] Rasiah SV, Ewer AK, Miller P, Kilby MD. Prenatal diagnosis, management and outcome of fetal dysrhythmia: A tertiary fetal medicine centre experience over an eight-year period. Fetal Diagnosis and Therapy. 2011;**30**(2):122-127

[5] McLaughlin ES, Schlosser BA, Border WL. Fetal diagnostics and Fetal intervention. Clinics in Perinatology. 2016 Mar;**43**(1):23-38

[6] Yuan SM. Fetal cardiac interventions. Pediatrics and Neonatology. 2015 Apr;**56**(2):81-87

[7] Schidlow DN, Tworetzky W, Wilkins-Haug LE. Percutaneous fetal cardiac interventions for structural heart disease. American Journal of Perinatology. 2014 Aug;**31**(7):629-636

[8] Chiappa E. The impact of prenatal diagnosis of congenital heart disease on pediatric cardiology and cardiac surgery. Journal of Cardiovascular Medicine (Hagerstown, Md.). 2007 Jan;**8**(1):12-16

[9] Franklin O, Burch M, Manning N, Sleeman K, Gould S, Archer N. Prenatal diagnosis of coarctation of the aorta improves survival and reduces morbidity. Heart. 2002;**87**:67-69

[10] Mahle WT, Clancy RR, McGaurn SP, Goin JE, Clark BJ. Impact of prenatal diagnosis on survival and early neurologic morbidity in neonates with the hypoplastic left heart syndrome. Pediatrics. 2001;**107**:1277-1282

[11] Bonnet D, Coltri A, Butera G, Fermont L, Le Bidois J, Kachaner J, Sidi D. Detection of transposition of the great arteries in fetuses reduces neonatal morbidity and mortality. Circulation. 1999;**99**:916-918

[12] Jenkins KJ, Correa A, Feinstein JA, et al. Non-inherited risk factors and congenital cardiovascular defects: Current knowledge: A scientific statement from the American Heart Association Council on cardiovascular disease in the young: Endorsed by the American Academy of Pediatrics. Circulation. 2007;**15**:2995-3014

[13] Ferencz C, Correa-Villasenor A, Loffredo CA, editors. Genetic and Environmental Risk Factors of Major Cardiovascular Malformations: The Baltimore-Washington Infant Study: 1981-1989. Armonk, NY: Futura Publishing Co; 1997

[14] Williams LJ, Correa A, Rasmussen S. Maternal lifestyle factors and risk for ventricular septal defects. Birth Defects Research. Part A, Clinical and Molecular Teratology. 2004;**70**:59-64

[15] Shaw GM, Nelson V, Iovannisci DM, Finnell RH, Lammer EJ. Maternal occupational chemical exposures and biotransformation genotypes as risk factors for selected congenital anomalies. American Journal of Epidemiology. 2003;**157**:75-484

[16] Carmichael SL, Shaw GM. Maternal life event stress and congenital anomalies. Epidemiology. 2000;**11**:0-35

[17] Botto LD, Mulinare J, Erickson JD. Occurrence of congenital heart defects in relation to maternal multivitamin use. American Journal of Epidemiology. 2000;**151**:878-884

[18] International Society of Ultrasound in Obstetrics and Gynecology, Carvalho JS, Allan LD, Chaoui R, Copel JA, DeVore GR, Hecher K, Lee W, Munoz H, Paladini D, Tutschek B, Yagel S. ISUOG Practice Guidelines (updated): sonographic screening examination of the fetal heart. Ultrasound in Obstetrics & Gynecology. 2013 Mar;**41**(3):348-359

[19] American Institute of Ultrasound in Medicine. AIUM practice guideline for the performance of fetal echocardiography. Journal of Ultrasound in Medicine. 2013 Jun; **32**(6):1067-1082

[20] Small M, Copel JA. Indications for fetal echocardiography. Pediatric Cardiology. 2004; **25**:210-222

[21] Smrcek JM, Berg C, Geipel A, Fimmers R, Axt-Fliedner R, Diedrich K, Gembruch U. Detection rate of early Fetal echocardiography and in utero development of congenital heart defects. Journal of Ultrasound in Medicine. 2005;**25**:187-196

[22] Volpe P, De Robertis V, Campobasso G, Tempesta A. Diagnosis of congenital heart disease by early and second-trimester Fetal echocardiography. Journal of Ultrasound in Medicine. 2012;**31**:563-568

[23] Carvalho JS, Ho SY, Shinebourne EA. Sequential segmental analysis in complex fetal cardiac abnormalities: A logical approach to diagnosis. Ultrasound in Obstetrics & Gynecology. 2005;**26**:105-111

[24] Wood D, Respondek-Liberska M, Puerto B, Weiner S. Perinatal echocardiography: Protocols for evaluating the fetal and neonatal heart. World Association of Perinatal Medicine Ultrasonography Working Group. Journal of Perinatal Medicine. 2009;**37**(1):5-11

[25] Yagel S, Cohen SM, Achiron R. Examination of the fetal heart by five short-axis views: A proposed screening method for comprehensive cardiac evaluation. Ultrasound in Obstetrics & Gynecology. 2001 May;**17**(5):367-369

[26] Available from: http://www.smgebooks.com/echocardiography/chapters/ECHO-16-05.pdf. p. 7

[27] Crane JM, Ash K, Fink N, Desjardins C. Abnormal fetal cardiac axis in the detection of intrathoracic anomalies and congenital heart disease. Ultrasound in Obstetrics & Gynecology. 1997 Aug;**10**(2):90-93

[28] Abuhamad A, Chaoui R. A Practical Guide to Fetal Echocardiography, Normal and Abnormal Hearts. Philadelphia, United States: Lippincott Williams and Wilkins; 2009. ISBN: 0781797578

[29] Schneider C, McCrindle BW, Carvalho JS, Hornberger LK, McCarthy KP, Daubeney PE. Development of z-scores for fetal cardiac dimensions from echocardiography. Ultrasound in Obstetrics & Gynecology. 2005;**26**:599-605

[30] Lee W, Riggs T, Amula V, et al. Fetal echocardiography: z-Score reference ranges for a large patient population. Ultrasound in Obstetrics & Gynecology. 2010;**35**:28-34

[31] Chobot V, Hornberger LK, Hange-Ansert S, Sahn DJ. Prenatal detection of restrictive foramen ovale. Journal of the American Society of Echocardiography. 1990;**3**:15-19

[32] Sharland G, Lockhart S. Isolated pericardial effusion: An indication for fetal karyotyping? Ultrasound in Obstetrics & Gynecology. 1995 Jul;**6**(1):29-32

[33] Slesnick TC, Ayres NA, Altman CA, Bezold LI, Eidem BW, Fraley JK, Kung GC, McMahon CJ, Pignatelli RH, Kovalchin JP. Characteristics and outcomes of fetuses with pericardial effusions. The American Journal of Cardiology. 2005 Aug 15;**96**(4):599-601

[34] Tudorache S, Chiuţu LC, Iliescu DG, Georgescu R, Stoica GA, Simionescu CE, Georgescu EF, Nemeş RN. Prenatal diagnosis and perinatal outcome in congenital diaphragmatic hernia. Single tertiary center report. Romanian Journal of Morphology and Embryology. 2014;**55**(3):823-833

[35] Chaoui R. The four-chamber view: Four reasons why it seems to fail in screening for cardiac abnormalities and suggestions to improve detection rate. Ultrasound in Obstetrics & Gynecology. 2003;**22**:3-10

[36] Ultrasound Screening: Supplement to Ultrasound Screening for Fetal Abnormalities. Available form: http://www.rcog.org.uk/print/womenshealth/clinical-guidance/ultrasound-screeningRCOG2011

[37] Israel Society of Ultrasound in Obstetrics and Gynecology. Available form: http://www.isuog.org.il/main/siteNew/?page=&action=sidLink&stld=301

[38] DeVore GR. The aortic and pulmonary outflow tract screening examination in the human fetus. Journal of Ultrasound in Medicine. 1992;**11**:345-348

[39] Del Bianco A, Russo S, Lacerenza N, et al. Four-chamber view plus three-vessel and trachea view for a complete evaluation of the fetal heart during the second trimester [published erratum appears in J Perinat Med 2006; 34:509]. Journal of Perinatal Medicine. 2006;**34**:309-312

[40] Achiron R, Glaser J, Gelernter I, Hegesh J, Yagel S. Extended fetal echocardiographic examination for detecting cardiac malformations in low risk pregnancies. British Medical Journal. 1992;**304**(3828):671-674

[41] Tonni G, Rosignoli L, Cariati E, Martins W, Miyague A, Bruns R, Araujo Jr E. Fetal thymus: Visualization rate and volume by integrating 2D- and 3D-ultrasound during 2nd trimester echocardiography. The Journal of Maternal-Fetal & Neonatal Medicine. 2015 Sep;**11**:1-6

[42] Pasquini L, Mellander M, Seale A, Matsui H, Roughton M, Ho SY, Gardiner HM. Z-scores of the fetal aortic isthmus and duct: An aid to assessing arch hypoplasia. Ultrasound in Obstetrics & Gynecology. 2007 Jun;**29**(6):628-633

[43] Jowett V, Aparicio P, Santhakumaran S, Seale A, Jicinska H, Gardiner HM. Sonographic predictors of surgery in fetal coarctation of the aorta. Ultrasound in Obstetrics & Gynecology. 2012 Jul;**40**(1):47-54

[44] Iliescu DG, Comanescu AC, Tudorache S, Cernea N. Right aortic arch with patent right ductus arteriosus and normal heart. Ultrasound in Obstetrics & Gynecology. 2012 Jul; **40**(1):115-116

[45] Alves Rocha L, Araujo Júnior E, Rolo LC, Barros FS, Silva KP, Martinez LH, Nardozza LM, Moron AF. Screening of congenital heart disease in the second trimester of pregnancy: Current knowledge and new perspectives to the clinical practice. Cardiology in the Young. 2014 Jun;**24**(3):388-396

[46] Gembruch U, Chatterjee MS, Bald R, Redel DA, Hansmann M. Color Doppler flow mapping of fetal heart. Journal of Perinatal Medicine. 1991;**19**(1-2):27-32

[47] Espinoza J, Gonçalves LF, Lee W, Mazor M, Romero R. A novel method to improve prenatal diagnosis of abnormal systemic venous connections using three- and four-dimensional ultrasonography and "inversion mode". Ultrasound in Obstetrics & Gynecology. 2005;**25**:428-434

[48] Volpe P, Campobasso G, De Robertis V, Di Paolo S, Caruso G, Stanziano A, Volpe N, Gentile M. Two- and four-dimensional echocardiography with B-flow imaging and spatiotemporal image correlation in prenatal diagnosis of isolated total anomalous pulmonary venous connection. Ultrasound in Obstetrics & Gynecology. 2007;**30**:830-837

[49] Paladini D, Volpe P, Sglavo G, Vassallo M, De Robertis V, Marasini M, Russo MG. Transposition of the great arteries in the fetus: Assessment of the spatial relationships of the arterial trunks by four-dimensional echocardiography. Ultrasound in Obstetrics & Gynecology. 2008;**31**:271-276

[50] Volpe P, Tuo G, De Robertis V, Campobasso G, Marasini M, Tempesta A, Gentile M, Rembouskos G. Fetal interrupted aortic arch: 2D–4D echocardiography, associations and outcome. Ultrasound in Obstetrics & Gynecology. 2010;**35**:302-309

[51] Molina FS, Faro C, Sotiriadis A, Daklis T, Nicolaides KH. Heart stroke volume and cardiac output by four-dimensional ultrasound in normal fetuses. Ultrasound in Obstetrics & Gynecology. 2008;**32**:181-187

[52] DeVore GR. Assessing fetal cardiac ventricular function. Seminars in Fetal & Neonatal Medicine. 2005;**10**:515-541

[53] Larsen LU, Petersen OB, Norrild K, Sorensen K, Uldbjerg N, Sloth E. Strain rate derived for color Doppler myocardial imaging for assessment of fetal cardiac function. Ultrasound in Obstetrics & Gynecology. 2006;**27**:210-213

[54] Hernandez-Andrade E, López-Tenorio J, Figueroa-Diesel H, et al. A modified myocardial performance (Tei) index based on the use of valve clicks improves reproducibility of fetal left cardiac functionassessment. Ultrasound in Obstetrics & Gynecology. 2005;**26**:227-232

[55] Crane JP, LeFevre ML, Winborn RC, Evans JK, Ewigman BG, Bain RP, Frigoletto FD, McNellis D. A randomized trial of prenatal ultrasonographic screening: Impact on the detection, management, and outcome of anomalous fetuses. The RADIUS Study Group. American Journal of Obstetrics and Gynecology. 1994;**171**:392-399

[56] Wood D, Respondek-Liberska M, Puerto B, Weiner S. Perinatal echocardiography: Protocols for evaluating the fetal and neonatal heart. World Association of Perinatal Medicine Ultrasonography Working Group. Journal of Perinatal Medicine. 2009; **37**(1):5-11

[57] Simpson LL. Screening for congenital heart disease. Obstetrics and Gynecology Clinics of North America. 2004;**31**:51-59

[58] Ahmed B, Stanojevic M, Kopjar T. Accuracy of the Fetal echocardiography in the high risk pregnancies. Donald School Journal of Ultrasound in Obstetrics and Gynecology. 2007 Jan–Mar;**1**(1):86-95

[59] Huggon IC, Ghi T, Cook AC, Zosmer N, Allan LD, Nicolaides KH. Fetal cardiac abnormalities identified prior to 14 weeks' gestation. Ultrasound in Obstetrics & Gynecology. 2002;**20**:22-29

[60] Carvalho JS, Moscoso G, Tekay A, Campbell S, Thilaganathan B, Shinebourne EA. Clinical impact of first and early second trimester fetal echocardiography on high risk pregnancies. Heart. 2004;**90**:921-926

[61] Taipale P, Ammala M, Salonen R, Hilesmaa V. Two-stage ultrasonography in screening for fetal anomalies at 13-14 and 18-22 weeks of gestation. Acta Obstetricia et Gynecologica Scandinavica. 2004;**83**:1141-1146

[62] Souka AP, Pilalis A, Kavalakis Y, Kosmas Y, Antsaklis P, Antsaklis A. Assessment of fetal anatomy at the 11-14-week ultrasound examination. Ultrasound in Obstetrics & Gynecology. 2004;**24**:730-734

[63] Smrcek JM, Berg C, Geipel A, Fimmers R, Axt-Fliedner R, Diedrich K, Gembruch U. Detection rate of early Fetal echocardiography and in utero development of congenital heart defects. Journal of Ultrasound in Medicine. 2005;**25**:187-196

[64] Tudorache S, Cara M, Iliescu DG, Novac L, Nicolae C. First trimester two- and four-dimensional cardiac scan: Intra- and interobserver agreement, comparison between methods and benefits of color Doppler technique. Ultrasound Obstetrics & Gynecology. 2013 Dec;**42**(6):659-68

[65] Tudorache S, Cara M, Iliescu DG, Novac L, Cernea N. First trimester two- and four-dimensional cardiac scan: Intra- and interobserver agreement, comparison between methods and benefits of color Doppler technique. Ultrasound in Obstetrics & Gynecology. 2013 Dec;**42**(6):659-668

[66] Chelemen T, Syngelaki A, Maiz N, Allan L, Nicolaides KH. Contribution of ductus venosus Doppler in first-trimester screening for major cardiac defects. Fetal Diagnosis and Therapy. 2011;**29**(2):127-134

[67] Borrell A, Perez M, Figueras F, Meler E, Gonce A, Gratacos E. Reliability analysis on ductus venosus assessment at 11-14 weeks' gestation in a high-risk population. Prenatal Diagnosis. May 2007;**27**(5):442-446

[68] Huggon IC, DeFigueiredo DB, Allan LD. Tricuspid regurgitation in the diagnosis of chromosomal anomalies in the fetus at 11-14 weeks of gestation. Heart. 2003;**89**:1071-1073

[69] Faiola S, Tsoi S, Huggon IC, Allan LD, Nicolaides KH. Likelihood ratio for trisomy 21 in fetuses with tricuspid regurgitation at the 11 to 13+6-week scan. Ultrasound in Obstetrics & Gynecology. 2005;**26**:22-27

[70] Maiz N, Nicolaides KH. Ductus Venosus in the first trimester: Contribution to screening of chromosomal, cardiac defects and monochorionic twin complications. Fetal Diagnosis and Therapy. 2010;**28**:65-71

[71] Oh C, Harman C, Baschat A. Abnormal first-trimester ductus venosus blood flow: A risk factor for adverse outcome in fetuses with normal nuchal translucency. Ultrasound in Obstetrics & Gynecology. 2007;**30**:192-196

[72] Papatheodorou S, Evangelou E, Makrydimas G, Ioannidis J. First-trimester ductus venosus screening for cardiac defects: A meta-analysis. BJOG : An International Journal of Obstetrics and Gynaecology. 2011;**118**:1438-1445

[73] Volpe P, De Robertis V, Campobasso G, Tempesta A. Diagnosis of congenital heart disease by early and second-trimester Fetal echocardiography. Journal of Ultrasound in Medicine. 2012;**31**:563-568

[74] Becker R, Albig M, Gasiorek-Wiens A, Entezami M, Knoll U, Wegner RD. The potential of first trimester anomaly scan and first trimester fetal echocardiography as screening procedures in a medium risk population. The Journal of Obstetrics and Gynecology of India. 2005 May/June;**55**(3):228-230

[75] Iliescu D, Tudorache S, Comanescu A, Antsaklis P, Cotarcea S, Novac L, Cernea N, Antsaklis A. Improved detection rate of structural abnormalities in the first trimester using an extended examination protocol. Ultrasound in Obstetrics & Gynecology. 2013 Sep;**42**(3):300-309

[76] Nemescu D, Berescu A. Acoustic output measured by thermal and mechanical indices during fetal echocardiography at the time of the first trimester scan. Ultrasound in Medicine & Biology. 2015 Jan;**41**(1):35-39

[77] Iliescu D, Cara M, Tudorache S, Antsaklis P, Ceausu I, Paulescu D, Novac L, Cernea N, Antsaklis A. Challenges in sonographic detection of fetal major structural abnormalities at the first trimester anomaly scan. Donald School Journal of Ultrasound in Obstetrics & Gynecology. 2015;**9**(3):239-259

[78] Roxana D, Florea M, Iliescu D, Cotarcea S, Tudorache S, Liliana N, Cernea N. The contribution and the importance of modern ultrasound techniques in the diagnosis of major structural abnormalities in the first trimester. Current Health Sciences Journal. 2012;**38**:1

[79] Rasiah SV, Publicover M, Ewer AK, Khan KS, Kilby MD, Zamora J. A systematic review of the accuracy of first-trimester ultrasound examination for detecting major congenital heart disease. Ultrasound in Obstetrics & Gynecology. 2006;**28**:110-111

[80] Smrcek JM, Berg C, Geipel A, Fimmers R, Axt-Fliedner R, Diedrich K, Gembruch U. Detection rate of early Fetal echocardiography and in utero development of congenital heart defects. Journal of Ultrasound in Medicine. 2005;**25**:187-196

[81] Syngelaki A, Chelemen T, Dagklis T, Allan L, Nicolaides KH. Challenges in the diagnosis of fetal non-chromosomal abnormalities at 11-13 weeks. Prenatal Diagnosis. 2011; **31**(1):90-102

[82] Khalil A, Nicolaides KH. Fetal heart defects: Potential and pitfalls of first-trimester detection. Seminars in Fetal & Neonatal Medicine. 2013 Oct;**18**(5):251-260

[83] Simpson JM, Jones A, Callaghan N, Sharland GK. Accuracy and limitation of transabdominal fetal echocardiography at 12-15 weeks of gestation in a population at high risk of congenital heart disease. BJOG: An International Journal of Obstetrics and Gynaecology. 2000;**107**:1492-1497

[84] Souka AP, von Kaisenberg CS, Hyett JA, Sonek JD, Nicolaides KH. Increased nuchal translucency with normal karyotype. American Journal of Obstetrics and Gynecology. 2005:1005-1021

[85] Makrydimas G, Sotiriadis A, Huggon IC, Simpson J, Sharland, Carvalho JS, Daubeney PE, Ioannidis JPA. Nuchal translucency and fetal cardiac defects: A pooled analysis of major fetal echocardiography centers. American Journal of Obstetrics and Gynecology. 2005;192:89-95

[86] Clur SA, Ottenkamp J, Bilardo CM. The nuchal translucency and the fetal heart: A literature review. Prenatal Diagnosis. 2009;**29**:739-748

[87] Souka AP, von Kaisenberg CS, Hyett JA, Sonek JD, Nicolaides KH. Increased nuchal translucency with normal karyotype. American Journal of Obstetrics and Gynecology. 2005:1005-1021

[88] Bilardo CM, Timmerman E, Pajkrt E, van Maarle M. Increased nuchal translucency in euploid fetuses – what should we be telling the parents? Prenatal Diagnosis. 2010;**30**:93-102

[89] Mavrides E, Cobian-Sanchez F, Tekay A, Moscoso G, Campbell S, Thilaganathan B, Carvalho JS. Limitations of using first-trimester nuchal translucency measurement in routine screening for major congenital heart defects. Ultrasound in Obstetrics & Gynecology. 2001;**17**:106-110

[90] Simpson LL, Malone FD, Bianchi DW, Ball RH, Nyberg DA, Comstock CH, et al. Nuchal translucency and the risk of congenital heart disease. Obstetrics and Gynecology. 2007 Feb;**109**(2 Pt 1):376-383

[91] Maiz N, Nicolaides KH. Ductus Venosus in the first trimester: Contribution to screening of chromosomal, cardiac defects and monochorionic twin complications. Fetal Diagnosis and Therapy. 2010;**28**:65-71

[92] Faiola S, Tsoi S, Huggon IC, Allan LD, Nicolaides KH. Likelihood ratio for trisomy 21 in fetuses with tricuspid regurgitation at the 11 to 13+6-week scan. Ultrasound in Obstetrics & Gynecology. 2005;**26**:22-27

[93] Grande M, Arigita M, Borobio V, Jimenez JM, Fernandez S, Borrell A. First-trimester detection of structural abnormalities and the role of aneuploidy markers. Ultrasound in Obstetrics & Gynecology. 2012 Feb;**39**(2):157-163

7

Fetal Central Nervous System Abnormalities

Andreea Ceausescu, Andreea Docea, Marina Dinu,
Stefan Degeratu, Dominic Iliescu and Monica Cara

Abstract

Central nervous system (CNS) is one of the most frequent sites for prenatal diagnosed congenital abnormalities (10 per 1000 live births, much higher than the heart—eight per 1000, kidneys—four per 1000, and other fetal systems). Due to the evolving pattern, ultrasound screening for fetal brain malformations is usually performed at 19–22 weeks' gestation, but severe congenital anomalies can be diagnosed much earlier. This chapter is a short review, structured in eight subchapters: the first one is dedicated to the normal ultrasound aspect of different CNS segments, and the following ones are to detect pathology in prenatal life. We used many ultrasound images and tried to correlate the prenatal findings with the ones obtained postpartum/postabortum for each case, by means of pathology/imaging techniques.

Keywords: cortex, spine, cerebellum, brain stem, malformations, development

1. Introduction

It has been said that the central nervous system (CNS) is the most complex among the fetal and adult systems. This is one of the most common sites of congenital malformation, both in fetuses with and without chromosomal abnormality. It is extremely difficult to diagnose structural abnormalities or mild ultrasound (US) abnormalities that have been linked to major functional problems. Just the opposite, major anatomic defects may not lead to significant malfunctioning of the system. It is extremely important to study the structure, in an attempt to understand the function of the normal and abnormal fetal central nervous system [1, 2]. The detection of CNS anomalies in fetal life is feasible using modern ultrasound equipment. Many anomalies of the central nervous system develop early, and nowadays, we have the tools to detect some conditions at 11–13 weeks [3–8] or even earlier. The first-trimester detection of CNS anomalies is probably the most important advance in modern sonoembriology. Later in pregnancy, neurosonography is a powerful tool in diagnosing CNS pathology.

The following chapter is structured as follows:

1. Normal findings
2. Ventricular system (ventriculomegaly, aqueduct stenosis)
3. Neural tube defects (NTDs) (anencephaly, encephalocele, myelomeningocele)
4. Cortical formation abnormalities (schizencephaly, lissencephaly, heterotopia, microcephaly)
5. Midline abnormalities (holoprosencephaly, complete/partial agenesis of corpus callosum or abnormal corpus callosum, absent cavum septum)
6. Posterior fossa abnormalities (mega cisterna magna, Blake's pouch cyst, Dandy-Walker or variant cerebellar, vermian hypoplasia)
7. Vascular abnormalities (hemorrhage, hematoma, dural fistula, aneurysms)
8. Destructive lesions (hydranencephaly, tumors/mass lesions, cysts, periventricular leukomalacia, infections, dysplasias, other lesions).

2. Normal findings

Some intracranial segments of CNS are seen on ultrasound *extremely early* in development, especially when using high-resolution probes and modern electronic tools. Although many features are indeed recognizable, the clinical utility of such studies is yet to be proven (**Figures 1–3**).

In the *late first trimester*, current guidelines recommend checking for present cranial bones, for normal midline falx, and for the presence of choroid plexus and filled ventricles [9]. The most recommended planes for assessing the head anatomy are the axial ones. In terms of spine assessment, the guidelines state that "longitudinal and axial views should be obtained to show normal vertebral alignment and integrity, and an attempt should be made to show intact overlying skin" [9] (**Figure 4**).

From the early *second trimester* onwards, the commendation is to obtain in standard assessment three standard axial planes (transventricular, transthalamic, and transcerebellar), and, if technically feasible, the fetal profile [10] (**Figures 5** and **6**).

The measurements for fetal head *biometry* (the biparietal diameter—BPD and the head circumference—HC) are possible when using the transventricular (biventricular) and the transthalamic plane. In the most commonly used technique, the calipers are placed from the outer edge to the

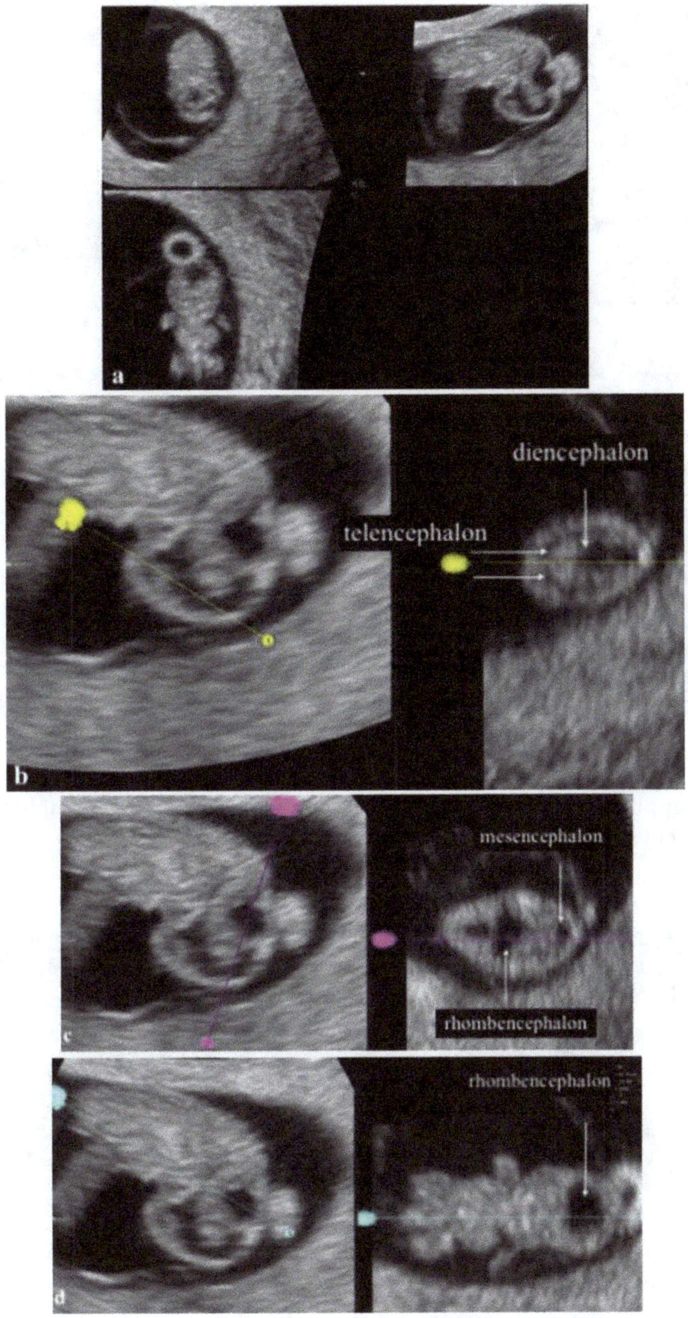

Figure 1. Dating ultrasound scan at 8 weeks of amenorrhea (WA) and 3 days (d). Volumetric ultrasound: sectional planes in the multiplanar mode (a). Subsequently, OmniView facility was used, the line mode (b, c, and d). The embryonic central nervous primitive vesicles can be observed.

inner edge (the "leading edge" technique), at the widest part of the skull, using a perpendicular angle to the midline falx. The HC is measured on the external contour. The cranial bones describe on axial planes a regular *ovoid* shape. The *midline* must be continuous, having no deviations, and the intracranial structures must be symmetrical, mirroring each other's half. Usually, the proximal hemisphere to the probe has a lower visibility, and only the distal one is described by the operator. On the *transthalamic plane*, the anatomic landmarks are (from anterior to posterior) the frontal horns of the lateral ventricles (LVs), the cavum septi pellucidi (CSP), located between

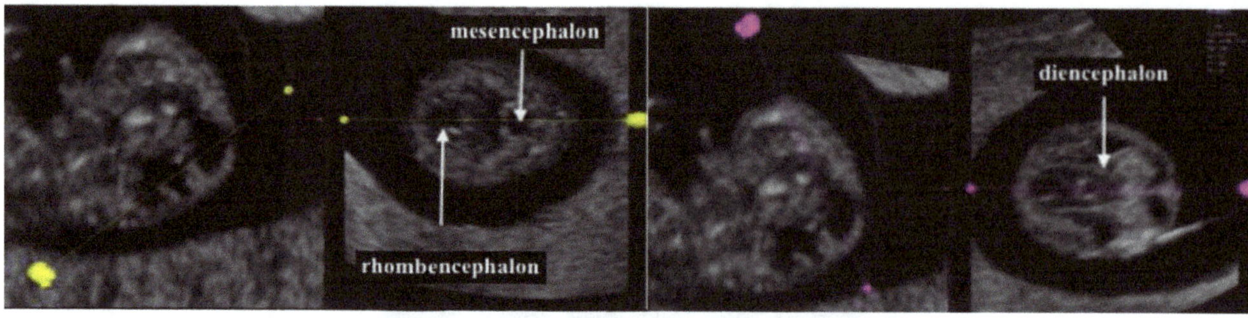

Figure 2. The same case, at 10 WA 1d. The same technique was used, after acquiring a static 3D volume.

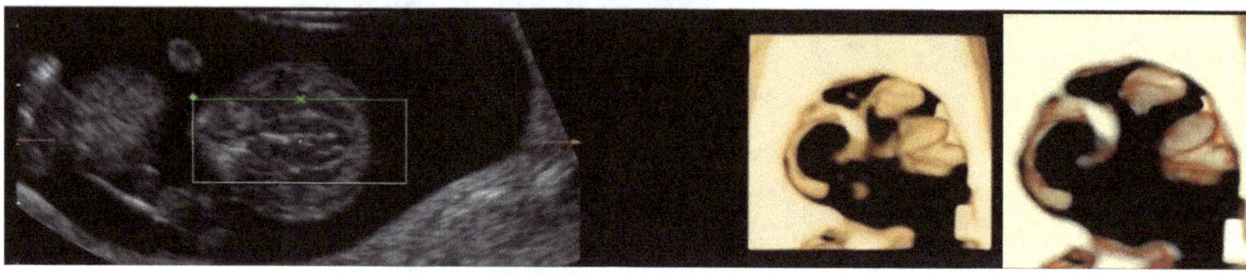

Figure 3. The same case, at 10 WA 1d. The region of interest is placed inside the head, and HD (high-definition) inversion mode surface rendering is applied. This imaging technique acts like a matrix, or a "mold," bringing forth fluid-filled cavities: the early ventricular system.

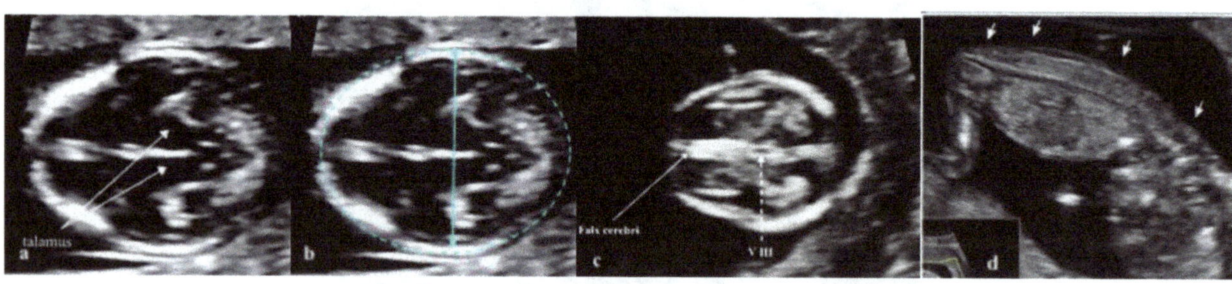

Figure 4. The thalamic plane (a and b), the third ventricle plane (c), and the longitudinal image of the spine, in a prone position (d). In b, the head biometry is represented (measurement of BPD and HC).

them as a fluid-filled structure, the two thalami (resembling together a "heart image"), the third ventricle between them, and the hippocampal gyrus. The *biventricular plane* is found just above the previous one and allows the visualization of the lateral ventricles, with the choroid plexus inside them. The width of the posterior horn of the lateral ventricle must be measured using the exact mark of the parieto-occipital sulcus, inside the echoes generated by the ventricular walls, by a direction aligned perpendicularly to the long axis of the ventricle. Before 25 WA, the measurement must be smaller than 8 mm. The *transcerebellar plane* is obtained just below the transthalamic one, in an oblique fashion. The slight posterior tilting allows the visualization of the frontal horns of the lateral ventricles, CSP, thalami, cerebellum, and cisterna magna [1, 10]. The transversal diameter of the cerebellum (in mm) equals roughly the gestational age (in weeks). In

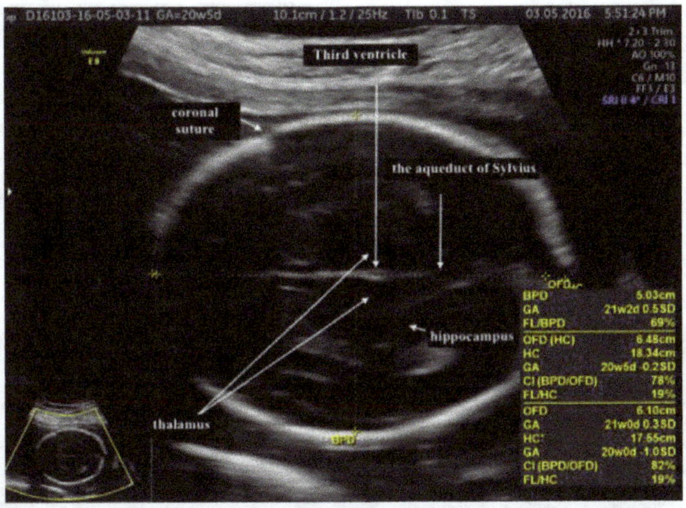

Figure 5. The thalamic plane.

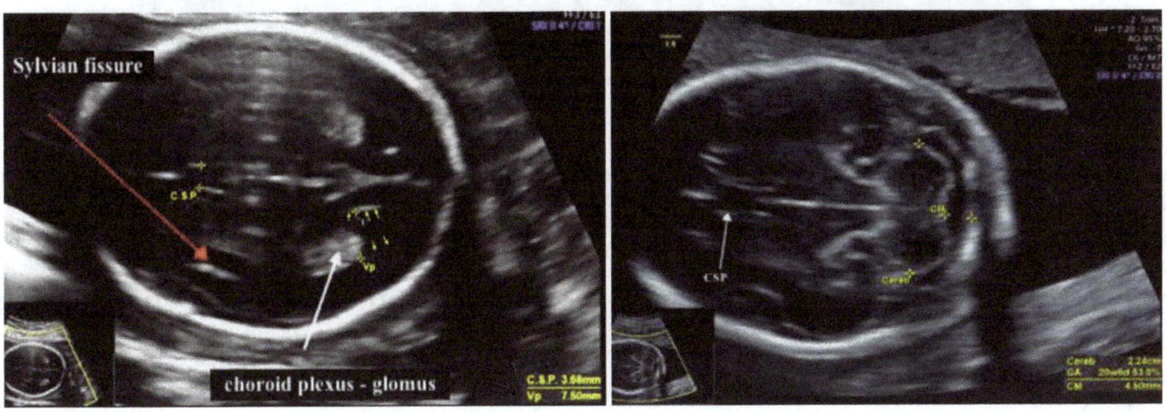

Figure 6. The biventricular (transventricular) and the transcerebellar plane.

the second half of gestation, the depth of the cisterna magna (measured between the cerebellar vermis and the intern margin of the occipital bone) is stable and should not exceed 10 mm.

The *neurosonogram* implies obtaining four more coronal planes and three sagittal/parasagittal planes and assessing the evolving cerebral fissures, gyrations, and circumvolutions [1]. The coronal planes are displayed in **Figure 7**.

The *transfrontal* plane is obtained through the anterior fontanelle. The interhemispheric fissure (IEF) in the median plane and the anterior horns of the lateral ventricles on both sides can be seen. This plane passes anterior to the genu of the corpus callosum (CC), and this is why the IEF appears uninterrupted. The *transcaudate* plane passes at the level of caudate nuclei and the genu of the CC. It interrupts the continuity of the IEF. CSP appears as an anechogenic triangular structure under the CC. Lateral ventricles are seen, surrounded by the cortex. Also, the Sylvian fissures may be identified, laterally. In the *transthalamic* plane, the thalami are seen adjoining. In some cases, the third ventricle is seen in the median plane. In this plane, at the base of the skull, the vessels of the circle of Willis and the optic chiasma

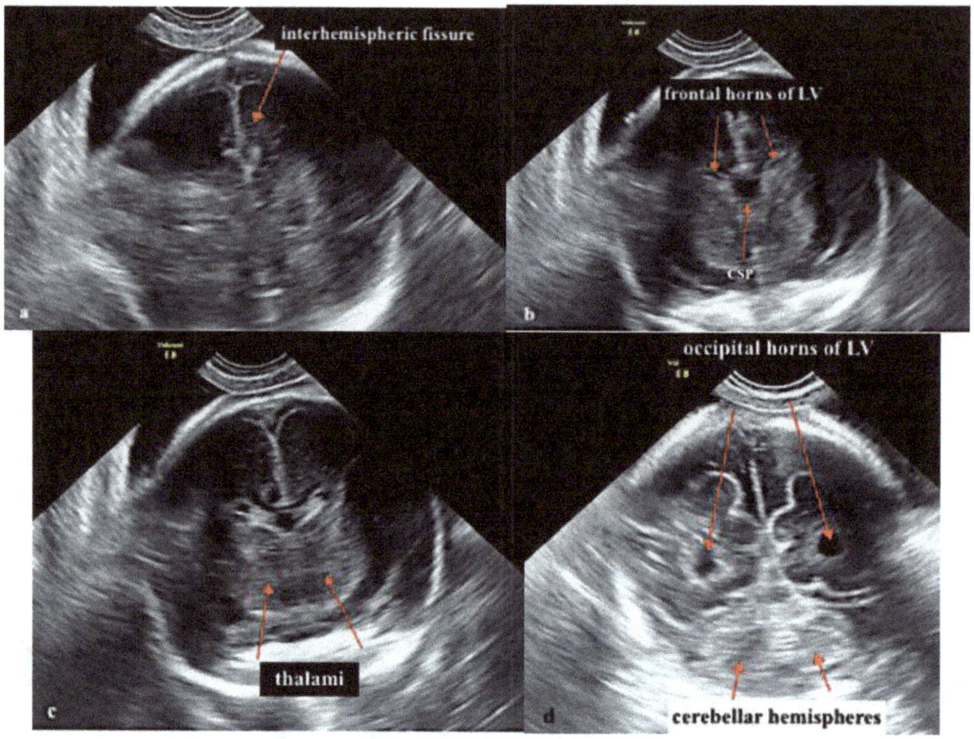

Figure 7. The transfrontal plane (the frontal-2), the transcaudate plane (mid-coronal-1), the transthalamic plane (mid-coronal-2), and the transcerebellar plane (occipital-1 and 2).

may be recognized. The *transcerebellar* plane is obtained through the posterior fontanelle. The occipital horns of the LV and IEF are seen, also the cerebellar hemispheres and the vermis.

The antero-posterior planes are displayed in **Figures 8** and **9**.

In the *midsagittal* (median) plane, all components of the CC (rostrum, genu, body, splenium) may be seen. Also, the CSP, the brain stem, pons, vermis, and posterior fossa. The parasagittal planes (right and left) depict the entire LV, the choroid plexus, the periventricular tissue, and the cortex.

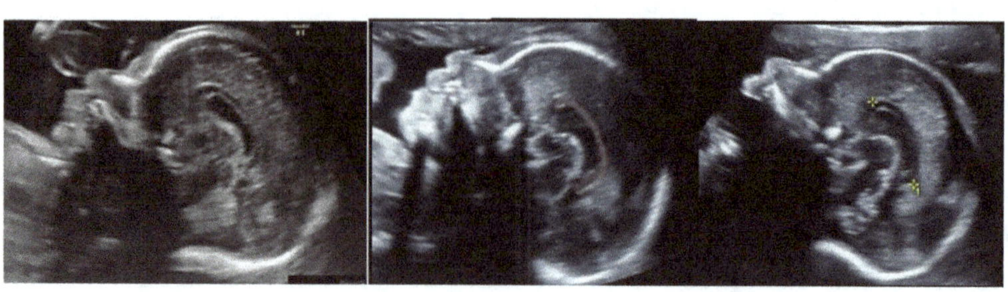

Figure 8. The sagittal plane. The corpus callosum is highlighted in the middle image.

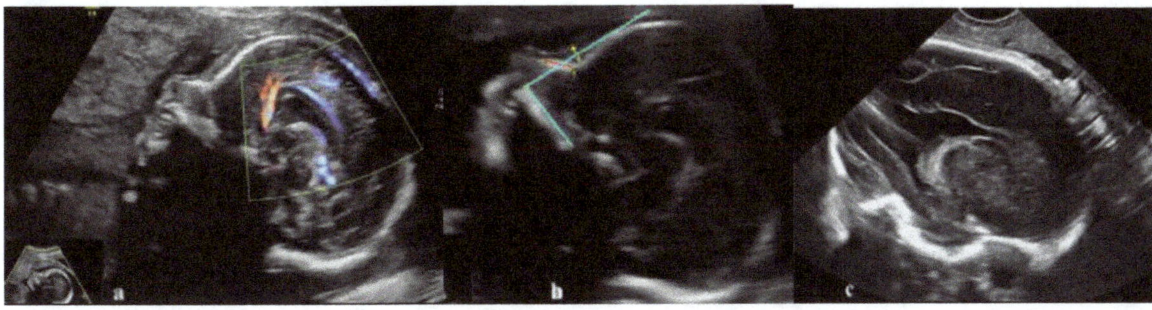

Figure 9. The sagittal plane with HD flow applied, displaying the pericallosal artery (a), the measurement of the nasal bone and the fronto-maxillary facial angle, and the parasagittal or oblique plane-1 (c).

2.1. The spine

In the sagittal and parasagittal planes, the ossification centers of the vertebral body and posterior arches form two parallel lines that converge in the sacrum, in the prone position of the fetus. Efforts must be made to demonstrate the integrity of the overlying skin.

In the second and third trimesters, these planes allow imaging of the spinal canal and of the spinal cord within it. The conus medullaris is usually found at the level of L2–L3 vertebrae (**Figure 10**).

In transverse planes or axial planes, the vertebrae have different shapes at different levels [1]. Fetal thoracic and lumbar vertebrae have a triangular shape, the first cervical vertebrae are quadrangular in shape, and sacral vertebrae are flat.

The normalcy of the vertebrae and ribs' arches may be very easily demonstrated in the coronal plane, using the 3D technique, skeletal mode. Both can be readily numbered (**Figure 11**).

In the prenatal scanning, many normal and abnormal structures may vary and evolve intensively. Thus, using descriptive terms is advisable. The observer may use a thorough detailed depiction of the visualized structures and features, may note the absent normal structure/ structures, and may signalize an abnormal structure. This approach is preferred to issuing a specific diagnosis.

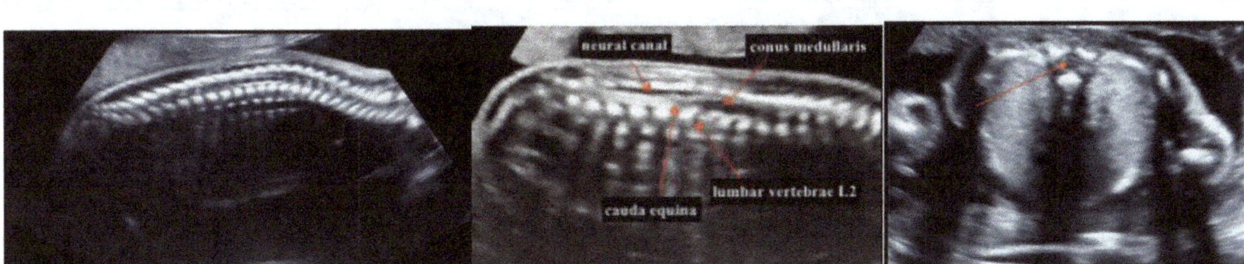

Figure 10. The imaging of the spine and the distal region of the spinal canal. Axial thoracic vertebrae.

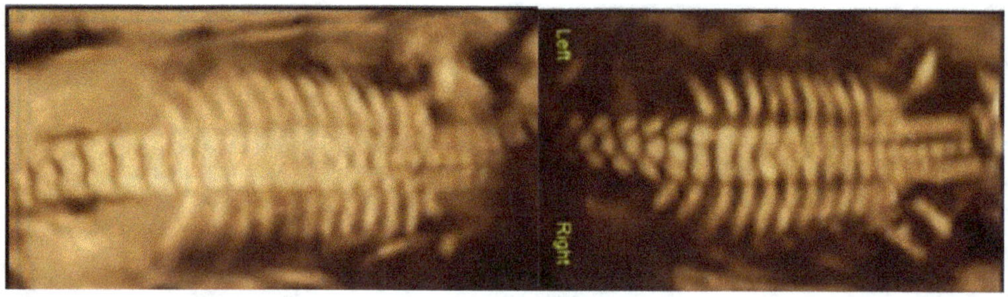

Figure 11. Imaging the spine in the coronal plane. In left image, a supernumerary lumbar rib case is shown.

3. Abnormalities of the ventricular system

Ventriculomegaly is the most frequent abnormal CNS finding diagnosed in utero and is the most common indication for second-level neurosonography and fetal magnetic resonance imaging (MRI) [11].

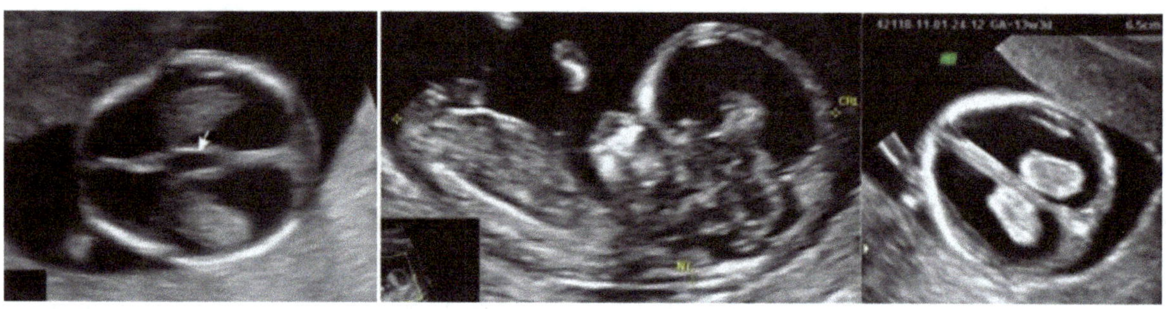

Figure 12. Early ventriculomegaly cases.

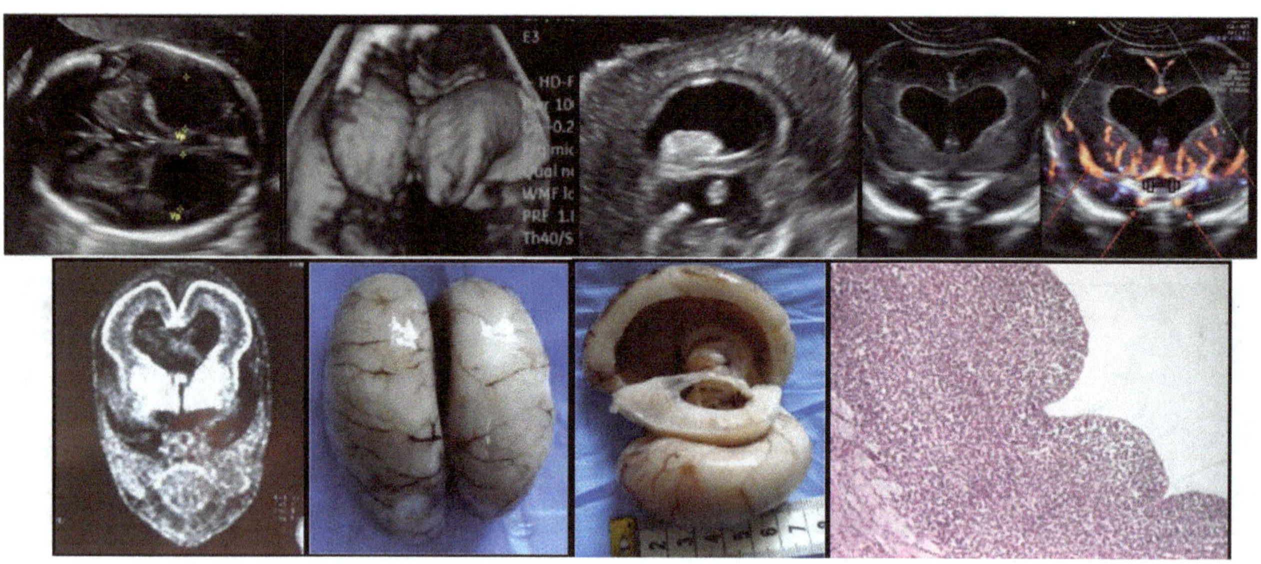

Figure 13. Severe obstructive ventriculomegaly, with unknown origin. Pathologic differentiation of diencephalon and mesencephalon. Conventional necropsy confirms the enlarged ventricles. Microscopy: marked astrocyte cell line proliferation, neuronal migration defects, and cortical fibrosis (stained with hematoxylin and eosin, ob. 40×).

Establishing its class of severity is based on the width of the atrium of the lateral ventricle measurement: ventriculomegaly is considered to be mild when the atrial width is 10–12 mm, moderate between12 and 15 mm, and severe if larger than 15 mm.

In rare cases, ventriculomegaly is accessible in early pregnancy (**Figure 12**).

Yet, this is usually a second- and third-trimester diagnosis. The prevalence of mild ventriculomegaly, based on current criteria, is estimated to be around 0.7% [12]. The finding of ventriculomegaly should trigger a thorough analysis of the fetal brain to investigate all associations (malformative, clastic, tumoral, and syndromic). If no underlying pathophysiology and etiology are found, ventriculomegaly is referred to as "isolated." Melchiorre et al. [13] demonstrated the particularly difficult counseling in such cases. Aqueductal stenosis is the most common cause of ventriculomegaly and its extreme form—fetal hydrocephalus. Published studies of neonates with aqueductal stenosis have noted variable outcomes, with normal development seen in 24–86% of cases [14] (**Figures 13–15**).

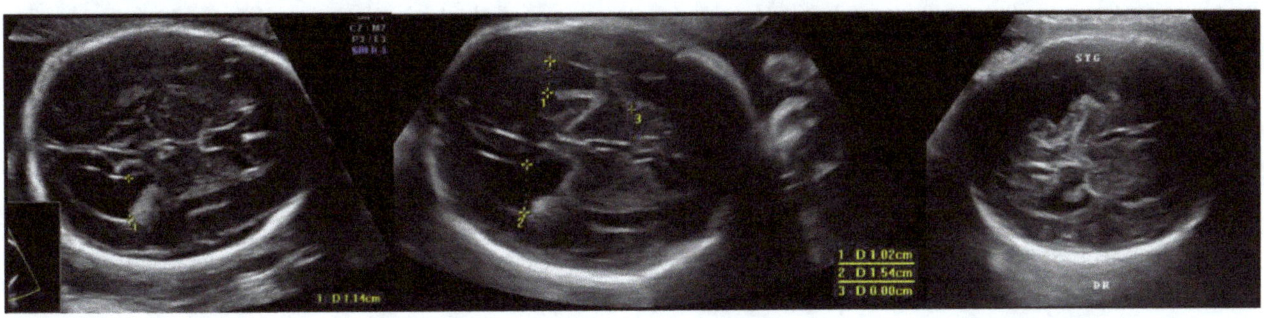

Figure 14. Different cases of unilateral borderline isolate ventriculomegaly, symmetric, and asymmetric.

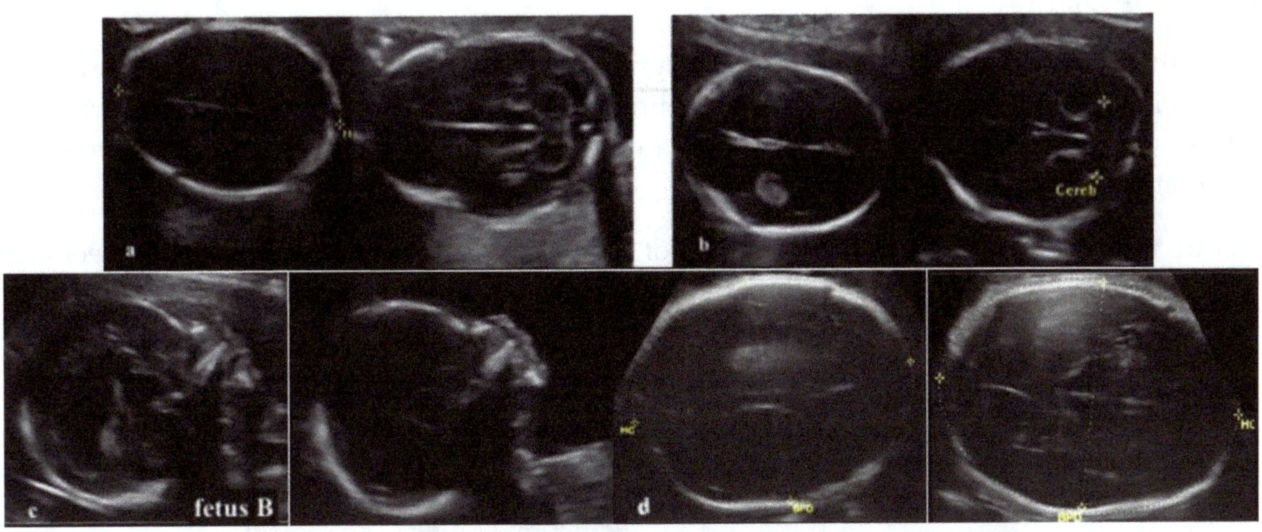

Figure 15. Twin monochorionic diamniotic pregnancy, with discordant major SNC anomaly: severe ventriculomegaly due to aqueductal stenosis. The images display comparatively the same planes: the transthalamic (a) and transcerebellar plane (b), the fetal profile (c) at 17 WA. The transthalamic plane at 25 WA (d). The long-term evolution of fetus B was favorable (after ventriculo-peritoneal shunt).

4. Neural tube defects

Neural tube defects (NTDs) are a frequent group of severe anomalies of the central nervous system. The most frequent conditions are anencephaly, spina bifida, and cephalocele [15]. The open NTDs occur as a result of a primary failure of the neural tube closure between the 17th and 30th postfertilization days. They have a rather stable prevalence. This highlights the importance of primary prevention by folic acid supplementation and the paramount meaning of accurate prenatal diagnosis. In rare cases, some forms of NTDs may be recognized very early in pregnancy (**Figure 16**).

Yet, the vast majority of cases are approached in the late first trimester (11–13 WA), due to the fact that the role of this scan has evolved [5, 7, 8, 16–18]. The technique has grown, no longer being a screening for aneuploidy tool [19–22]—but a method to almost assess the complete fetal anatomy. This became the first anomaly scan in many units [4, 5, 18, 23–25].

In terms of central nervous system, the newest area of debate is the significance of posterior fossa ultrasound semiology. At 11–14 weeks of gestation, it is possible to visualize and measure many spaces in the posterior brain: the brainstem (BS), the fourth ventricle or intracranial translucency (IT), and the cisterna magna (CM). In some settings, such anatomical spaces are assessed routinely by ultrasound in parasagittal or oblique views of the fetal face, as part of the nuchal translucency (NT) scan [26, 27]. Abnormalities of the posterior brain spaces or deviations of their measurements have been proposed as markers of congenital malformations of the posterior fossa [26–29]. Subsequently, the correlation between the decreased amount of intracranial fluid and open spina bifida (OSB) has been established [16, 30]. More recently, it has been suggested that increased fluid may indicate the presence of cystic posterior fossa anomalies such as Dandy-Walker malformation (DWM) and Blake's pouch cyst (BPC) [31–35].

Also, the axial planes offer many indirect signs of OSB and have competed with the sagittal planes in the efficacy of first-trimester screening for OSB [36–38]. It seems that in experienced hands, OSB may reach 100% early detection rates, being reliably diagnosed at 11–14 weeks of screening [39].

In our view, both sagittal and axial planes of the fetal head may be used in OSB screening, depending on the operator's skills and the equipment used. Also, the small BPD may be useful [40, 41].

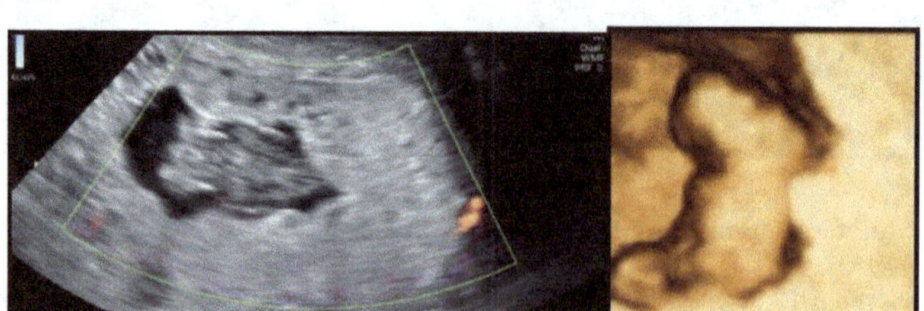

Figure 16. Early embryonic demise, in a case of suspected exencephaly.

2D planes and markers for fetal central nervous system (CNS) morphologic assessment at the first-trimester ultrasound scan are shown in **Figure 17**: left column, a normal fetus; right column, isolated OSB fetus.

In the thalamic plane, the regularity of the skull and the bone ossification should be assessed. Also, measurements may be performed: the biparietal diameter (BPD), the head circumference (HC), and optional—the occipito-frontal diameter (OFD). Thalamus, the third ventricle (red arrow), and symmetry of the intracranial structures may be subjectively assessed. In this plane, the "crash sign" may be subjectively evaluated (the aqueduct of Sylvius position) or the distance between this feature and the occipital bone may be measured (the aqueduct—indicated by the blue quadrant, and mesencephalon—normal by the yellow contour and pathologic by the red contour).

In the lateral third-ventricle plane, aside from the regularity of the skull and the bone ossification assessment, the following structures should be visualized: the midline falx echo, the choroid plexuses, the interhemispheric fissure, the posterior horns of the lateral ventricles (LVs), the lateral walls of the anterior horns of the LV, and the thin brain mantle. In this plane, the "dry brain phenomenon" is usually present in OSB cases: the subjective large choroid plexus for the skull (**Figure 18**).

In the sagittal plane (often called the *mid-sagittal* plane), many CNS structures may be identified and measured: the thalamus (T), the brain stem (BS), the medulla oblongata (MO), the midbrain (M), and the future cisterna magna (CM). In OSB cases, some mild signs may be found: the alteration of the BS (brainstem diameter)/BSOS (brainstem to occipital bone diameter) ratio and the decreased frontomaxillary facial (FMF) angle. The most valuable in screening seems to be the alteration of the cisterna magna (**Figure 19**).

Along with the mild early signs of spinal neural tube defects, other major malformations reach 100% detection rates in many reports. **Figures 20–22** show several such cases, showing correlations between the ultrasound data and the specimen aspects.

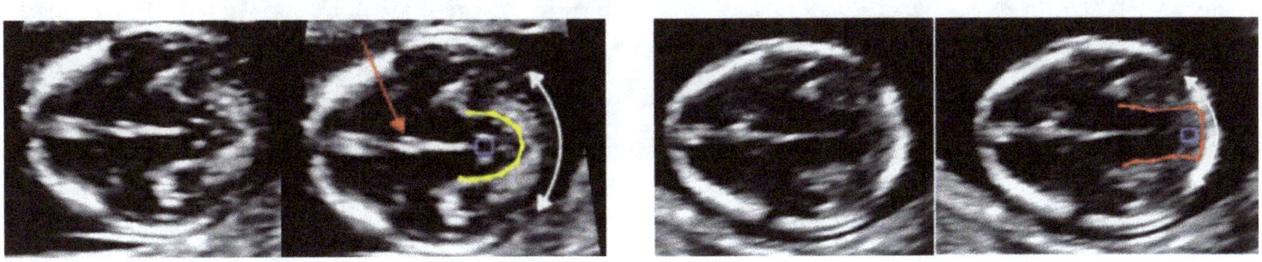

Figure 17. The transthalamic view of cranium in a normal (left) and an OSB case (right).

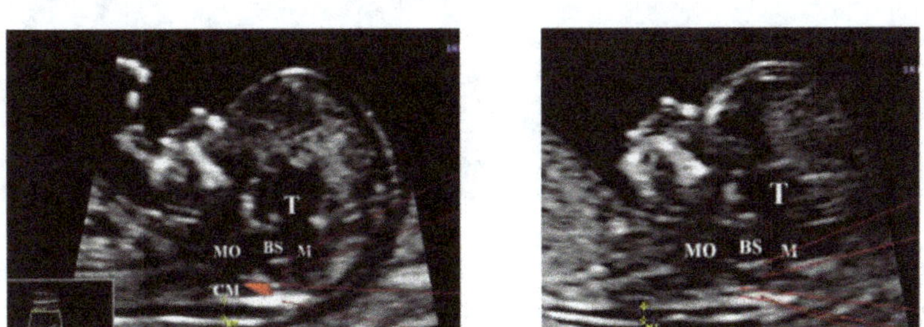

Figure 18. The sagittal plane of cranium in a normal (left) and an OSB case (right).

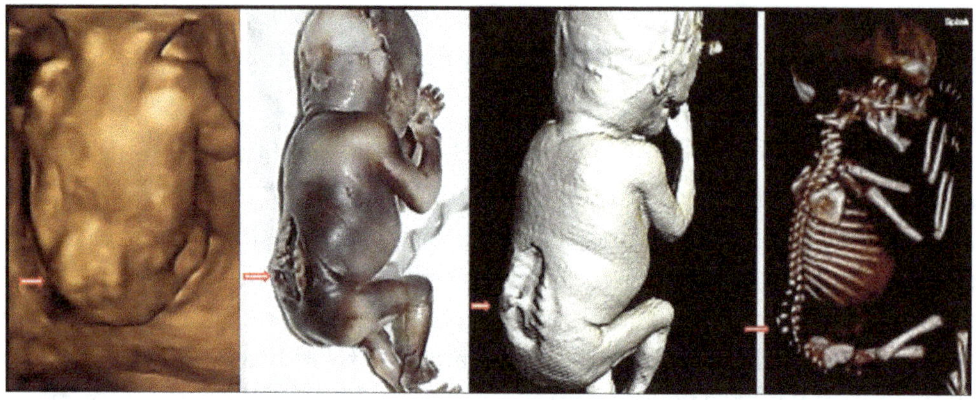

Figure 19. Rachischisis. Medical termination of pregnancy at 16 WA. 3D ultrasound in a surface-rendering mode (a), pathologic specimen (schisis of the lumbar skin, with exposing the meninges and the spinal canal structures) and MRI details of specimen, confirming the hemivertebra suspected on US.

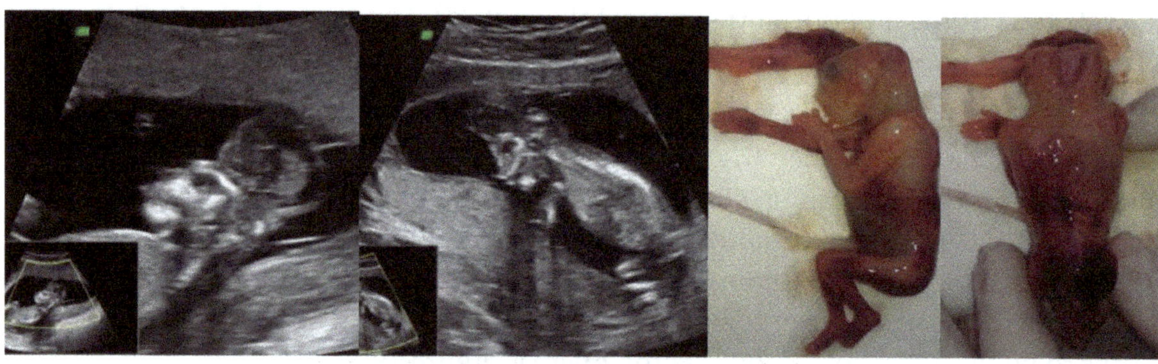

Figure 20. Exencephaly. Ultrasound images and the pathologic specimen at 12 WA.

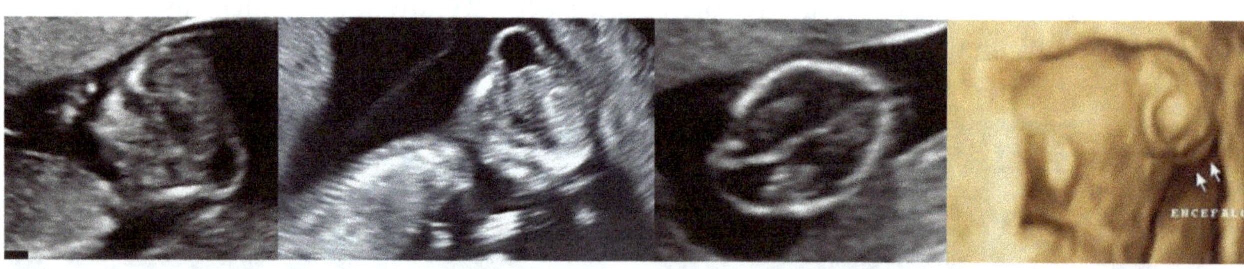

Figure 21. Encephalocele at 12 W. Conventional 2D ultrasound and 3D surface rendering.

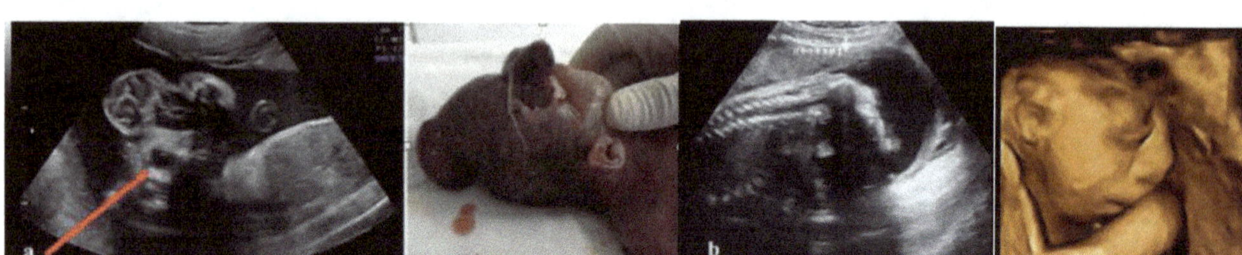

Figure 22. Complex lethal facial and cerebral anomaly. The red arrow indicates the single orbit. The pathologic specimen confirms ciclopy, proboscis, exencephaly (a). Second-trimester case of anencephaly: 2D conventional and 3D ultrasound (b).

5. Cortical formation abnormalities

The cerebral *cortex development* implies evolvement through three steps: neuronal precursor proliferation and differentiation; migration of immature neurons; and cortical maturation (the laminar organization and occurrence of synapsis). Neurons migrate from the ventricular zone (called the germinal matrix) toward the pial surface, along radially oriented glial scaffolds [42–44]. Gyration and sulcation occur afterword, beyond 32 WA. Disruption of any of these steps in cerebral development, due to inherited or acquired causes, can result in a wide spectrum of abnormalities.

Schizencephaly is a congenital cerebral defect in clefting, where clefts extend through the hemispheres from the ventricles to the pial surface [45]. Having two clinical types (open and closed), it seems to be caused by a primary failure of development of the cerebral mantle in early pregnancy. The condition is different from *porencephaly*, being characterized by the presence of heterotopic gray matter lining the cleft. Although primary, it has also been reported as a destructive process mediated by vascular injury also.

Lissencephaly means literally "smooth brain." This is a rare brain malformation, gene-linked, characterized by the absence of normal convolutions in the cerebral cortex, leading to *microcephaly*. In most cases, neonates have usually a normal sized head at birth. The "cobblestone lissencephaly" is characterized by the irregular surface of the brain on the pathological specimen. This is due to aberrant neuroglial overmigration into the subarachnoid space. The formation of an extracortical agyric neuroglial layer occurs. It seems that the primary cause is the deficit of glycosylation of dystroglycans, resulting in neuroglial overmigration [44–50].

The presence of neurons in any position other than the cortex is called *neuronal heterotopia*. This is caused by an abnormal phenomenon of migration during fetal development. The most frequent type is *periventricular* heterotopia, given by an abnormal development of the neuroependyma [44, 50]. It consists of groups of disorganized neurons and glial cells that are located along the walls of the lateral ventricles. They may be isolated (X-linked and non-X-linked forms) or associated with other CNS malformations. The prevalence in the general population is unknown, but it has been related with epilepsy, seizures, and/or developmental delay, with different grades of severity. The prenatal diagnosis has been reported, but the condition is underdiagnosed in the vast majority of screening settings. The true *microcephaly* is considered part of a complex disorder [48–51], occurring in syndromes (with or without chromosomal anomalies). It may be associated exclusively with cerebral anomalies (due to either primary cerebral maldevelopment or clastic events like the ischemohemorrhagic ones) or infectious diseases; the latter has gained a particular interest lately, in light of the recent emergence of microcephaly related to Zika virus infection [48–51]. *Macrocephaly* may result from macrocrania, hydrocephalus, or a major subarachnoid space abnormality. If not associated with other conditions, macrocephaly is synonymous with megalencephaly, meaning an increase in the weight and size of the brain [52] (**Figure 23**).

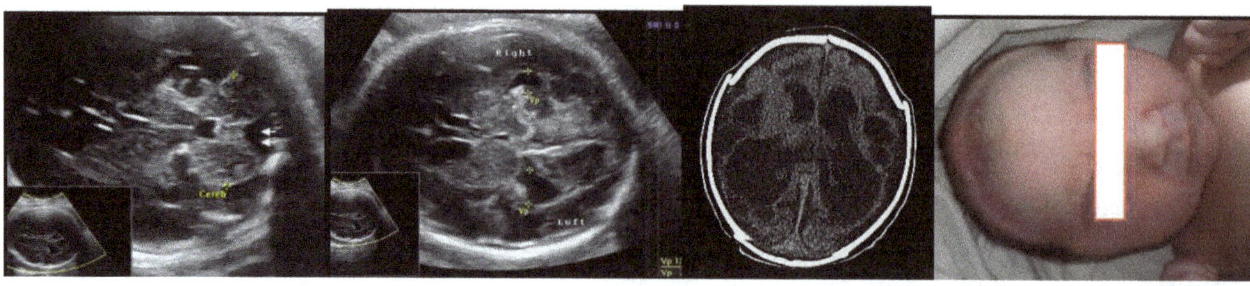

Figure 23. Complex cortical anomaly. Nodular periventricular heterotopia seen. Cortical hypoplasia. Microcephaly. Periventricular leukomalacia. The postpartum image highlights the abnormal excessive ossification of the coronal suture and the dysmorphic facial features of the neonate.

6. Midline abnormalities

Holoprosencephaly is a congenital induction disorder, occurring extremely early in pregnancy (3–6 WA), with failing the segmentation of the neural tube [53–57]. This leads to incomplete separation of the prosencephalon. It has been classified into four subtypes: alobar, semilobar, lobar, and a middle interhemispheric fusion variant (syntelencephaly).

The alobar holoprosencephaly is the most severe type, having a complete lack of separation of the cerebral hemispheres; this lead to a single ventricle, absence of the CC and IEF, and fused thalami. In the semilobar type, the cerebral hemispheres are fused anteriorly. In lobar holoprosencephaly, the fusion of the cerebral hemispheres is present at the frontal lobes. The middle interhemispheric fusion variant results from nonseparation of posterior frontal and parietal lobes.

The *corpus callosum* is the largest commissure of the brain, and its development is accelerated between 8 and 20 WA. Any disturbance of this process may lead to CC agenesis or partial agenesis (hypogenesis or dysgenesis). Many CC abnormalities (in terms of dimensions and shape) are frequently diagnosed during pregnancy although their significance is still debated [58–67]. Abnormal CC has been described among patients assessed for mental retardation.

In a similar way, the absence of fluid in the CSP (with or without intact *septum pellucidum* and corpus callosum) may indicate subtle or severe midline brain abnormalities. All these conditions may have significant implications for postnatal neurological development [58, 61, 63–68] (**Figures 24** and **25**).

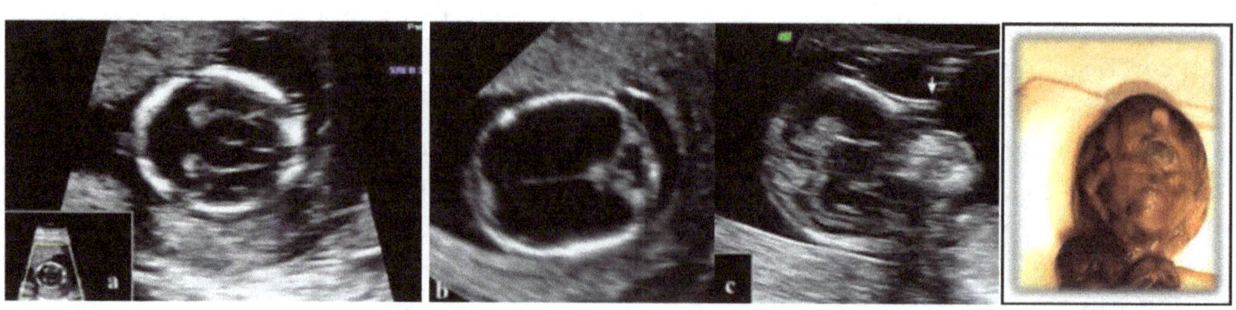

Figure 24. Different cases of holoprosencephaly in the first trimester (a,b). c. a case which associates proboscis.

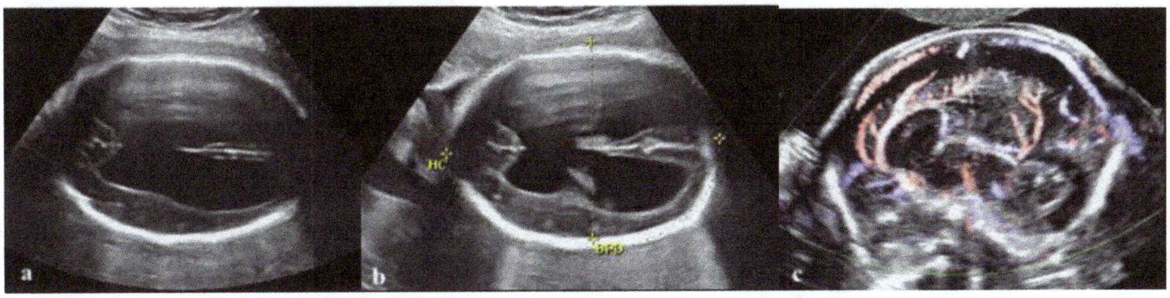

Figure 25. Second-trimester alobar holoprosencephaly (a and b). Short and thick corpus callosum (c).

7. Posterior fossa abnormalities

Posterior fossa abnormalities include the Dandy-Walker malformation (complete or partial agenesis of the cerebellar vermis, cystic dilatation of the fourth ventricle, and enlarged posterior fossa, with upward displacement of the tentorium, torcula, and transverse sinuses); the mega cisterna magna (a CM measuring more than 10 mm and a normal vermis); the Blake's pouch cyst (the presence of an upwardly displaced normal cerebellar vermis, normal appearance of the fastigium, tentorium, and size of the cisterna magna); and isolated vermian hypoplasia (a normally formed vermis but of smaller size, with an otherwise normal size and anatomy of the posterior fossa) [69, 70]. It seems that the Dandy-Walker malformation, even if apparently isolated on ultrasound imaging, carries a high risk for chromosomal and associated structural anomalies. Isolated mega CM and Blake's pouch cyst have a low risk for aneuploidy and associated structural anomalies. The isolated vermian hypoplasia is extremely rare; thus, the literature does not offer definite conclusions about its significance. This needs to be further assessed (**Figure 26**).

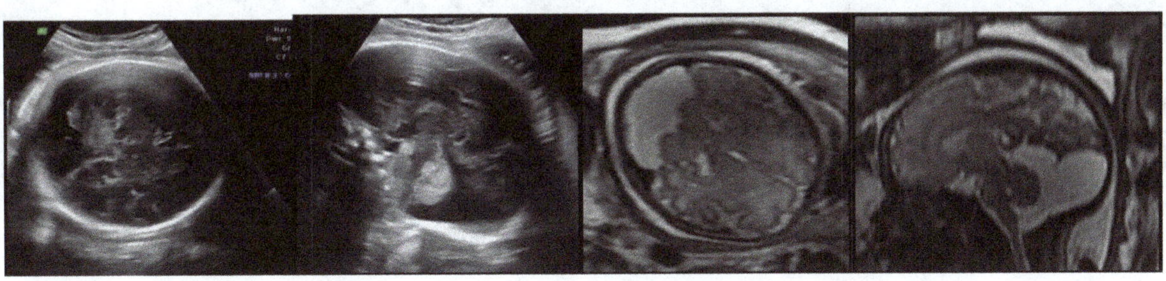

Figure 26. Isolated mega cisterna magna. US and MRI images of the same third-trimester case.

8. Vascular abnormalities

Possible causes of hemorrhage include arteriovenous malformation, benign or malignant, intracranial tumors, fetal infection, drug toxicity, and clotting disorders, such as isoimmune or alloimmune thrombocytopenia [71–79].

Fetal *hemorrhagic* and *hypoxic-ischemic* insults can lead to antenatal brain damage and fetal stroke. These are associated with fetal death, postnatal seizures, mental retardation, psychomotor delays, and cerebral palsy [72]. Fetal intracranial hemorrhages and strokes can be prenatally diagnosed by ultrasound and MRI. The classification of intracranial hemorrhages includes five major types: intraventricular hemorrhage, cerebellar, subdural, primary subarachnoid hemorrhages, and other intraparenchymal hemorrhages. Intraventricular hemorrhage is the most common variety of neonatal intracranial hemorrhages and is characteristic of the immature brain. Intraventricular hemorrhages are subdivided according to their severity into four grades: the first three grades are limited to the ventricles, while the fourth grade includes parenchymal involvement.

The outcome of bleeding into the ventricles ranges from hemorrhage absorption and resolution without residual deficit, to brain damage, with neurological and mental deficits, epilepsy and in extreme cases to fetal or neonatal death. Different scoring systems have been developed to predict the prognostic significance of fetal intraventricular hemorrhage. They depend upon ventricular enlargement and the presence or absence of brain parenchymal damage [72–79].

Spontaneous antenatal subdural hemorrhage is rare [71].

Vein of Galen aneurysmal malformation is a rare congenital malformation (1% of all abnormalities of the fetal cerebral arteriovenous system [80]. It occurs in isolation, although there have been reported cases related to cardiac abnormalities or cystic hygroma. The current hypothesis is the early occurrence (between the 6 and 11 WA), as a result of the persistence of an abnormal connection between the primitive choroidal vessels and the proximal region of the prosencephalic median vein. The persistence of the connection leads to the appearance of some abnormal arteriovenous shunts and the formation of the vein of Galen (**Figures 27** and **28**).

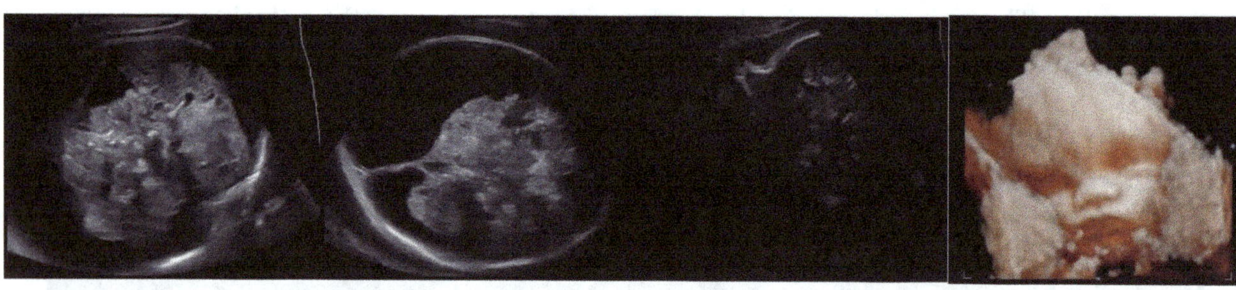

Figure 27. Massive intraparenchymatous hemorrhage in a case of fetal/neonatal alloimmune thrombocytopenia.

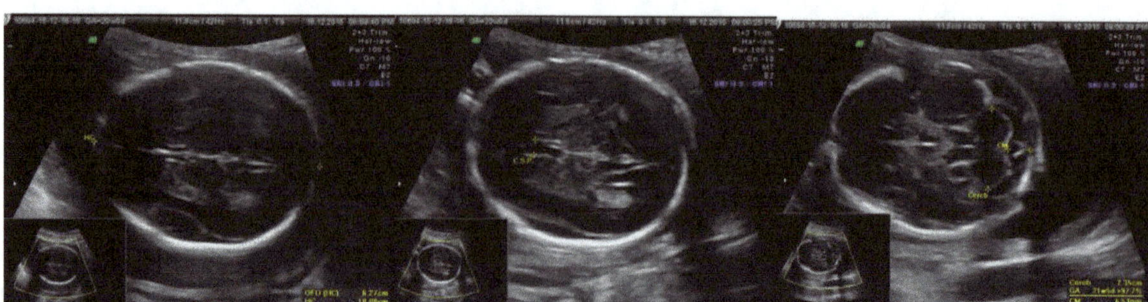

Figure 28. The same case. The fetus has had a complete normal neurosonogram in mid-trimester.

9. Destructive cerebral lesions

The destructive lesions may include an extremely wide range of conditions: hydranencephaly, tumors/mass lesions, cysts, periventricular leukomalacia, infections, dysplasias, intracranial hemorrhage, and other lesions. Identification of these abnormalities can be extremely helpful in providing the patients with management options. Moreover, it has the potential to modulate the neonatal therapy [81–85].

Hydranencephaly is a severe congenital condition: most of the cerebral hemispheres are replaced by a membranous sac. The pathogenic mechanism and the prognosis remain controversial. Still, fetal and postnatal neuroimaging data and histopathologic findings suggest an early bilateral internal carotid artery occlusion occurring at 8–12 WA [81].

Fetal brain *tumors* are rare and have a different histologic pattern [84]. The definitive diagnosis relies on histopathology. The distinction between potentially curable tumors and tumors rapidly fatal after birth is extremely difficult. Moreover, some intracranial masses are not real tumors. Among the histological structure, we mention teratoma, glioblastoma, fetus-in-fetu, craniopharyngioma, and hemangioma.

The acronym TORCH is used to refer to congenital *infections*: toxoplasmosis, other infections (syphilis, varicella zoster, and parvovirus B19), cytomegalovirus, and herpes simplex virus. Zika virus has emerged as an important worldwide congenital infection. Many maternal and fetal symptoms are common. All mentioned infections may cause neurologic damage (ventriculomegaly, intraventricular adhesions, subependymal cysts, intracerebral calcifications, and microcephaly). The Zika virus leads to a more severe spectrum of CNS abnormalities and affects mildly other organ systems [85]. All congenital infections have rather nonspecific ultrasound findings. For the imagist professional, the awareness of imaging features of common congenital infections may facilitate early diagnosis and may, at times, lead to prompt initiation of therapy.

Periventricular leukomalacia has been reported in preterm and growth-restricted fetuses and neonates, and in monochorionic complicated pregnancies. It manifests as punctate white matter lesions or focal white matter necrosis. In clinical settings, cranial US has a limited sensitivity in detecting them. MRI is a more useful tool [78, 86].

Unfortunately, *cortical dysplasias*, involved as an epileptogenic substrate, are the most subtle lesions to identify, diagnose, and characterize [87, 88]. Improved MRI techniques with a multimodality approach (magnetoencephalography, positron emission tomography) will probably increase sensitivity and specificity for identifying them.

The most used classification [88] tried to unify the terminology of cortical dysplasias, which are seen as a subset of all malformations of cortical development. This proposal is based on histopathologic data, clinical and imaging findings, being currently under review [87] (**Figures 29–31**).

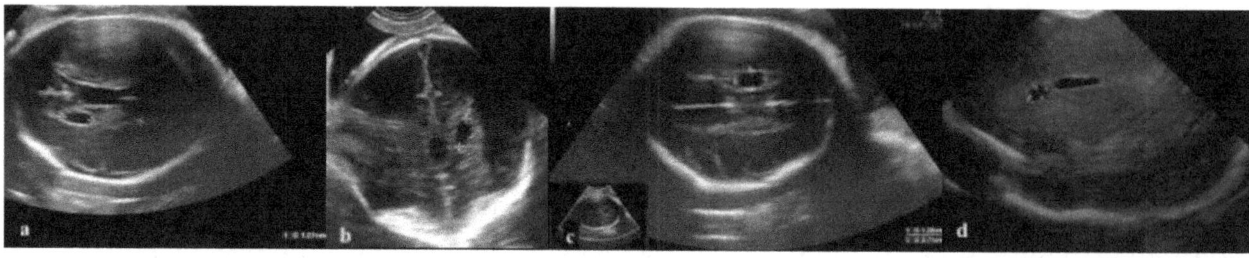

Figure 29. Benign, small dimensions, non-evolving intracerebral cyst: 28 WA (a and b), 30 WA (c), and postpartum, by means of transfontanellar ultrasound assessment (d).

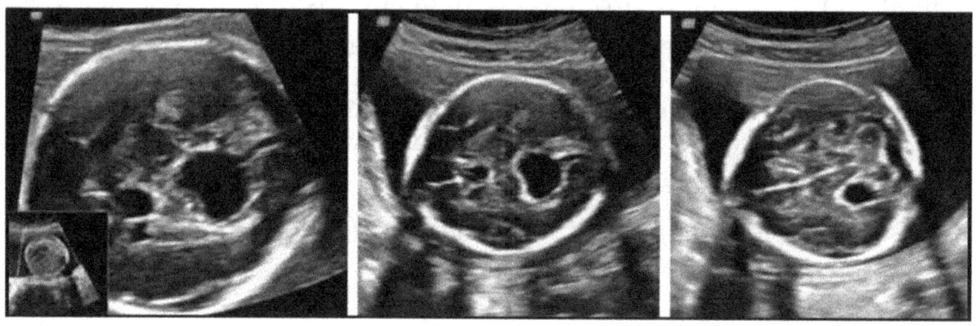

Figure 30. Porencephaly.

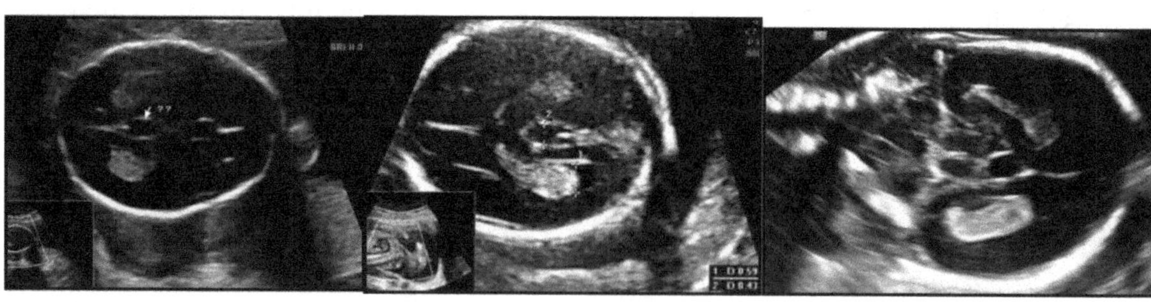

Figure 31. Arachnoid cyst.

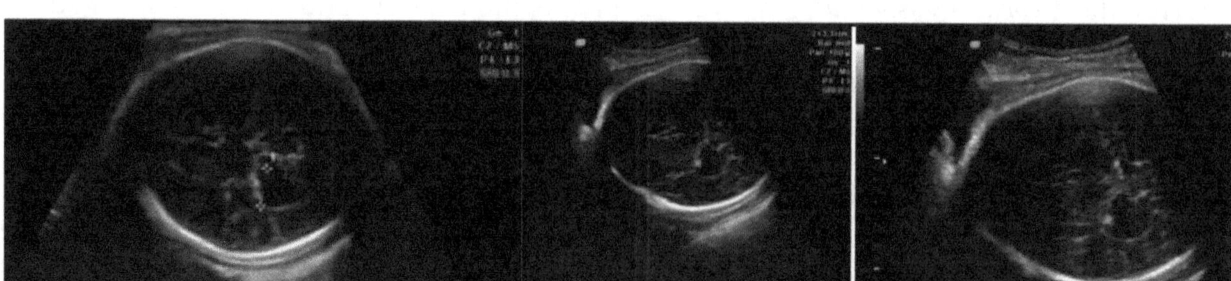

Figure 32. Midline abnormality and unilateral asymmetric borderline ventriculomegaly.

The above division of CNS congenital anomalies is an arbitrary one. In the most severe cases, several types of cortical malformation may be found simultaneously. Moreover, many types succed one another, or overlap in time.

Figures 32–34 show several examples of such associated abnormalities.

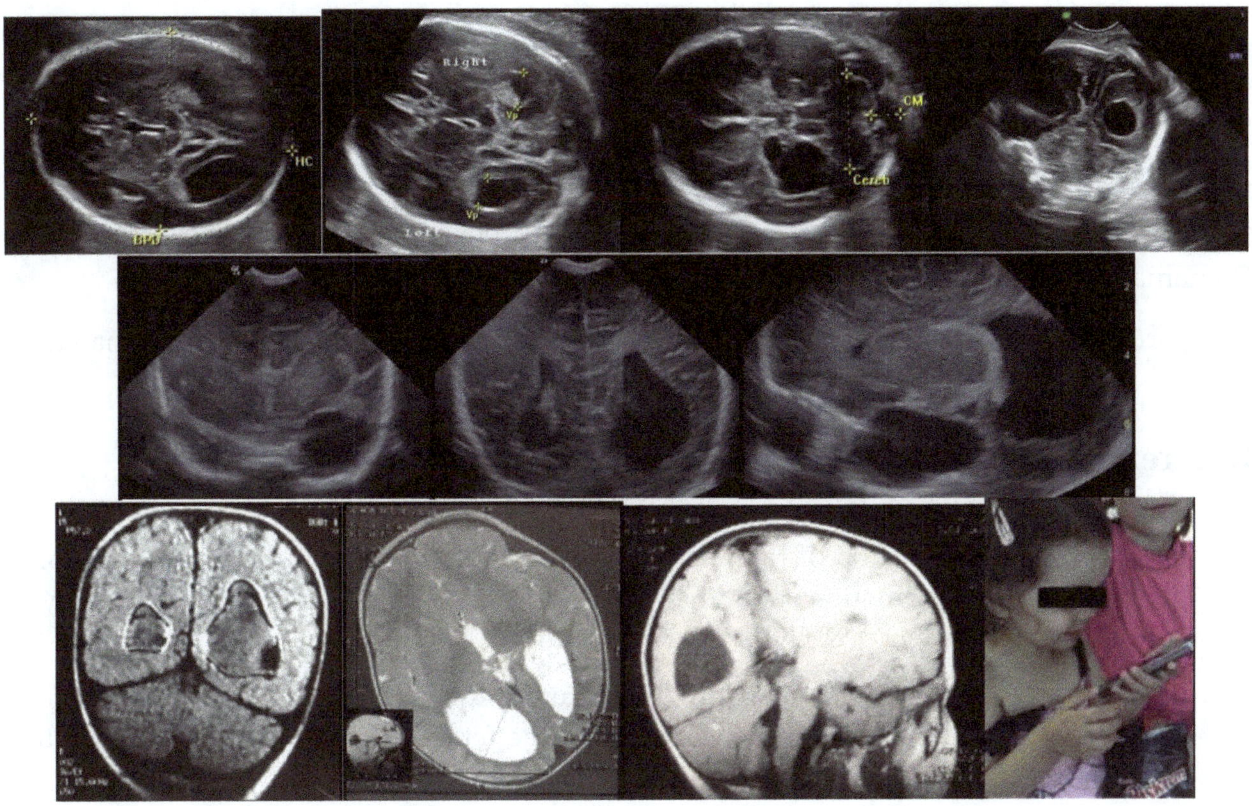

Figure 33. Complete agenesis of the corpus callosum. Unilateral voluminous intracerebral cyst. Severe unilateral asymmetric ventriculomegaly. Subsequently, the short-term and long-term evolution was completely normal.

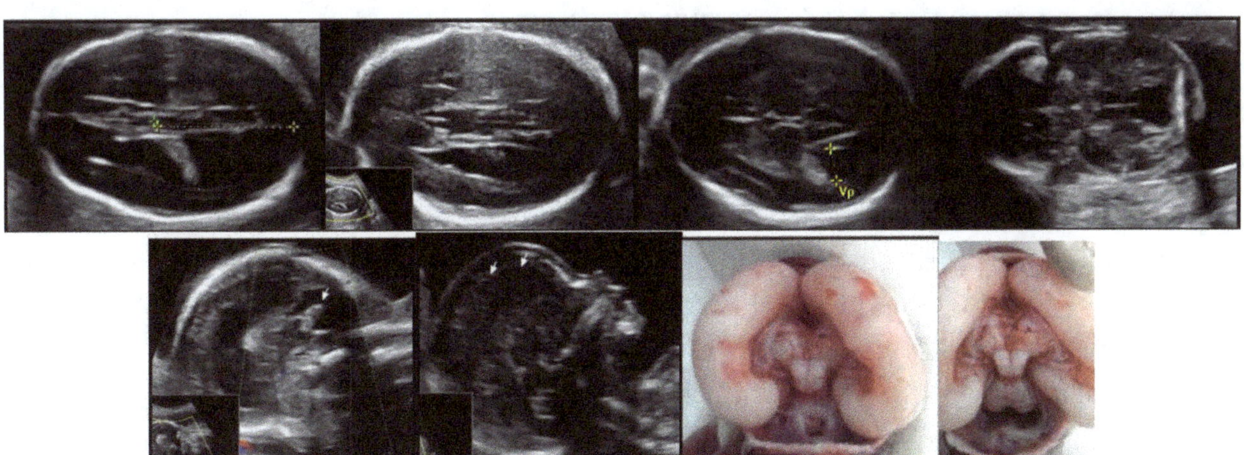

Figure 34. Complete agenesis of the corpus callosum. Cystic dilatation of the fourth ventricle and enlarged posterior fossa, with upward displacement of the tentorium, torcula, and transverse sinuses. Confirmation of the absence of CC by means of conventional autopsy.

Author details

Andreea Ceausescu[1*], Andreea Docea[1], Marina Dinu[1], Stefan Degeratu[2], Dominic Iliescu[3] and Monica Cara[4]

*Address all correspondence to: and_deea2006@yahoo.com

1 Department of Obstetrics and Gynecology, Emergency University Hospital, Craiova, Romania

2 Department of Obstetrics and Gynecology, University Hospital, Craiova, Romania

3 Prenatal Diagnostic Unit, University of Medicine and Pharmacy of Craiova, Craiova, Romania

4 Department of Public Health, University of Medicine and Pharmacy, Craiova, Romania

References

[1] Sonographic examination of the fetal central nervous system: Guidelines for performing the 'basic examination' and the 'fetal neurosonogram'. International Society of Ultrasound in Obstetrics & Gynecology Education Committee. 2007;**29**:109-116

[2] Kurjak A, Antsaklis P, Stanojevic M, Vladareanu R, Vladareanu S, Neto RM, Barisic LS, Porovic S, Delic T. Multicentric studies of the fetal neurobehavior by KANET test. Journal of Perinatal Medicine. 2017;**45**(6):717-727

[3] Iliescu D, Comănescu A, Antsaklis P, Tudorache S, Ghiluşi M, Comănescu V, Paulescu D, Ceauşu I, Antsaklis A, Novac L, Cernea N. Neuroimaging parameters in early open spina bifida detection. Further benefit in first trimester screening? Romanian Journal of Morphology and Embryology. 2011;**52**(3):809-817

[4] Syngelaki A, Chelemen T, Dagklis T, Allan L, Nicolaides KH. Challenges in the diagnosis of fetal non-chromosomal abnormalities at 11-13 weeks. Prenatal Diagnosis. 2011;**31**:90-102

[5] Iliescu D, Tudorache S, Comanescu A, Antsaklis P, Cotarcea S, Novac L, Cernea N, Antsaklis A. Improved detection rate of structural abnormalities in the first trimester using an extended examination protocol. Ultrasound in Obstetrics & Gynecology. 2013;**42**(3):300-309

[6] Şorop-Florea M, Ciurea RN, Ioana M, Stepan AE, Stoica GA, Tănase F, Comănescu MC, Novac MB, Drăgan I, Pătru CL, Drăguşin RC, Zorilă GL, Cărbunaru OM, Oprescu ND, Ceauşu I, Vlădăreanu S, Tudorache Ş, Iliescu DG. The importance of perinatal autopsy. Review of the literature and series of cases. Romanian Journal of Morphology and Embryology. 2017;**58**(2):323-337

[7] Nemescu D, Dumitrescu A, Navolan D, Onofriescu M. First trimester three-dimensional ultrasound diagnosis of iniencephaly. A case report with review of literature. Gineco.eu. 2015;**11**:114-118. DOI: 10.18643/gieu.2015.114

[8] Dragusin R, Florea M, Iliescu D, Cotarcea S, Tudorache S, Novac L, Cernea N. The contribution and the importance of modern ultrasound techniques in the diagnosis of major structural abnormalities in the first trimester—Case reports. Current Health Sciences Journal. 2012;**38**(1):20-24

[9] Salomon LJ, Alfirevic Z, Bilardo CM, Chalouhi GE, Ghi T, Kagan KO, Lau TK, Papageorghiou AT, Raine-Fenning NJ, Stirnemann J, Suresh S, Tabor A, Timor-Tritsch IE, Toi A, Yeo G, International Society of Ultrasound in Obstetrics. ISUOG practice guidelines: Performance of first-trimester fetal ultrasound scan. Ultrasound in Obstetrics & Gynecology. 2013;**41**(1):102-113

[10] Salomon LJ, Alfirevic Z, Berghella V, Bilardo C, Hernandez-Andrade E, Johnsen SL, Kalache K, Leung K-Y, Malinger G, Munoz H, Prefumo F, Toi A, Lee W, on behalf of the ISUOG Clinical Standards Committee. Practice guidelines for performance of the routine mid-trimester fetal ultrasound scan. Ultrasound in Obstetrics & Gynecology. 2011;**37**:116-126

[11] Guibaud L, Lacalm A. Etiological diagnostic tools to elucidate 'isolated' ventriculomegaly. Ultrasound in Obstetrics & Gynecology. 2015;**46**(1):1-11

[12] Vergani P, Locatelli A, Strobelt N, Cavallone M, Ceruti P, Paterlini G, Ghidini A. Clinical outcome of mild fetal ventriculomegaly. American Journal of Obstetrics and Gynecology. 1998;**178**:218-222

[13] Melchiorre K, Bhide A, Gika AD, Pilu G, Papageorghiou AT. Counseling in isolated mild fetal ventriculomegaly. Ultrasound in Obstetrics & Gynecology. 2009;**34**:212-224

[14] Levitsky DB, Mack LA, Nyberg DA, Shurtleff DB, Shields LA, Nghiem HV, Cyr DR. Fetal aqueductal stenosis diagnosed sonographically: How grave is the prognosis? AJR. American Journal of Roentgenology. 1995;**164**(3):725-730

[15] Timbolschi D, Schaefer E, Monga B, Fattori D, Dott B, Favre R, Kohler M, Nisand I, Viville B, Astruc D, Kehrli P, Gasser B, Lindner V, Marcellin L, Flori E, Girard-Lemaire F, Dollfus H, Doray B. Neural tube defects: The experience of the registry of congenital malformations of Alsace, France, 1995-2009. Fetal Diagnosis and Therapy. 2015;**37**(1):6-17

[16] Garcia-Posada R, Eixarch E, Sanz M, Puerto B, Figueras F, Borrell A. Cisterna magna width at 11-13 weeks in the detection of posterior fossa anomalies. Ultrasound in Obstetrics & Gynecology. 2013;**41**(5):515-520

[17] Vladareanu R. Update in obstetrics and gynecology. Maedica (Buchar). 2011;**6**(1):66-67

[18] Tudorache S, Iliescu DG, Turcu A, Florea M, Dragusin R, Novac L, Cernea N, Cernea D. First trimester anomaly scan—The last redoubt won: Open Spina bifida. Donald School Journal of Ultrasound in Obstetrics and Gynecology. 2015;**9**(1):80-90

[19] Nicolaides KH. Screening for fetal aneuploidies at 11 to 13 weeks. Prenatal Diagnosis. 2011;**31**:7-15

[20] Burada F, Sosoi S, Iliescu D, Ioana M, Cernea D, Tudorache S. A rare occurrence of three consecutive autosomal trisomic pregnancies in a couple without offspring. Clinical and Experimental Obstetrics & Gynecology. 2016;**43**(2):287-290

[21] Sosoi S, Streata I, Tudorache S, Burada F, Siminel M, Cernea N, Ioana M, Iliescu DG, Mixich F. Prenatal and postnatal findings in a 10.6 Mb interstitial deletion at 10p11.22-p12.31. Journal of Human Genetics. 2015;**60**(4):183-185

[22] Calin FD, Ciobanu AM, Dimitriu MCT, Pacu I, Banacu M, Popescu I, Tarcomnicu IM, Ceauşu Z, Socea B, Paunica-Paunea G, Furau CG, Furau GO, Bacalbaşa N, Gheorghiu D, Ionescu CA. Edwards' syndrome diagnosis-between first trimester screening and ultrasound minor markers. Archives of the Balkan Medical Union. 2016;**51**(3):445-450

[23] Volpe P, Ubaldo P, Volpe N, Campobasso G, De Robertis V, Tempesta A, Volpe G, Rembouskos G. Fetal cardiac evaluation at 11-14 weeks by experienced obstetricians in a low-risk population. Prenatal Diagnosis. 2011;**31**:1054-1061

[24] Tudorache S, Cara M, Iliescu DG, Novac L, Cernea N. First trimester two- and four-dimensional cardiac scan—intra and interobserver agreement. Ultrasound in Obstetrics & Gynecology. 2013;**42**(6):659-668

[25] Becker R, Wegner RD. Detailed screening for fetal anomalies and cardiac defects at the 11-13-week scan. Ultrasound in Obstetrics & Gynecology. 2006;**27**:613-618

[26] Chaoui R, Benoit B, Heling KS, Kagan KO, Pietzsch V, Sarut Lopez A, Tekesin I, Karl K. Prospective detection of open spina bifida at 11-13 weeks by assessing intracranial translucency and posterior brain. Ultrasound in Obstetrics & Gynecology. 2011;**38**:722-726

[27] Egle D, Strobl I, Weiskopf-Schwendinger V, Grubinger E, Kraxner F, Mutz-Dehbalaie IS, Strasak A, Scheier M. Appearance of the fetal posterior fossa at 11+3 to 13+6 gestational weeks on transabdominal ultrasound examination. Ultrasound in Obstetrics & Gynecology. 2011;**38**:620-624

[28] Lachmann R, Picciarelli G, Moratalla J, Greene N, Nicolaides KH. Frontomaxillary facial angle in fetuses with spina bifida at 11-13 weeks' gestation. Ultrasound in Obstetrics & Gynecology. 2010;**36**:268-271. DOI: 10.1002/uog.7718

[29] Loureiro T, Ushakov F, Montenegro N, Gielchinsky Y, Nicolaides KH. Cerebral ventricular system in fetuses with open spina bifida at 11-13 weeks' gestation. Ultrasound in Obstetrics & Gynecology. 2012;**39**:620-624. DOI: 10.1002/uog.11079

[30] Volpe P, Contro E, Fanelli T, Muto B, Pilu G, Gentile M. Appearance of fetal posterior fossa at 11-14 weeks in fetuses with Dandy-Walker malformation or chromosomal anomalies. Ultrasound in Obstetrics & Gynecology. 2016;**47**(6):720-725

[31] Lachmann R, Sinkovskaya E, Abuhamad A. Posterior brain in fetuses with Dandy-Walker malformation with complete agenesis of the cerebellar vermis at 11-13 weeks: A pilot study. Prenatal Diagnosis. 2012;**32**:765-769

[32] Lee MY, Won HS, Hyunetal MK. One case of increased intracranial translucency during the first trimester associated with the Dandy-Walker variant. Prenatal Diagnosis. 2012;**32**:602-603

[33] Lafouge A, Gorincour G, Desbriere R, Quarello E. Prenatal diagnosis of Blake's pouch cyst following first-trimester observation of enlarged intracranial translucency. Ultrasound in Obstetrics & Gynecology. 2012;**40**:479-480

[34] Gandolfi Colleoni G, Contro E, Carletti A, Ghi T, Campobasso G, Rembouskos G, Volpe G, Pilu G, Volpe P. Prenatal diagnosis and outcome of fetal posterior fossa fluid collections. Ultrasound in Obstetrics & Gynecology. 2012;**39**:625-631

[35] Volpe P, Contro E, De Musso F, Ghi T, Farina A, Tempesta A, Volpe G, Rizzo N, Pilu G. Brainstem-vermis and brainstem-tentorium angles allow accurate categorization of fetal upward rotation of cerebellar vermis. Ultrasound in Obstetrics & Gynecology. 2012;**39**:632-635

[36] Tudorache S, Stiolica Turcu A, Iliescu DG, Florea M, Dragusin R, Cernea D. Modelling isolated spina bifida screening performance using axial and sagittal views of the brain and spine anatomy at the 11-13 week scan. Ultrasound in Obstetrics & Gynecology. 2015;**46**(S1):67

[37] Mangione R, Dhombres F, Lelong N, Amat S, Atoub F, Friszer S, Khoshnood B, Jouannic J-M. Screening for fetal spina bifida at the 11-13-week scan using three anatomical features of the posterior brain. Ultrasound in Obstetrics & Gynecology. 2013;**42**:416-420. DOI: 10.1002/uog.12463

[38] Ushakov F, Fernandez M, Lesmes Heredia C, Pandya P. OP06.08: "Crash sign": Displacement and deformation of mesencephalon against occipital bone in the diagnosis of spina bifida at 11-13 weeks. Ultrasound in Obstetrics & Gynecology. 2014;**44**:80. DOI: 10.1002/uog.13693

[39] Chen FC, Gerhardt J, Entezami M, Chaoui R, Henrich W. Detection of Spina bifida by first trimester screening—Results of the prospective multicenter berlin IT-study. Ultraschall in der Medizin. 2017;**38**(2):151-157

[40] Karl K, Benoit B, Entezami M, Heling KS, Chaoui R. Small biparietal diameter in fetuses with spina bifida on 11-13-week and mid-gestation ultrasound. Ultrasound in Obstetrics & Gynecology. 2012;**40**:140-144. DOI: 10.1002/uog.11175

[41] Simon EG, Arthuis CJ, Haddad G, Bertrand P, Perrotin F. A biparietal/transverse abdominal diameter (BPD/TAD) ratio ≤1: A potential hint for open spina bifida at 11-13 weeks scan. Ultrasound in Obstetrics & Gynecology. Mar 2015;**45**(3):267-272. DOI: 10.1002/uog.13406

[42] Malinger G, Ben-Sira L, Lev D, Ben-Aroya Z, Kidron D, Lerman-Sagie T. Fetal brain imaging: A comparison between magnetic resonance imaging and dedicated neurosonography. Ultrasound in Obstetrics & Gynecology. 2004;**23**(4):333-340

[43] Pugash D, Hendson G, Dunham CP, Dewar K, Money DM, Prayer D. Sonographic assessment of normal and abnormal patterns of fetal cerebral lamination. Ultrasound in Obstetrics & Gynecology. 2012;**40**(6):642-651

[44] Blondiaux E, Sileo C, Nahama-Allouche C, Moutard ML, Gelot A, Jouannic JM, Ducou le Pointe H, Garel C. Periventricular nodular heterotopia on prenatal ultrasound and magnetic resonance imaging. Ultrasound in Obstetrics & Gynecology. 2013;**42**(2):149-155

[45] Howe DT, Rankin J, Draper ES. Schizencephaly prevalence, prenatal diagnosis and clues to etiology: A register-based study. Ultrasound in Obstetrics & Gynecology. 2012;**39**(1):75-82

[46] Tonni G, Pattacini P, Bonasoni MP, Araujo Júnior E. Prenatal diagnosis of lissencephaly type 2 using three-dimensional ultrasound and fetal MRI: Case report and review of the literature. Revista Brasileira de Ginecologia e Obstetrícia. 2016;**38**(4):201-206

[47] Lacalm A, Nadaud B, Massoud M, Putoux A, Gaucherand P, Guibaud L. Prenatal diagnosis of cobblestone lissencephaly associated with Walker-Warburg syndrome based on a specific sonographic pattern. Ultrasound in Obstetrics & Gynecology. 2016;**47**(1):117-122

[48] Guibaud L, Lacalm A. Diagnostic imaging tools to elucidate decreased cephalic biometry and fetal microcephaly: A systematic analysis of the central nervous system. Ultrasound in Obstetrics & Gynecology. 2016;**48**(1):16-25

[49] Leibovitz Z, Daniel-Spiegel E, Malinger G, Tamarkin M, Gindes L, Schreiber L, Ben-Sira L, Lev D, Shapiro I, Bakry H, Weizman B, Zreik A, Egenburg S, Arad A, Tepper R, Kidron D, Lerman-Sagie T. Prediction of microcephaly at birth using three reference ranges for fetal head circumference: Can we improve prenatal diagnosis? Ultrasound in Obstetrics & Gynecology. 2016;**47**(5):586-592

[50] Vinurel N, Van Nieuwenhuyse A, Cagneaux M, Garel C, Quarello E, Brasseur M, Picone O, Ferry M, Gaucherand P, des Portes V, Guibaud L. Distortion of the anterior part of the interhemispheric fissure: Significance and implications for prenatal diagnosis. Ultrasound in Obstetrics & Gynecology. 2014;**43**(3):346-352

[51] Chibueze EC, Parsons AJQ, Lopes KDS, Yo T, Swa T, Nagata C, Horita N, Morisaki N, Balogun OO, Dagvadorj A, Ota E, Mori R, Oladapo OT. Diagnostic accuracy of ultrasound scanning for prenatal microcephaly in the context of Zika virus infection: A systematic review and meta-analysis. Scientific Reports. 2017;**7**(1):2310

[52] Biran-Gol Y, Malinger G, Cohen H, Davidovitch M, Lev D, Lerman-Sagie T, Schweiger A. Developmental outcome of isolated fetal macrocephaly. Ultrasound in Obstetrics & Gynecology. 2010;**36**(2):147-153

[53] Grande M, Arigita M, Borobio V, Jimenez JM, Fernandez S, Borrell A. First-trimester detection of structural abnormalities and the role of aneuploidy markers. Ultrasound in Obstetrics & Gynecology. 2012;**39**(2):157-163

[54] Chaoui R, Heling KS, Thiel G, Karl K. Agnathia-otocephaly with holoprosencephaly on prenatal three-dimensional ultrasound. Ultrasound in Obstetrics & Gynecology. 2011;**37**(6):745-748

[55] Malinger G, Lev D, Kidron D, Heredia F, Hershkovitz R, Lerman-Sagie T. Differential diagnosis in fetuses with absent septum pellucidum. Ultrasound in Obstetrics & Gynecology. 2005;**25**(1):42-49

[56] Blin G, Rabbé A, Mandelbrot L. Prenatal diagnosis of lobar holoprosencephaly using color Doppler: Three cases with the anterior cerebral artery crawling under the skull. Ultrasound in Obstetrics & Gynecology. 2004;**24**(4):476-478

[57] Muresan D, Popa R, Stamatian F, Rotar IC. The use of modern ultrasound tridimensional techniques for the evaluation of fetal cerebral midline structures—A practical approach. Medical Ultrasonography. 2015;**17**(2):235-240

[58] Shen O, Gelot AB, Moutard ML, Jouannic JM, Sela HY, Garel C. Abnormal shape of the cavum septi pellucidi: An indirect sign of partial agenesis of the corpus callosum. Ultrasound in Obstetrics & Gynecology. 2015;**46**(5):595-599

[59] Viñals F, Correa F, Gonçalves-Pereira PM. Anterior and posterior complexes: A step towards improving neurosonographic screening of midline and cortical anomalies. Ultrasound in Obstetrics & Gynecology. 2015;**46**(5):585-594

[60] Cagneaux M, Lacalm A, Huissoud C, Allias F, Ville D, Massardier J, Guibaud L. Agenesis of the corpus callosum with interhemispheric cyst, associated with aberrant cortical sulci and without underlying cortical dysplasia. Ultrasound in Obstetrics & Gynecology. 2013;**42**(5):603-605

[61] Cagneaux M, Guibaud L. From cavum septi pellucidi to anterior complex: How to improve detection of midline cerebral abnormalities. Ultrasound in Obstetrics & Gynecology. 2013;**42**(4):485-486

[62] Paladini D, Pastore G, Cavallaro A, Massaro M, Nappi C. Agenesis of the fetal corpus callosum: Sonographic signs change with advancing gestational age. Ultrasound in Obstetrics & Gynecology. 2013;**42**(6):687-690

[63] Pugash D, Langlois S, Power P, Demos M. Absent cavum with intact septum pellucidum and corpus callosum may indicate midline brain abnormalities. Ultrasound in Obstetrics & Gynecology. 2013;**41**(3):343-344

[64] Santo S, D'Antonio F, Homfray T, Rich P, Pilu G, Bhide A, Thilaganathan B, Papageorghiou AT. Counseling in fetal medicine: Agenesis of the corpus callosum. Ultrasound in Obstetrics & Gynecology. 2012;**40**(5):513-521

[65] Lerman-Sagie T, Ben-Sira L, Achiron R, Schreiber L, Hermann G, Lev D, Kidron D, Malinger G. Thick fetal corpus callosum: An ominous sign? Ultrasound in Obstetrics & Gynecology. 2009;**34**(1):55-61

[66] Shinar S, Har-Toov J, Lerman-Sagie T, Malinger G. Thick corpus callosum in the second trimester can be transient and is of uncertain significance. Ultrasound in Obstetrics & Gynecology. 2016;**48**(4):452-457

[67] Malinger G, Lev D, Oren M, Lerman-Sagie T. Non-visualization of the cavum septi pellucidi is not synonymous with agenesis of the corpus callosum. Ultrasound in Obstetrics & Gynecology. 2012;**40**(2):165-170

[68] Li Y, Estroff JA, Khwaja O, Mehta TS, Poussaint TY, Robson CD, Feldman HA, Ware J, Levine D. Callosal dysgenesis in fetuses with ventriculomegaly: Levels of agreement between imaging modalities and postnatal outcome. Ultrasound in Obstetrics & Gynecology. 2012;**40**(5):522-529

[69] D'Antonio F, Khalil A, Garel C, Pilu G, Rizzo G, Lerman-Sagie T, Bhide A, Thilaganathan B, Manzoli L, Papageorghiou AT. Systematic review and meta-analysis of isolated posterior fossa malformations on prenatal ultrasound imaging (part 1): Nomenclature, diagnostic accuracy and associated anomalies. Ultrasound in Obstetrics & Gynecology. 2016;**47**(6):690-697

[70] D'Antonio F, Khalil A, Garel C, Pilu G, Rizzo G, Lerman-Sagie T, Bhide A, Thilaganathan B, Manzoli L, Papageorghiou AT. Systematic review and meta-analysis of isolated posterior fossa malformations on prenatal imaging (part 2): Neurodevelopmental outcome. Ultrasound in Obstetrics & Gynecology. 2016;**48**(1):28-37

[71] Meagher SE, Walker SP, Choong S. Mid-trimester fetal subdural hemorrhage: Prenatal diagnosis. Ultrasound in Obstetrics & Gynecology. 2002;**20**(3):296-298

[72] Elchalal U, Yagel S, Gomori JM, Porat S, Beni-Adani L, Yanai N, Nadjari M. Fetal intracranial hemorrhage (fetal stroke): Does grade matter? Ultrasound in Obstetrics & Gynecology. 2005;**26**(3):233-243

[73] Vergani P, Strobelt N, Locatelli A, Paterlini G, Tagliabue P, Parravicini E, Ghidini A. Clinical significance of fetal intracranial hemorrhage. American Journal of Obstetrics and Gynecology. 1996;**175**:536-543

[74] Malinger G, Lerman-Sagie T, Watemberg N, Rotmensch S, Lev D, Glezerman M. A normal second-trimester ultrasound does not exclude intracranial structural pathology. Ultrasound in Obstetrics & Gynecology. 2002;**20**:51-56

[75] Ghi T, Simonazzi G, Perolo A, Savelli L, Sandri F, Bernardi B, Santini D, Bovicelli L, Pilu G. Outcome of antenatally diagnosed intracranial hemorrhage: Case series and review of the literature. Ultrasound in Obstetrics & Gynecology. 2003;**22**:121-130

[76] Aziz NA, Peeters-Scholte CM, de Bruine FT, Klumper FJ, Adama van Scheltema PN, Lopriore E, Steggerda SJ. Fetal cerebellar hemorrhage: Three cases with postnatal follow-up. Ultrasound in Obstetrics & Gynecology. 2016;**47**(6):785-786

[77] Garel C, Rosenblatt J, Moutard ML, Heron D, Gelot A, Gonzales M, Miné E, Jouannic JM. Fetal intracerebral hemorrhage and COL4A1 mutation: Promise and uncertainty. Ultrasound in Obstetrics & Gynecology. 2013;**41**(2):228-230

[78] Cruz-Martinez R, Tenorio V, Padilla N, Crispi F, Figueras F, Gratacos E. Risk of ultrasound-detected neonatal brain abnormalities in intrauterine growth-restricted fetuses born between 28 and 34 weeks' gestation: Relationship with gestational age at birth and fetal Doppler parameters. Ultrasound in Obstetrics & Gynecology. 2015;**46**(4):452-459

[79] Buca D, Pagani G, Rizzo G, Familiari A, Flacco ME, Manzoli L, Liberati M, Fanfani F, Scambia G, D'Antonio F. Outcome of monochorionic twin pregnancy with selective intrauterine growth restriction according to umbilical artery Doppler flow pattern of smaller twin: Systematic review and meta-analysis. Ultrasound in Obstetrics & Gynecology. 2017;**50**(5):559-568

[80] Herghelegiu D, Ionescu CA, Pacu I, Bohiltea R, Herghelegiu C, Vladareanu S. Antenatal diagnosis and prognostic factors of aneurysmal malformation of the vein of Galen: A case report and literature review. Medicine (Baltimore). 2017;**96**(30):e7483

[81] Cecchetto G, Milanese L, Giordano R, Viero A, Suma V, Manara R. Looking at the missing brain: Hydranencephaly case series and literature review. Pediatric Neurology. 2013;**48**(2):152-158

[82] Scher MS, Belfar H, Martin J, Painter MJ. Destructive brain lesions of presumed fetal onset: Antepartum causes of cerebral palsy. Pediatrics. 1991;**88**(5):898-906

[83] Pretorius DH, Russ PD, Rumack CM, Manco-Johnson ML. Diagnosis of brain neuropathology in utero. Neuroradiology. 1986;**28**(5-6):386-397

[84] Desvignes F, Beaufrère AM, Biard M, Déchelotte P, Laurichesse-Delmas H, Lemery D, Gallot D. Prenatal diagnosis of cerebral tumors and differential diagnosis. Journal de Gynécologie, Obstétrique et Biologie de la Reproduction. 2013;**42**(3):290-296

[85] Levine D, Jani JC, Castro-Aragon I, Cannie M. How does imaging of congenital Zika compare with imaging of other TORCH infections? Radiology. 2017;**285**(3):744-761

[86] Panigrahy A, Wisnowski JL, Furtado A, Lepore N, Paquette L, Bluml S. Neuroimaging biomarkers of preterm brain injury: Toward developing the preterm connectome. Pediatric Radiology. 2012;**42**(Suppl 1):S33-S61

[87] Madan N, Grant PE. New directions in clinical imaging of cortical dysplasias. Epilepsia. 2009;**50**(Suppl. 9):9-18

[88] Palmini A, Najm I, Avanzini G, Babb T, Guerrini R, Foldvary-Schaefer N, Jackson G, L_ders HO, Prayson R, Spreafico R, Vinters HV. Terminology and classification of the cortical dysplasias. Neurology. 2004;**62**(6 suppl 3):S2-S8

8

Congenital Anomalies in Human Embryos

Shiori Nakano, Haruyuki Makishima and
Shigehito Yamada

Abstract

Morphogenesis mainly occurs during embryonic stage, and congenital anomalies also occur at that time. The Kyoto Collection, one of the largest collections of human embryos, including a lot of those with congenital anomalies, is significantly helpful for analyzing embryonic growth. From the collection, normal and abnormal embryos have been selectively presented in this chapter. Recently developed imaging technology enabled three-dimensional (3D) imaging of embryos and fetuses in high resolution. The devices available for embryonic and fetal imaging and the results obtained therefrom are introduced in this chapter. In addition, new strategies for diagnosing congenital anomalies, such as autopsy imaging and genetic analyses, are discussed.

Keywords: human embryo, congenital anomalies, three-dimensional (3D) imaging, genetic analyses, autopsy imaging

1. Introduction

Congenital anomalies occur during the embryonic period, in which morphogenesis happens. The Kyoto Collection, one of the largest collections of human embryos, consists of over 40,000 human embryos and fetuses, including a large number of embryos with anomalies. Here we introduce embryonic cases with congenital anomalies, supplemented with valuable pictures, and discuss about the diagnoses of these anomalies at an early embryonic age using new 3D imaging modalities.

2. Normal development of human embryos

2.1. Staging of human embryonic development

Carnegie stage 13: Four limb buds and optic vesicle appear

32 days after fertilization

CRL (crown-rump length): 5 mm

At this stage, two upper and two lower limb buds become visible. The optic vesicle can be easily recognized and the lens placode begins to differentiate. Although more than 30 pairs of somites have formed by this time, the number of somites becomes increasingly difficult to determine and therefore will no longer be used for staging henceforth.

Carnegie stage 14: Lens pit and optic cup appear

34 days after fertilization

CRL: 6 mm

The lens pit begins to invaginate into the optic cup, although its closure remains incomplete at this stage. On the other hand, the optic vesicle emerges from the endolymphatic appendage and becomes easy to define. The upper limb buds elongate and taper, while the cephalic and cervical flexures become prominent in terms of the internal features; the future cerebral hemispheres and cerebellar plates differentiate at this point. The dorsal and ventral pancreatic buds have become noticeable, along with the development of the ureteric bud, which acquires a metanephrogenic blastema.

Carnegie stage 15: Lens vesicles are covered by surface ectoderm, nasal pit and hand plates form

34 days after fertilization

CRL: 8 mm

Lens vesicles have closed and are covered by the surface ectoderm at this time, while the nasal plate invaginates forming a nasal pit. At this stage, auricular hillocks arise, and hand plates begin to form. In the meantime, the foramen secundum develops in the heart while the lung buds begin to branch into lobar buds. The primary urogenital sinus completes its formation by the end of this stage.

Carnegie stage 16: Nasal pit faces ventrally, retinal pigment becomes visible, foot plates emerge

38 days after fertilization

CRL: 10 mm

Nasal pits deepen and start to face ventrally, while the retinal pigment becomes externally visible. In the meantime, hand plates become distinct and foot plates start to emerge. Furthermore, the nasolacrimal groove forms between the frontal and maxillary processes.

Carnegie stage 17: Nasofrontal groove become distinct, and finger rays exhibited

40 days after fertilization

CRL: 11 mm

In comparison with the previous stage, the auricular hillocks and nasofrontal (nasolacrimal) grooves have become more distinct, and the trunk has straightened. The hand plates have come to exhibit conspicuous digital rays, and the foot has acquired a rounded digital plate by this stage.

Carnegie stage 18: Elbows become discernible, toe rays appear, and eyelid folds appear

42 days after fertilization

CRL: 13 mm

The body shape has become more cuboidal by this time. Both cervical and lumbar flexures are denoted, the elbows are discernible and interdigital notches begin to appear in the hand plates. Toe rays are observed in the foot plate. As for the facial features, eyelid folds start appearing, and the auricular hillocks transform into specific parts of the external ear. Furthermore, ossification may begin in some skeletal structures.

Carnegie stage 19: Trunk elongation and straightening

44 days after fertilization

CRL: 16 mm

The trunk begins its elongation and straightening. Simultaneously, the eyes and external ears become distinct. As a result of the growing size of the brain, the eyes get positioned in the front part of the face. The upper and lower limbs are approximately parallel, with preaxial borders being cranial, and postaxial borders caudal. Moreover, intestines have developed and parts of them can be observed in normal umbilical cord (physiological umbilical hernia).

Carnegie stage 20: Longer upper limb bends at elbow

46 days after fertilization

CRL: 19 mm

The angle of the cervical flexure becomes smaller, and the head is directed upwards. Vascular plexus starts to appear in the superficial tissues of the head. Meanwhile, the coiled intestine finishes its development. Spontaneous movements are recognized at this stage. The upper limbs have increased in length at this time, and it is flexed at the elbows and hand joints. Fingers can be observed over the chest, in a slight curve.

Carnegie stage 21: Fingers grow longer, hands approach each other

48 days after fertilization

CRL: 21 mm

The head becomes round and the superficial vascular plexus spreads to surround the head. Meanwhile, the tail becomes rudimentary. At this time, the hands are slightly flexed at the wrists and are placed closely over the cardiac prominence.

Carnegie stage 22: Eyelids and external ears develop

50 days after fertilization

CRL: 23 mm

The vascular plexus of the head becomes more distinct at this stage. The eyelids start to thicken and encroach into the eyes. In the meantime, the tragus and antitragus of the external ear assume a more definite form, as the external ear repositions higher on the head. The tail is about to disappear.

Carnegie stage 23: The end of embryonic period

52 days after fertilization

CRL: 30 mm

At this stage, the head would be observed with a more rounded appearance and the trunk with a more mature shape. The eyelids and ear auricles have become conspicuous, the limbs have increased in length, and the forearms have ascended toward the level or higher than that of the shoulders. Meanwhile, the vascular plexus approaches the vertex of the head. Although external sex differences are not yet apparent, the external genitalia have developed relatively well by this time. The tail is no longer observed at this stage.

2.2. Facial development

At Carnegie stage 12, three pharyngeal arches appear. The first pharyngeal arch emerges from the maxillary and mandibular prominences (stage 13, **Figure 1**), which will later constitute the lateral and caudal boundaries of the stomodeum (i.e., primitive oral cavity), respectively.

The sides and front of the neck arise from the second pharyngeal arch, also known as the hyoid arch. Meanwhile, the frontonasal prominence (FNP) grows and covers the ventral part of the forebrain (stage 13), which will eventually form the forehead (frontal part of the FNP) and the primordial mouth and nose (nasal part of the FNP).

By the end of the fourth developmental week, nasal placodes (thickening of surface ectoderm that later becomes peripheral neural tissue) develop on the frontolateral aspects of the FNP (stage 13). The mesenchyme swells around the nasal placodes, which leads to the formation of medial and lateral nasal prominences (stage 16). The maxillary prominence merges with the medial nasal prominence, leading to its fusion. The fused medial nasal prominence will not only form the primary palate (stage 16–18), but also the midline of the nose and that of the upper lip.

The nasolacrimal groove divides the lateral nasal prominence from the maxillary prominence (observed in stages 16, 17).

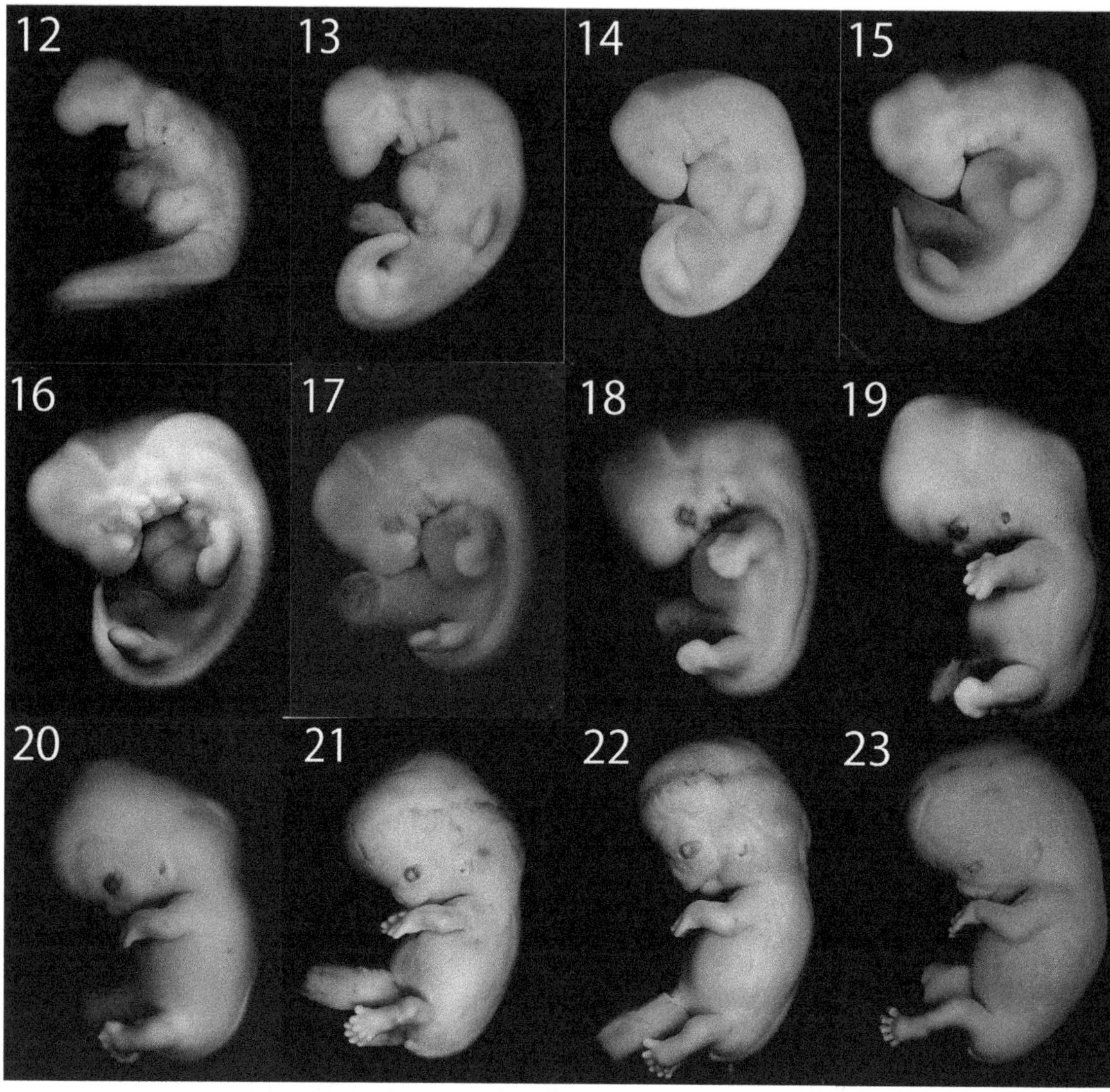

Figure 1. Development of human embryo, Carnegie stages 12–23.

During the fifth developmental week, primordial ear auricles form around the first pharyngeal groove, at the interface between the mandibular prominences and the hyoid arches (stage 16). While the auricle emerges from the auricular hillocks, the external acoustic meatus arises from the first pharyngeal groove. At an early stage of ear development, the external ears are located in the neck region, which then start to ascend toward the level of the eyes on either side of the head, simultaneously with the development of the mandible.

The maxillary and lateral nasal prominences fuse with the nasolacrimal groove during the sixth developmental week, which enables the nose and cheek to be continuous (stage 18).

The seventh developmental week is marked by the fusion of the medial nasal prominence and the maxillary and lateral nasal prominences (stage 19~). Merging of the maxillary and medial nasal prominences creates continuity between the upper jaw and lip, leading to the segregation of the nasal cavity and oral cavity.

2.3. Development of upper and lower extremities

The embryonic development of the limbs [1] is illustrated here using computer graphics [2].

- Carnegie stage 12: The upper limb buds begin to develop.
- Carnegie stage 13: The upper limb buds gain more definite shape, while the lower limb buds start to develop.
- Carnegie stage 14: The upper limb buds grow and taper toward the tip, which forms the hand plate later on. In the upper limbs, innervation and blood supply begin at this stage. The development of the lower limb buds is delayed with respect to the upper limb buds.
- Carnegie stage 15: The hand plates in the upper limb buds have become distinct. In the lower limbs, the rostral half is rounded, whereas the caudal half is tapered. At this stage, innervation begins in the lower limb buds as well.
- Carnegie stage 16: The hand plates form a central part, a carpal part, and a digital flange, whereas the lower limb buds form a femoral part, a crural part, and a foot plate.
- Carnegie stage 17: Finger rays can be recognized in the hand plate while the rim of the hand plate becomes crenated due to the appearance of individual fingers in some advanced specimens. The lower limb buds have increased in size and a rounded digital plate is set off from the crurotarsal region.
- Carnegie stage 18: The upper limbs have lengthened and are slightly bent at the elbow. Finger rays are distinct. As for the lower limb bud, toe rays begin to appear, although the notch on the rim of the foot plate is still incomplete.
- Carnegie stage 19: The upper limbs rotate medially, as if to hold the chest. Apoptoses occur in the mesenchymal tissues of interdigital areas to create deeper interdigital notches in the foot plate. Toe rays become prominent, and knees and ankles become noticeable.
- Carnegie stage 20: The upper limbs are bent at the elbow and hand joints, resulting in a pronated position. Meanwhile, the lower limbs are also bent at the knee joints, and notches are present between the toe rays in the foot plate.
- Carnegie stage 21: Elbows and knees become distinct in the upper and lower limbs, respectively. Hands are crossed over the chest. Meanwhile, fingers grow longer and distal phalangeal portions become slightly swollen, indicating the beginning of palmar pads. The feet are approaching each other at this stage.
- Carnegie stage 22: Hands get larger in front of the body and fingers elongate, which may clasp over with those of the other hand. Although toe digits are still webbed, feet approach closer.
- Carnegie stage 23: The upper and lower limbs have lengthened, well formed, and bent at joints. Fingers grow longer and toes cease to be webbed; all the digits are separate and distinct.

3. Representative external anomalies of human embryos

3.1. CNS anomalies

3.1.1. Holoprosencephaly (HPE)

Holoprosencephaly (HPE) refers to an anomaly in which the differentiation of the prosencephalon from the neural tube is defective, thus leading to malformations of the forebrain, midface, and occasionally limbs. It can be recognized as early as CS12 or 13.

HPE can be classified into three categories, depending on the degree of defect in the development of prosencephalon: alobar holoprosencephaly, semi lobar holoprosencephaly, and lobar prosencephaly.

Alobar holoprosencephaly is the most severe, which usually associates with cyclopia, ethmocephaly, and cebocephaly. Cyclopia (**Figure 2A**) is characterized by a single eye centered in the middle of the face, caused by the fusion of the optic vesicles due to the lack of midline tissue. The name of this malformation is derived from the cyclops (or cyclopes) in Greek mythology, first mentioned in Homer's epic poem, "Odyssey" in the seventh century B.C. There are cases of cyclopia with incomplete fusion of optic vesicles, but either with the nose absent or complicated further with proboscis located above the orbit [3]. The cyclopic embryo presented in **Figure 1** shows single eye in the center of the face, without any nose.

Ethmocephaly is morphologically similar to cyclopia, except that both eyes exist with distinct orbits, although marked by hypotelorism, with proboscis located between the eyes (**Figure 2B**) [4]. Cebocephaly is also an anomaly that exhibits hypotelorism in the two distinct orbits, characterized by a single nostril, occasionally complicated by cleft lip and/or palate [5].

HPE is one of the most common lethal congenital anomalies that occur at embryonic stages, and the prevalence rate is approximately 1/250. However, most of them cannot survive to develop into a fetus, which makes it a rare anomaly in newborns (1/10,000–20,000) [6].

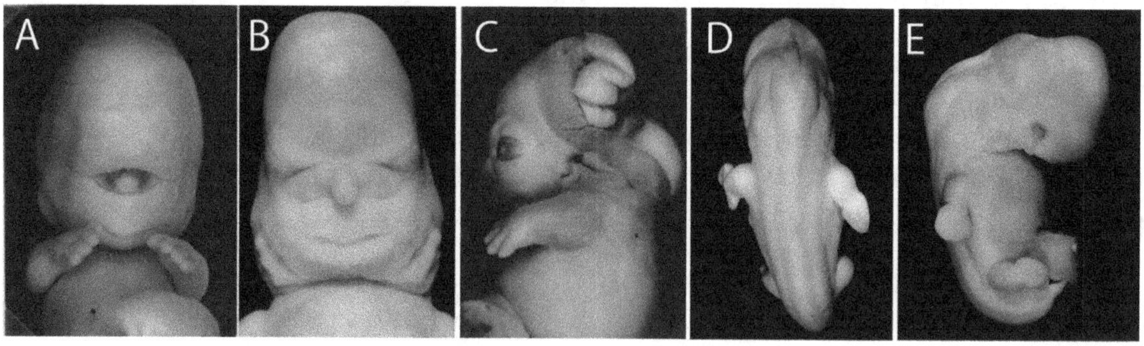

Figure 2. Congenital anomalies in the CNS. (A) Embryo presenting cyclopia, (B) embryo presenting ethmocephaly, with proboscis located between the eyes, (C) exencephaly presenting the opening in the neural tube, (D) spina bifida occulta observed dorsally, and (E) spina bifida occulta observed laterally.

Although it is yet to be proved, four main genes: *SHH*, *ZIC2*, *SIX3*, and *TGIF* are suggested to be associated with the onset of HPE, along with the aneuploidies in chromosomes 13 and 18. The existence of environmental factors is suggested, and a strong positive correlation of the occurrence with maternal age is noted [7, 8].

3.1.2. *Exencephaly*

The morphological characteristics of exencephaly are exposed brain and absence of the skull and scalp. This condition arises due to the failure to close the cephalic part of the neural tube, occasionally due to the overgrowth of neural tissue [9] (**Figure 2C**). Exencephaly can be recognized at CS 12 at the earliest, much ahead of the stage at which the development of the neural tube completes.

Neural tube defects such as exencephaly, anencephaly, and spina bifida are extremely common lethal congenital anomalies, and the prevalence rate is approximately 1/1000 [10]; most of these survive for only few hours, and all cases lead to death within a few days. Although the understanding remains unclear, folic acid deficiency is a suggested factor for anencephaly, along with the *MTHFD 1* gene, which is significant in folate metabolism [11].

3.1.3. *Spina bifida*

Spina bifida is the most common congenital anomaly of the CNS, resulting from the incomplete fusion of the vertebrae and hence exposure of the spinal cord. It can be classified into spina bifida occulta (**Figure 2D** and **E**), and spina bifida cystica (or aperta), which can be further classified into meningocele, meningomyelocele, and myelocele [12]. Spina bifida occulta is the mildest form, caused by the malformation of the bony arch that extends caudally, failing to fuse dorsal midline to the spinal cord. The spinal cord itself, however, is unaffected, extended caudally, or duplicated at the end, with no neurological damage. The bone defect is covered by skin, although sometimes patches of hair or pigment may be observed in the area covering the defect. **Figures 4** and **5** exhibit an embryo with spina bifida occulta, presenting a malformation of the bony arch, with neither neurological defect nor swelling.

On the other hand, spina bifida cystica refers to the malformation of the bony arch as well as the neural tube that has failed to close. Meningocele has a fluid-containing cystic swelling, emerging from a defect in the vertebral arch; the spinal cord is completely confined to the spinal canal, but may exhibit myelodysplasia.

Meningomyelocele and myelocele also refer to cystic swellings emerging dorsally through a vertebral arch, although the spinal cord (located inside the sac) bears its fundus. Myelocele is different from meningomyelocele in the following aspects: spinal cord is exposed to the external surface, often in the lumbosacral area; neutral folds stay flat, and will not elevate; not only the spinal cord, the brain is also often malformed, which may result in hydrocephalus, Chiari 2 malformation, and other defects [13].

Although spina bifida can be recognized as early as CS 12, it becomes observable earliest by CS 13, when the closure of the neural tube is supposed to be completed.

A significant amount of folic acid is known to prevent spina bifida; early postnatal treatments, including the closure of the spinal lesion within 48 h after birth, and medical management are essential for life henceforth [14].

3.2. Facial anomalies

3.2.1. Cleft lip

Cleft lip, often accompanied by cleft palate, is the most common congenital facial anomaly that causes dental defects, yielding defective speech and feeding disorders, and sometimes ear infections. The prevalence among the Asian and American Indian populations is as high as 1 in 500 births, which is relatively higher than that in European-derived or African-derived population, where prevalence rates are at approximately 1/1000 and 1/2500, respectively [15].

The morphological characteristic of cleft lip is the opening in the upper lip to the roof of the mouth, either located in the center (median cleft lip) (**Figure 3A**) or left and/or right side (bilateral/ unilateral cleft lip, **Figure 3B** and **C**), as a result of failed fusion of various processes. Median cleft lip is the rarest, and is commonly associated with mental retardation, attributed to the loss of midline structures.

As for lateral cleft lips, 80% of them are unilateral, out of which 70% are left-sided. Cleft lip can be recognized as early as CS 18, and is considered a multifactorial defect, involving genetic factors, environmental factors, teratogens, and maternal conditions. There are over 50 recognized syndromes that include this malformation, often caused by mutant genes [16].

The occurrence of isolated cleft lip is higher in male, whereas the occurrence of isolated cleft palate is higher in females [15].

3.2.2. Micrognathia

Micrognathia is a facial malformation characterized by an underdeveloped and receded mandible, thus presenting a bird-like face, as shown in **Figure 3D**. It was first mentioned in the clay tablets of ancient Babylonia, back in 1700 BC [17].

Micrognathia is often a part of chromosomal disorder; it is commonly seen in patients of Pierre Robin syndrome, and is associated with trisomy 13, trisomy18, Treacher-Collins syndrome,

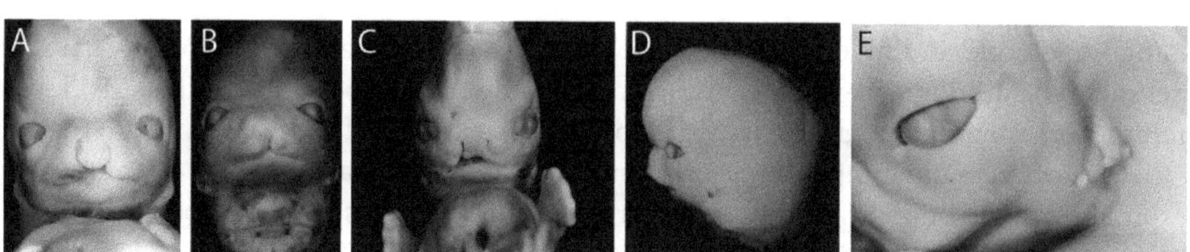

Figure 3. Congenital anomalies of face. (A) Median cleft lip, (B) left-sided unilateral cleft lip, (C) right-sided unilateral cleft lip, (D) micrognathia from lateral view, and (E) malformed pinna.

and Nager syndrome [18, 19]. The frequency of Pierre Robin syndrome is approximately 1 in 8500–14,000 births [20], and signs of micrognathia can be observed as early as CS 18. It is also often observed in association with cleft palate [21].

Because of the undersized jaw, most have feeding problems after birth and some may have major respiratory obstruction; however, there is usually no need for surgical treatment, since it can be naturally corrected through growth. However, micrognathia leads to dental anomalies, breathing problems, and tongue growth defect, which need close observation.

3.2.3. Low-set ears

Low-set ears refer to malpositioned auricles, located anteriorly to the horizontal line drawn at the level of the inner canthus (**Figure 3E**).The size of a low-set ear is usually smaller compared to that in a normally developed embryo, with the angle posteriorly rotated [22]. Low-set ears accompany a variety of congenital chromosomal defects, including Turner's syndrome, Patau syndrome, Treacher-Collins syndrome, trisomy 18, trisomy 13, Cri du chat syndrome, and Down syndrome. It is often observed along with micrognathia.

Malformations of the ear can be recognized earliest at CS 18, although it can be estimated earlier by observing the auricle hill. Besides being low-set, the auricles may also be malformed as shown in **Figure 3E**.

3.3. Anomalies of extremities

3.3.1. Polydactyly

Polydactyly is a limb malformation, characterized by additional digit(s) in the limbs (**Figure 4A** and **B**) [23]. There can be preaxial, postaxial, or median polydactyly, corresponding to extra digits on the radial or tibial sides, ulnar or fibular sides, or in between medial fingers, respectively [24].This malformation is more likely to occur in the hands than in the feet, and can be estimated at CS 16 [25]. The prevalence varies across races, and occurs more frequently in the right hand than the left, among the Japanese. Its frequency on each finger may also vary; the highest to lowest being in the order: thumb, little finger, middle finger, ring finger, and index finger in the Japanese population. Polydactyly is one of the most common hereditary malformations of the extremities, with *GLI3* and *SHH* genes being responsible [23]. The extra digit in preaxial polydactyly may be surgically treated after 8–12 months of birth, whereas that of postaxial polydactyly is dissected shortly after birth.

3.3.2. Cleft hand/foot

Cleft hand/foot, also known as split-hand/split-foot malformation (SHFM), is a limb malformation that imparts an appearance resembling a lobster claw, due to the absence of the middle finger and hence an abnormal gap between the second and fourth metacarpal bones and soft tissues (**Figure 4C**). The two fingers on either side of the cleft in a cleft hand may be fused, which would make it appear as if there are only two digits on one hand [26].

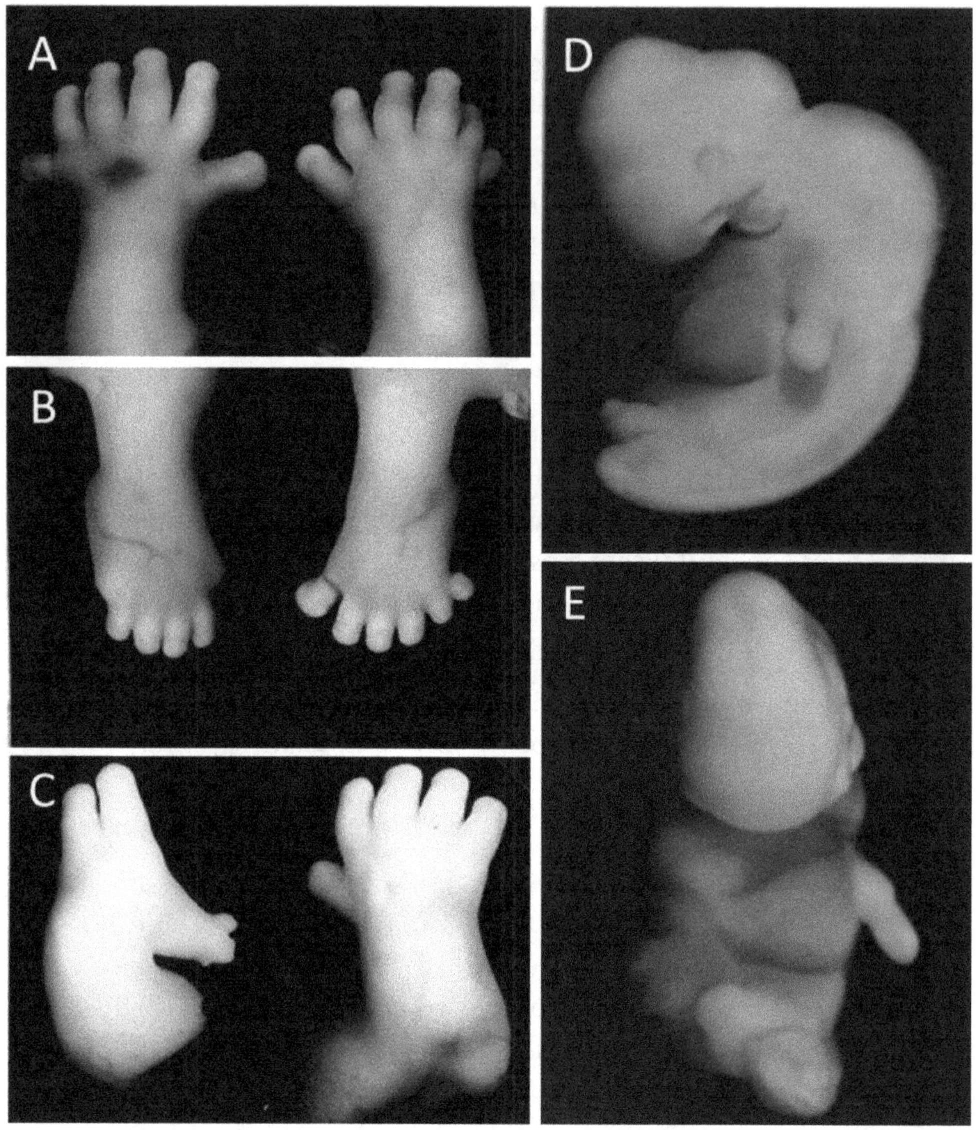

Figure 4. Congenital anomalies of extremities. (A) Polydactyly in hand; (B) polydactyly in foot; (C) cleft hand, (D) sirenomelia, lateral view, and (E) sirenomelia, anterior view.

Ectrodactyly, or oligodactyly refers to malformations of the limb such that there are digits less than 5, arising from either ulnar deficiency, radial deficiency, or median deficiency (cleft hand/foot) [26]. **Figure 4C** shows a cleft hand with four distinct digits, with a large gap in between the second and third digits, presenting a lobster claw-like feature.

The inheritance of cleft hand is autosomal dominant, caused by deletions or mutations in autosomes such as chromosomes 2, 3, 7, and 10. For example, the deletion in chromosome 2 results not only in ectrodactyly, but also in microcephaly, micrognathia, low-set ears, and mental retardation. Although ectrodactyly is often associated with other malformations, a single family has been reported for the inheritance of isolated ectrodactyly resulting from X-linked recessive inheritance [26]. Another well-known syndrome that is associated with this malformation is EEC (ectrodactyly-ectodermal dysplasia-cleft lip/palate) syndrome, which comprises of ectodermal dysplasia and cleft lip, occasionally accompanied by cleft palate, due to an autosomal dominant inheritance [27]. The prevalence is approximately 1 in 18,000 births [28], and can be observed as early as CS 18, at the stage when the finger rays develop. There is no difference between females and males in terms of occurrence, and surgical treatment is scheduled when the child is 1 or 2 years old.

3.3.3. Sirenomelia (meromelia)

Sirenomelia, named after the Sirens (half-bird women in Greek mythology, often confused with mermaids), is an extremely rare form of malformation of the extremities, characterized by fused lower limbs hence resembling "merpeople" (**Figure 4D** and **E**) [29]. With only a single umbilical artery and vein, it is difficult for both limbs to develop, resulting in the formation of fused lower limbs [30]. It can be divided into categories, based on the degree of development of the lower limb: sympus apus, sympus monopus, and sympus dipus, referring to absence of feet, short feet, and a pair of feet, respectively. Anomalies of the kidneys, large intestine, and external genitalia are commonly observed as accompanying complications.

This lethal congenital anomaly begins to show up at CS 13, with an occurrence rate of approximately 1.5–4.2 in 100,000 births, with more than half of them born dead. All such cases lead to death within 5 h after birth [29]. Although chromosomal aneuploidy is not associated, maternal diabetes mellitus and monozygotic twins are considered important factors for increasing the risk of sirenomelia [31].

4. Diagnostic strategies for human embryos

4.1. Imaging modalities

4.1.1. Ultrasound

Fetal ultrasound was developed as A-mode in the late 1950s, then modified to B-mode in the 1970s, followed by real-time imaging in the 1980s, and 3D imaging [32, 33] in the 1990s. Currently, ultrasonography is applied throughout pregnancy. Transvaginal ultrasonography is useful for examining the gestational sac at approximately 5 weeks, the yolk sac at 5.5 weeks, flickering cardiac motion at 6 weeks, etc. Embryos and early fetuses within 12 weeks of gestation are usually examined by transvaginal ultrasonography, whereas those beyond 12 weeks of gestation are examined by transabdominal ultrasonography. Ultrasonography is used for examining embryos and fetuses for several reasons, one of them is to determine the gestational age and estimate the fetal weight. A formula for estimating the latter was first suggested in the late 1970s [34]. Since then, a number of formulae have been proposed and accepted [35–39], while new formulae for the estimation have also been frequently promoted [40, 41]. Another purpose of ultrasonography is to detect (and occasionally, to assess) congenital fetal anomalies. Ultrasonography was first applied to evaluate anencephaly [42], but now it is able to detect a wide range of anomalies. The definition of optimal fetal anatomy survey has been published as guidelines by the International Society of Ultrasound in Obstetrics and Gynecology (ISUOG) [43] for performing effective screening of morphological anomalies. Meanwhile, studies conducted during the 1980s–1990s made it clear that soft markers in ultrasonography indicate an elevated risk of chromosomal abnormalities [44–46], even though they may not be directly harmful by themselves. Soft markers combined with maternal serum is capable of detecting aneuploidy with high precision [47].

4.1.2. Magnetic resonance imaging

Magnetic resonance (MR) microscopy refers to MR imaging for screening small samples. It is significantly useful for the 3D measurement of chemically fixed human embryos, due to the large amount of mobile or NMR responsive protons existing in the preservation fluid (formalin) [48]. Being a non-invasive and non-destructive imaging process, it has been applied to a number of animal models for understanding developmental embryology [49–52]. MR imaging provides highly beneficial features [50, 53, 54], reaching a resolution of 40 μm/pixel or higher when scanning a sample for an extended amount of time. Superconducting magnets with field strength of 1.0–9.4 T [52, 54, 55] have been used for describing human embryo using MR imaging. **Figure 5C–D** and **E–F** is obtained with MR microscopes equipped with 7.0 and 2.34 T magnets, respectively.

4.1.3. Phase-contrast X-ray computed tomography

X-rays are electromagnetic waves with characteristic amplitude and phase. When X-rays penetrate a sample, its amplitude decreases and the phase gets shifted. Conventional X-ray imaging (radiography) is based on absorption contrast (i.e. amplitude imaging) and represented by the internal mass density distribution within the sample (**Figure 6A** and **B**). Unfortunately, only sensitivity to X-ray distribution is not enough for a detailed analysis of the samples containing biological soft tissues such as embryos, unless it is either combined with contrast agents or performed at higher X-ray doses. Another way of solving this issue is by exploiting the phase information of X-rays. Since lighter elements, such as hydrogen, carbon, nitrogen, and oxygen are 1000 times more sensitive to phase-shift compared to the actual absorption [56], they can be used to detect the phase-shift. To that end, it is essential to convert the phase shift into a change in X-ray intensity, which can be measured easily by current-detecting devices. Conversion methods, such as interferometry and diffractometry, are applied for the

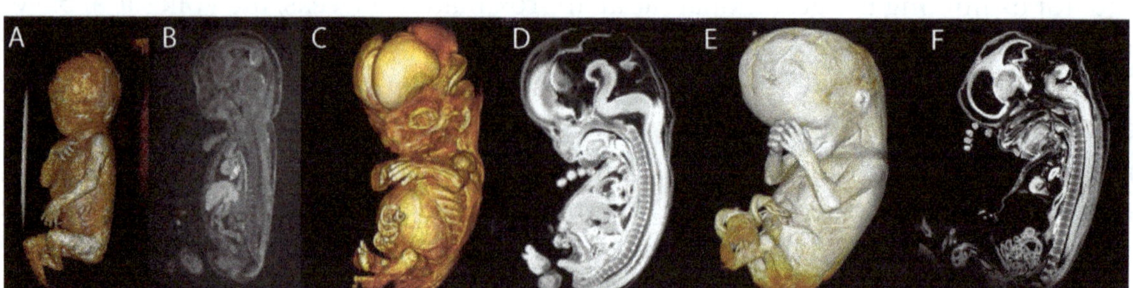

Figure 5. The results of MRI from several imaging devices. A, B: 2.34 T super parallel MRM (MR microscope), developed by Prof. Kose et al. in the University of Tsukuba. C, D: Pre-clinical MRI (Bruker BioSpin, 7 T) in the Human Health Sciences, Kyoto University Graduate School of Medicine, Japan. E, F: Clinical MRI (Siemens Magnetom, 3 T) in the Kyoto University Hospital, Japan.

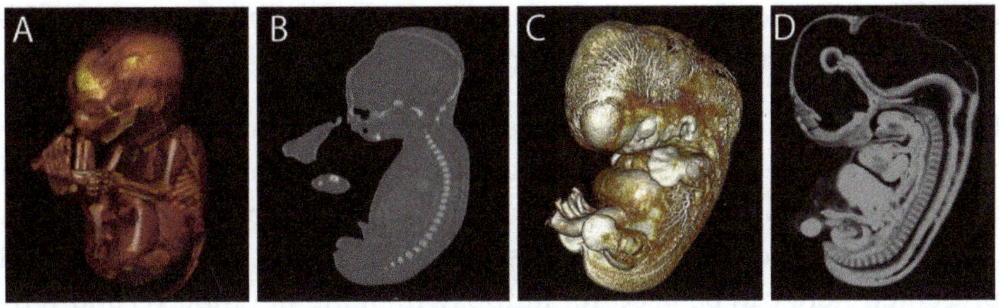

Figure 6. The results of X-ray CT. A, B: Clinical CT (Toshiba Alexion) in the Laboratory of Physical Anthropology, Graduate School of Science, Kyoto University, Japan. C, D: Phase contrast CT, Photon Factory of the KEK (High Energy Accelerator Research Organization) in Tsukuba, Japan. A, C: Surface reconstruction and B, D: midsagittal section.

generation of 2D and 3D images using synchrotron radiations from appropriate devices [57, 58]. An image of a human embryo at CS 17, obtained by applying a two-crystal X-ray interferometer [59], is displayed in **Figure 6C** and **D**.

4.2. New strategies for diagnosis of congenital anomalies

4.2.1. Autopsy imaging of human embryos and fetuses

Additional imaging modalities can be applied for dead embryos and fetuses. Classically, solid reconstruction and fine drawing were primarily the approaches used; the first 3D morphological imaging technique was the wax plate technique, using serial histological sections of human embryos, which was developed by Born [60]. Recently, the 3D reconstruction of serial sections has been carried out by using computer graphic methods, which has made the 3D reconstruction much easier and quicker than before. The 2D image stacks generated from serial sections have a high resolution, although the issues of section registration and distortion remain unsolved. A solution to this problem is a novel imaging modality for the generation of high-resolution 3D reconstructed images [61], which uses episcopic fluorescence image capture (EFIC). In EFIC imaging, tissue autofluorescence is used to image the block face prior to cutting any section. Although the samples are sliced and some lost during the procedure, the optical resolution of EFIC is reported to reach approximately 5–6 μm [62].

MRI is a useful imaging modality, not only for living prenatal embryos and fetuses, but also for dead embryos and fetuses in autopsy imaging. Despite the longer time taken to capture images, the higher resolution is definitely an advantage; the time required for a high-resolution imaging ranges from several hours to days. MR devices should be selected depending on the sample size; specially, MR microscopy, clinical MRI, and experimental MRI are suitable for small-sized embryos, larger fetuses, and embryos/fetuses with an intermediate size, respectively [39] (**Figure 5**) [2, 63, 64].

X-ray imaging is also used for dead embryos and fetuses. Since there is no need to consider the impact of radiation exposure on the tissue, longer time may be devoted to capture high resolution images. Conventional (absorption-contrast) X-ray CT (cCT) is used for fetal skeletal imaging (**Figure 6A** and **B**). Phase-contrast X-ray CT (pCT) is another method of X-ray imaging [40]. Since X-rays are electromagnetic waves, phase-contrast X-ray imaging is capable of recording the phase-shift of X-rays while passing through the samples and reconstructing

2D/3D images of the samples in combination with CT. An embryo or an early fetus, mostly composed of soft tissue, is suitable for pCT imaging (**Figure 6C** and **D**).

Ultrasonography of living embryos and fetuses is very commonly performed nowadays, and many malformations can be diagnosed during the early prenatal period. In the cases of pregnancy termination, not all the aborted fetuses are dissected and pathologically diagnosed, due to technical difficulties associated with the dissection of small fetuses. However, the imaging modalities presented here can be used for autopsy imaging of embryos and fetuses, regardless of their size. If any clue to the fetal anomaly (that might have led to the abortion) could be identified by using these imaging modalities, supplemented by appropriate genetic tests, then a final accurate diagnosis can be obtained. Based on the final diagnosis, parents would be provided with sufficient detailing of their lost pregnancy, which would enable them to receive a genetic counseling prior to the next pregnancy.

The imaging modalities described in this section are summarized in **Figures 5** and **6**. The appropriate modalities for imaging dead embryos or fetuses should be used depending on the stage of pregnancy.

4.2.2. Genetic analysis of the human embryo and fetus

Amniotic fluid, chorionic villi, and umbilical cord blood are used for genetic analyses of human embryos and fetuses. Recently, a new approach for prenatal testing was proposed in the name of noninvasive prenatal testing (NIPT) that uses DNA fragments derived from maternal villus cells to determine the genetic information of the fetus. In comparison to maternal serum analysis, NIPT has considerably higher sensitivity and specificity for aneuploidy [65]. However, due to the infrequent derivation of cell-free DNA (cfDNA) from multiple sources such as in placental mosaicism, maternal conditions including cancer, or fetal and/or maternal copy number variation (CNV) [66], NIPT has a risk of predicting false-positive and false-negative results.

The cell samples obtained from amniotic fluid and chorionic villi may be used for both screening and diagnostic tests. Traditional karyotype analysis is the most commonly used method to examine cells, obtained from chorionic villus sampling (CVS) and amniocentesis (AC), for the diagnosis of aneuploidies and large rearrangements. The diagnostic accuracy of traditional karyotype analysis is higher than 99% for aneuploidy and for chromosomal abnormalities larger than 5–10 Mb [67]. On the other hand, fluorescence in-situ hybridization (FISH) analysis can detect specific chromosomes or chromosomal regions by using fluorescently labeled probes. The turnaround for FISH results (usually within 2 days) is faster than that of conventional karyotyping results (7–14 days, including the cell culture period). Due to the existence of false-positive and false-negative reports, FISH [68–70] is considered as a mere screening test, although still commonly used to screen chromosomes 13, 18, 21, X, and Y. Therefore, clinical diagnosis using FISH results should be supplemented by other clinical and laboratory analyses such as abnormal ultrasonography, positive screening test using maternal serum and/or soft markers, confirmatory traditional metaphase chromosome analysis, or chromosomal microarray analysis (CMA).

CMA is capable of detecting small chromosomal aneuploidies that cannot otherwise be identified by conventional karyotyping [71]. Since CMA can be performed without cell or tissue culture, the results can be obtained within 3–7 days. Since CMA can also be carried out with nonviable cells, which are not suitable for conventional karyotyping analysis, this technique [71] is applicable to the cases of fetal death or stillbirth. CMA can identify almost all the abnormalities, except for balanced translocations and triploidy. While the results of conventional karyotyping in the detection of structural abnormalities, seen in prenatal ultrasonography, did not show anything notable, approximately 6% of the fetuses were identified for chromosomal defects by CMA [72, 73]; CMA qualifies as the primary test, in case a structural abnormality is detected by fetal ultrasonography, as also recommended by the American Congress of Obstetricians and Gynecologists (ACOG) [71].

In the late 1980s, single gene disorders were diagnosed from fetal samples. Although only prenatal diagnosis of β-thalassemia was done using amplified fetal DNA [74] initially, the number of diagnosable diseases or genes has increased thereafter. Thus, the whole-genome sequencing, using DNA samples from amniotic fluid, was developed in the next-generation sequencing (NGS) era [75]. In fact, whole-exome sequencing (WES) is more appropriate for fetal genetic analysis, because the coding exons in WES contain 85% of disease-coding mutations, even though it accounts for only 2% of the entire genome. Prenatal WES, using fetal blood samples, has been performed since 2013 [76]. Meanwhile, massive parallel sequencing (MPS) using NGS opened the way to NIPT [77] in the late 2000s. Now, NIPT is widely used for aneuploidy, throughout the world [78], and even some of the fetal single-gene diseases can be detected using cell-free fetal DNA (cffDNA) obtained from maternal blood [79, 80]. Although the number of diseases detectable using cffDNA is gradually increasing, cffDNA analyses are merely screening tests and would not replace the diagnostic testing, as mentioned in the guidelines of professional societies [81–86].

Author details

Shiori Nakano, Haruyuki Makishima and Shigehito Yamada*

*Address all correspondence to: shyamada@cac.med.kyoto-u.ac.jp

Congenital Anomaly Research Center, Kyoto University Graduate School of Medicine, Japan

References

[1] O'Rahilly R, Gardner E. The timing and sequence of events in the development of the limbs in the human embryo. Anatomy and Embryology (Berlin). 1975;**148**:1-23

[2] Yamada S, Uwabe C, Nakatsu-Komatsu T, Minekura Y, Iwakura M, Motoki T, Nishimiya K, Iiyama M, Kakusho K, Minoh M, Mizuta S, Matsuda T, Matsuda Y, Haishi T, Kose K, Fujii S, Shiota K. Graphic and movie illustrations of human prenatal development and their application to embryological education based on the human embryo specimens in the Kyoto collection. Developmental Dynamics. 2006;**235**:468-477

[3] Sharma D, Yadav J, Garg E. Cyclopia syndrome. BMJ Case Reports. 2014;**2014**:bcr2014 203535

[4] Goldstein I, Weissman A, Brill-Zamir R, Laevsky I, Drugan A. Ethmocephaly caused by de novo translocation 18;21—Prenatal diagnosis. Prenatal Diagnosis. 2003;**23**:788-790

[5] Callahan J, Harmon C, John Aleshire J, Hickey B, Jones B. Alobar holoprosencephaly with cebocephaly. Journal of Diagnostic Medical Sonography. 2017;**33**:39-42

[6] Matsunaga E, Shiota K. Holoprosencephaly in human embryos: Epidemiologic studies of 150 cases. Teratology. 1977;**16**:261-272

[7] Dubourg C, Bendavid C, Pasquier L, Henry C, Odent S, David V. Holoprosencephaly. Orphanet Journal of Rare Diseases. 2007;**2**:8

[8] Yamada S, Uwabe C, Fujii S, Shiota K. Phenotypic variability in human embryonic holoprosencephaly in the Kyoto collection. Birth Defects Research. Part A, Clinical and Molecular Teratology. 2004;**70**:495-508

[9] Tonni G, Azzoni D, Pizzi C, Bonasoni MP, Cavalli P, Pattacini P, Ventura A. Anencephaly-exencephaly sequence and congenital diaphragmatic hernia in a fetus with 46, XX karyotype: Early prenatal diagnosis, necropsy, and maternal folate pathway genetic analysis. Fetal and Pediatric Pathology. 2010;**29**:69-80

[10] Katsanis N. Ciliary proteins and exencephaly. Nature Genetics. 2006;**38**:135-136

[11] Copp AJ, Stanier P, Greene ND. Neural tube defects: Recent advances, unsolved questions, and controversies. Lancet Neurology. 2013;**12**:799-810

[12] Cameron AH. The spinal cord lesion in spina bifida cystica. Lancet. 1956;**271**:171-174

[13] Detrait ER, George TM, Etchevers HC, Gilbert JR, Vekemans M, Speer MC. Human neural tube defects: Developmental biology, epidemiology, and genetics. Neurotoxicology and Teratology. 2005;**27**:515-524

[14] Mitchell LE, Adzick NS, Melchionne J, Pasquariello PS, Sutton LN, Whitehead AS. Spina bifida. Lancet. 2004;**364**:1885-1895

[15] Dixon MJ, Marazita ML, Beaty TH, Murray JC. Cleft lip and palate: Understanding genetic and environmental influences. Nature Reviews. Genetics. 2011;**12**:167-178

[16] Fraser FC. The genetics of cleft lip and cleft palate. American Journal of Human Genetics. 1970;**22**:336-352

[17] Poswillo D. The aetiology and surgery of cleft palate with micrognathia. Annals of the Royal College of Surgeons of England. 1968;**43**:61-88

[18] Bromley B, Benacerraf BR. Fetal micrognathia: Associated anomalies and outcome. Journal of Ultrasound in Medicine. 1994;**13**:529-533

[19] Mandell DL, Yellon RF, Bradley JP, Izadi K, Gordon CB. Mandibular distraction for micrognathia and severe upper airway obstruction. Archives of Otolaryngology—Head & Neck Surgery. 2004;**130**:344-348

[20] Collins B, Powitzky R, Robledo C, Rose C, Glade R. Airway management in pierre robin sequence: Patterns of practice. The Cleft Palate-Craniofacial Journal. 2014;**51**:283-289

[21] Price KE, Haddad Y, Fakhouri WD. Analysis of the relationship between micrognathia and cleft palate: A systematic review. The Cleft Palate-Craniofacial Journal. 2016;**53**:e34-e44

[22] Sivan Y, Merlob P, Reisner SH. Assessment of ear length and low set ears in newborn infants. Journal of Medical Genetics. 1983;**20**:213-215

[23] Malik S. Polydactyly: Phenotypes, genetics and classification. Clinical Genetics. 2014; **85**:203-212

[24] Nishimura H, Okamoto N. Sequential Atlas of Human Congenital Malformations: Observations of Embryos, Fetuses, and Newborns. Tokyo: Igaku Shoin; 1976. p. 242

[25] Yasuda M. Pathogenesis of preaxial polydactyly of the hand in human embryos. Journal of Embryology and Experimental Morphology. 1975;**33**:745-756

[26] Ogino T. Clinical features and teratogenic mechanisms of congenital absence of digits. Development, Growth & Differentiation. 2007;**49**:523-531

[27] Ianakiev P, Kilpatrick MW, Toudjarska I, Basel D, Beighton P, Tsipouras P. Split-hand/split-foot malformation is caused by mutations in the p63 gene on 3q27. American Journal of Human Genetics. 2000;**67**:59-66

[28] van Bokhoven H, Hamel BC, Bamshad M, Sangiorgi E, Gurrieri F, Duijf PH, Vanmolkot KR, van Beusekom E, van Beersum SE, Celli J, Merkx GF, Tenconi R, Fryns JP, Verloes A, Newbury-Ecob RA, Raas-Rotschild A, Majewski F, Beemer FA, Janecke A, Chitayat D, Crisponi G, Kayserili H, Yates JR, Neri G, Brunner HG. p63 Gene mutations in eec syndrome, limb-mammary syndrome, and isolated split hand-split foot malformation suggest a genotype-phenotype correlation. American Journal of Human Genetics. 2001;**69**:481-492

[29] Banerjee A, Faridi MM, Banerjee TK, Mandal RN, Aggarwal A. Sirenomelia. Indian Journal of Pediatrics. 2003;**70**:589-591

[30] Ito T, Nowatari M, Kitsunezaki M, Isaka M, Kenmochi M, Ishii M. A case of sirenomelia sequence: The mermaid syndrome. The Kitasato Medical Journal. 2009;**39**:171-174

[31] Monteagudo A, Mayberry P, Rebarber A, Paidas M, Timor-Tritsch IE. Sirenomelia sequence: First-trimester diagnosis with both two- and three-dimensional sonography. Journal of Ultrasound in Medicine. 2002;**21**:915-920

[32] Benson CB, Doubilet PM. The history of imaging in obstetrics. Radiology. 2014;**273**:S92-S110

[33] Rao R, Platt LD. Ultrasound screening: Status of markers and efficacy of screening for structural abnormalities. Seminars in Perinatology. 2016;**40**:67-78

[34] Warsof SL, Gohari P, Berkowitz RL, Hobbins JC. The estimation of fetal weight by computer-assisted analysis. American Journal of Obstetrics and Gynecology. 1977;**128**:881-892

[35] Aoki M. Fetal weight calculation; Osaka University method. In: Ciba Y, editor. Ultrasound in Obstetrics and Gynaecology. Kyoto: Kinpoudo; 1990. pp. 95-107

[36] Hadlock FP, Harrist RB, Sharman RS, Deter RL, Park SK. Estimation of fetal weight with the use of head, body, and femur measurements—A prospective study. American Journal of Obstetrics and Gynecology. 1985;**151**:333-337

[37] Shepard MJ, Richards VA, Berkowitz RL, Warsof SL, Hobbins JC. An evaluation of two equations for predicting fetal weight by ultrasound. American Journal of Obstetrics and Gynecology. 1982;**142**:47-54

[38] Shinozuka N, Akamatsu N, Sato S, Kanzaki T, Takeuchi H, Natori M, Chiba Y, Okai T. Ellipse tracing fetal growth assessment using abdominal circumference: JSUM standardization committee for fetal measurements. Journal of Medical Ultrasound. 2000;**8**:87-94

[39] Shinozuka N, Okai T, Kohzuma S, Mukubo M, Shih CT, Maeda T, Kuwabara Y, Mizuno M. Formulas for fetal weight estimation by ultrasound measurements based on neonatal specific gravities and volumes. American Journal of Obstetrics and Gynecology. 1987;**157**:1140-1145

[40] Kalantari M, Negahdari A, Roknsharifi S, Qorbani M. A new formula for estimating fetal weight: The impression of biparietal diameter, abdominal circumference, mid-thigh soft tissue thickness and femoral length on birth weight. Iranian Journal of Reproductive Medicine. 2013;**11**:933-938

[41] Schild RL, Fell K, Fimmers R, Gembruch U, Hansmann M. A new formula for calculating weight in the fetus of < or = 1600 g. Ultrasound in Obstetrics & Gynecology. 2004;**24**:775-780

[42] Cunningham ME, Walls WJ. Ultrasound in the evaluation of anencephaly. Radiology. 1976;**118**:165-167

[43] Salomon LJ, Alfirevic Z, Berghella V, Bilardo C, Hernandez-Andrade E, Johnsen SL, Kalache K, Leung KY, Malinger G, Munoz H, Prefumo F, Toi A, Lee W, Committee ICS. Practice guidelines for performance of the routine mid-trimester fetal ultrasound scan. Ultrasound in Obstetrics & Gynecology. 2011;**37**:116-126

[44] Benacerraf BR, Frigoletto FD Jr, Cramer DW. Down syndrome: Sonographic sign for diagnosis in the second-trimester fetus. Radiology. 1987;**163**:811-813

[45] Benacerraf BR, Frigoletto FD Jr, Greene MF. Abnormal facial features and extremities in human trisomy syndromes: Prenatal US appearance. Radiology. 1986;**159**:243-246

[46] Benacerraf BR, Nadel A, Bromley B. Identification of second-trimester fetuses with autosomal trisomy by use of a sonographic scoring index. Radiology. 1994;**193**:135-140

[47] Dey M, Sharma S, Aggarwal S. Prenatal screening methods for aneuploidies. North American Journal of Medical Sciences. 2013;**5**:182-190

[48] Matsuda Y, Ono S, Otake Y, Handa S, Kose K, Haishi T, Yamada S, Uwabe C, Shiota K. Imaging of a large collection of human embryo using a super-parallel MR microscope. Magnetic Resonance in Medical Sciences. 2007;**6**:139-146

[49] Bone SN, Johnson GA, Thompson MB. Three-dimensional magnetic resonance microscopy of the developing chick embryo. Investigative Radiology. 1986;**21**:782-787

[50] Smith BR, Effmann EL, Johnson GA. MR microscopy of chick embryo vasculature. Journal of Magnetic Resonance Imaging. 1992;**2**:237-240

[51] Smith BR, Johnson GA, Groman EV, Linney E. Magnetic resonance microscopy of mouse embryos. Proceedings of the National Academy of Sciences of the United States of America. 1994;**91**:3530-3533

[52] Smith BR, Linney E, Huff DS, Johnson GA. Magnetic resonance microscopy of embryos. Computerized Medical Imaging and Graphics. 1996;**20**:483-490

[53] Effmann EL, Johnson GA, Smith BR, Talbott GA, Cofer G. Magnetic resonance microscopy of chick embryos in ovo. Teratology. 1988;**38**:59-65

[54] Haishi T, Uematsu T, Matsuda Y, Kose K. Development of a 1.0 T MR microscope using a Nd-Fe-B permanent magnet. Magnetic Resonance Imaging. 2001;**19**:875-880

[55] Smith BR. Visualizing human embryos. Scientific American. 1999;**280**:76-81

[56] Momose A, Fukuda J. Phase-contrast radiographs of nonstained rat cerebellar specimen. Medical Physics. 1995;**22**:375-379

[57] Becker P, Bonse U. The skew-symmetric two-crystal X-ray interferometer. Journal of Applied Crystallography. 1974;**7**:593-598

[58] Yoneyama A, Takeda T, Tsuchiya Y, Wu J, Thet Thet L, Koizumi A, Hyodo K, Itai Y. A phase-contrast X-ray imaging system—With a 60×30mm field of view—Based on a skew-symmetric two-crystal X-ray interferometer. Nuclear Instruments and Methods in Physics Research Section A: Accelerators, Spectrometers, Detectors and Associated Equipment. 2004;**523**:217-222

[59] Yoneyama A, Yamada S, Takeda T. Fine biomedical imaging using X-ray phase-sensitive technique. In: Gargiulo GD, McEwan A, editors. Advanced Biomedical Engineering. Rijeka: InTech; 2011. pp. 107-128

[60] Born G. Die Plattenmodelliermethode. Archiv für Mikroskopische Anatomie. 1883;**22**: 584-599

[61] Yamada S, Itoh H, Uwabe C, Fujihara S, Nishibori C, Wada M, Fujii S, Shiota K. Computerized three-dimensional analysis of the heart and great vessels in normal and holoprosencephalic human embryos. Anatomical Record (Hoboken). 2007;**290**:259-267

[62] Weninger WJ, Mohun T. Phenotyping transgenic embryos: A rapid 3-D screening method based on episcopic fluorescence image capturing. Nature Genetics. 2002;**30**:59-65

[63] Yamada S, Samtani RR, Lee ES, Lockett E, Uwabe C, Shiota K, Anderson SA, Lo CW. Developmental atlas of the early first trimester human embryo. Developmental Dynamics. 2010;**239**:1585-1595

[64] Yamaguchi Y, Miyazaki R, Kamatani M, Uwabe C, Makishima H, Nagai M, Katsube M, Yamamoto A, Imai H, Kose K, Togashi K, Yamada S. Three-dimensional models of the segmented human fetal brain generated by magnetic resonance imaging. Congenit Anom (Kyoto). 2017 May 11. DOI: 10.1111/cga.12229

[65] Palomaki GE, Deciu C, Kloza EM, Lambert-Messerlian GM, Haddow JE, Neveux LM, Ehrich M, van den Boom D, Bombard AT, Grody WW, Nelson SF, Canick JA. DNA sequencing of maternal plasma reliably identifies trisomy 18 and trisomy 13 as well as down syndrome: An international collaborative study. Genetics in Medicine 2012;**14**:296-305

[66] Snyder MW, Gammill HS, Shendure J. Copy-number variation and false positive results of prenatal screening. The New England Journal of Medicine. 2015;**373**:2585

[67] Jackson LG, Zachary JM, Fowler SE, Desnick RJ, Golbus MS, Ledbetter DH, Mahoney MJ, Pergament E, Simpson JL, Black S, et al. A randomized comparison of transcervical and transabdominal chorionic-villus sampling. The U.S. National Institute of Child Health and Human Development chorionic-villus sampling and amniocentesis study group. The New England Journal of Medicine. 1992;**327**:594-598

[68] Bryndorf T, Lundsteen C, Lamb A, Christensen B, Philip J. Rapid prenatal diagnosis of chromosome aneuploidies by interphase fluorescence in situ hybridization: A one-year clinical experience with high-risk and urgent fetal and postnatal samples. Acta Obstetricia et Gynecologica Scandinavica. 2000;**79**:8-14

[69] Tepperberg J, Pettenati MJ, Rao PN, Lese CM, Rita D, Wyandt H, Gersen S, White B, Schoonmaker MM. Prenatal diagnosis using interphase fluorescence in situ hybridization (FISH): 2-year multi-center retrospective study and review of the literature. Prenatal Diagnosis. 2001;**21**:293-301

[70] Toutain J, Epiney M, Begorre M, Dessuant H, Vandenbossche F, Horovitz J, Saura R. First-trimester prenatal diagnosis performed on pregnant women with fetal ultrasound abnormalities: The reliability of interphase fluorescence in situ hybridization (FISH) on mesenchymal core for the main aneuploidies. European Journal of Obstetrics, Gynecology, and Reproductive Biology. 2010;**149**:143-146

[71] American College of Obstetricians and Gynecologists Committee on Genetics. Committee opinion no. 581: The use of chromosomal microarray analysis in prenatal diagnosis. Obstetrics and Gynecology. 2013;**122**:1374-1377

[72] Aagaard-Tillery KM, Malone FD, Nyberg DA, Porter TF, Cuckle HS, Fuchs K, Sullivan L, Comstock CH, Saade GR, Eddleman K, Gross S, Dugoff L, Craigo SD, Timor-Tritsch IE, Carr SR, Wolfe HM, Bianchi DW, D'Alton ME, First and Second Trimester Evaluation of Risk Research Consortium. Role of second-trimester genetic sonography after Down syndrome screening. Obstetrics and Gynecology. 2009;**114**:1189-1196

[73] Baer RJ, Flessel MC, Jelliffe-Pawlowski LL, Goldman S, Hudgins L, Hull AD, Norton ME, Currier RJ. Detection rates for aneuploidy by first-trimester and sequential screening. Obstetrics and Gynecology. 2015;**126**:753-759

[74] Pirastu M, Ristaldi MS, Cao A. Prenatal diagnosis of beta thalassaemia based on restriction endonuclease analysis of amplified fetal DNA. Journal of Medical Genetics. 1989;**26**:363-367

[75] Talkowski ME, Ordulu Z, Pillalamarri V, Benson CB, Blumenthal I, Connolly S, Hanscom C, Hussain N, Pereira S, Picker J, Rosenfeld JA, Shaffer LG, Wilkins-Haug LE, Gusella JF, Morton CC. Clinical diagnosis by whole-genome sequencing of a prenatal sample. The New England Journal of Medicine. 2012;**367**:2226-2232

[76] Yang Y, Muzny DM, Reid JG, Bainbridge MN, Willis A, Ward PA, Braxton A, Beuten J, Xia F, Niu Z, Hardison M, Person R, Bekheirnia MR, Leduc MS, Kirby A, Pham P, Scull J, Wang M, Ding Y, Plon SE, Lupski JR, Beaudet AL, Gibbs RA, Eng CM. Clinical whole-exome sequencing for the diagnosis of mendelian disorders. The New England Journal of Medicine. 2013;**369**:1502-1511

[77] Chiu RW, Chan KC, Gao Y, Lau VY, Zheng W, Leung TY, Foo CH, Xie B, Tsui NB, Lun FM, Zee BC, Lau TK, Cantor CR, Lo YM. Noninvasive prenatal diagnosis of fetal chromosomal aneuploidy by massively parallel genomic sequencing of DNA in maternal plasma. Proceedings of the National Academy of Sciences of the United States of America. 2008;**105**:20458-20463

[78] Hui L, Bianchi DW. Recent advances in the prenatal interrogation of the human fetal genome. Trends in Genetics. 2013;**29**:84-91

[79] Lench N, Barrett A, Fielding S, McKay F, Hill M, Jenkins L, White H, Chitty LS. The clinical implementation of non-invasive prenatal diagnosis for single-gene disorders: Challenges and progress made. Prenatal Diagnosis. 2013;**33**:555-562

[80] Lewis C, Hill M, Chitty LS. Non-invasive prenatal diagnosis for single gene disorders: Experience of patients. Clinical Genetics. 2014;**85**:336-342

[81] Gregg AR, Gross SJ, Best RG, Monaghan KG, Bajaj K, Skotko BG, Thompson BH, Watson MS. ACMG statement on noninvasive prenatal screening for fetal aneuploidy. Genetics in Medicine. 2013;**15**:395-398

[82] Wilson KL, Czerwinski JL, Hoskovec JM, Noblin SJ, Sullivan CM, Harbison A, Campion MW, Devary K, Devers P, Singletary CN. NSGC practice guideline: Prenatal screening and diagnostic testing options for chromosome aneuploidy. Journal of Genetic Counseling. 2013;**22**:4-15

[83] Benn P, Borrell A, Chiu RW, Cuckle H, Dugoff L, Faas B, Gross S, Huang T, Johnson J, Maymon R, Norton M, Odibo A, Schielen P, Spencer K, Wright D, Yaron Y. Position statement from the chromosome abnormality screening committee on behalf of the Board of the International Society for Prenatal Diagnosis. Prenatal Diagnosis. 2015;**35**:725-734

[84] Gregg AR, Skotko BG, Benkendorf JL, Monaghan KG, Bajaj K, Best RG, Klugman S, Watson MS. Noninvasive prenatal screening for fetal aneuploidy, 2016 update: A position statement of the American College of Medical Genetics and Genomics. Genetics in Medicine. 2016;**18**:1056-1065

[85] Committee Opinion Summary No. 640: Cell-free DNA screening for fetal aneuploidy. Obstetrics and Gynecology. 2015;**126**:691-692

[86] Practice Bulletin No. 163 Summary: Screening for fetal aneuploidy. Obstetrics and Gynecology. 2016;**127**:979-981

9

Correlations between Ultrasound and Pathology in Fetal Ventricular System Anomalies

Tanya Kitova, Borislav Kitov, Denis Milkov and Aida Masmoudi

Abstract

A total of 113 cases of fetal hydrocephalus with a lethal outcome (FHLO) from the Embryo-Fetopathologic Clinic at the Center for Maternity and Neonatology, Tunis, Tunisia and Obstetrics and Gynecology Clinic at St. George EAD University Hospital, Plovdiv, Bulgaria were studied, 86 of which had syndrome malformations: neural tube defects (NTDs)—29.2%, chromosomal abnormalities—23.9%, skeletal dysplasias—9.8%, VACTERL association—5.3%, Dandy-Walker malformation—3.4%, Other—14.2%. Risk factors for FHLO are miscarriages (odds ratio (OR): 19.500; confidence interval (CI): 4.020-94.594), stillbirths (OR: 10.897; CI: 1.169-10.564) and previous birth of a malformative child (OR = 5.385; CI: 1.385–18.896). FHLO is significantly associated with a maternal age over 40 years and third degree consanguinity of the fetus (OR = 18.500; CI: 1.146–298.547). The trisomies in our study were 27 (23.9%) and are significantly associated with an age above 38 years and FHLO (OR = 13.689; CI: 3.952–52.122). In medical abortion, stillbirth, or neonatal death, a fetopathological study enriches our knowledge of malformations, complements and completes the ultrasound examination, modifies genetic counseling, and determines the medical behavior in subsequent pregnancies. Also, associated risk factors and fetopathological changes in FHLO must be studied to increase the ultrasound prenatal diagnosis success.

Keywords: congenital hydrocephalus, ultrasound, MRI, cerebral anomalies, risk factors

1. Introduction

Congenital hydrocephalus (CH) is a severe malformation which is often associated with other abnormalities. The prenatally diagnosed serious birth defects, especially those associated with a high risk of premature death, stillbirth, or neonatal death, are often referred to as "lethal," as it is assumed that their potential treatment will be unsuccessful, which is the basis for the decision for the interruption of pregnancy due to medical reasons [1, 2]. Depending on the clinical criteria used in the definition of the disease, its incidence varies from 1 to 32 per 10,000 live births [3]. An increase in the prenatal diagnosis of CH has been observed, whereas the incidence of stillbirths remains stable. The interruption of pregnancy due to medical reasons reduces by almost a half the rate of hydrocephalus in live births. Currently, prenatal ultrasound is able to visualize ventriculomegaly, which can be caused by a number of reasons. Knowledge of the risk factors associated with CH may increase the chances of an early prenatal ultrasound diagnosis. Animal experiments have found that a wide range of environmental factors can cause hydrocephalus. They include alcohol consumption, X-rays, infections, eating disorders, and exposure to chemicals during pregnancy [4]. It has been established that one gene (L1 of Xq28 encoded for L1CAM) is connected with CH in humans. Although X-linked CH has a frequency of about 2–7% of all cases, L1CAM is found in about 15% of sporadic cases [5]. L1CAM mutations are closely related to stenosis of the cerebral aqueduct, the major pathology causing hydrocephalus in these cases. Sipek et al., in their study of CH for the period 1961–2000 in the Czech Republic, found that a mother's age of over 37 years was statistically significantly related to CH, unlike the study by Van Landingham et al. [4, 6].

2. Aim of the study

To study the prenatally ultrasound diagnosed ventriculomegaly by fetopathological autopsy in fetuses, which ended in interruption of pregnancy due to medical reasons, stillbirth, or neonatal death, by searching associated with the congenital hydrocephalus isolated or syndromic malformations as well as the eventual risk factors for their occurrence.

3. Materials and methods

A total of 113 fetuses with CH were studied whose outcome was lethal. One hundred and three of them were received over a period of 3 years (2006–2009) and autopsied at the Embryo-Fetopathologic Clinic at the Center for Maternity and Neonatology, Tunis, Tunisia, out of a total of 21,316 births. Ten of the cases were from the Obstetrics and Gynecology Clinic at St. George EAD University Hospital, Plovdiv, Bulgaria, during the year 2016 out of a total of 2104 deliveries. The incidence of fetal hydrocephalus with a lethal outcome (FHLO) in both centers is almost identical—4.8 and 4.9 per 1000 births.

The fetuses are the result of interruption of pregnancy due to medical reasons, spontaneous abortions, and stillbirths. The maternal and fetal data were collected from the obstetric history, and a classical autopsy was performed immediately following the expulsion of the fetus, after authorization for macroscopic and microscopic examination. The autopsy includes observation, biometry of the fetus, and in situ examination of the body cavities. The examination of the brain was performed 6 months later, after conservation with 10% formalin. It began with biometrics, measurement of the biparietal and frontal-occipital diameters, and study of the relationship between ocular distance and eyelid length. After opening the cranial cavity, the meninx, brainstem, cerebellum, cerebral hemispheres, gyrification, and morphology were observed. The biometry of the brain—weight and bitemporal and fronto-occipital diameters of the encephalon, and weight and transverse diameter of the cerebellum—was also studied. The ventricular system was examined by horizontal or vertical hemispheric slices until the central part of the lateral ventricle was opened. The presence, shape, and thickness of corpus callosum were examined. With a linear meter, the ventricular width in the central part was measured. At a width of more than 10 mm, ventricular dilatation was diagnosed as hydrocephalus and at a diameter of over 15 mm—major hydrocephalus. In each study, material was taken for histological examination of the cerebral cortex, cerebellum, brainstem, choroid plexus, and cerebral meninx. SPSS version 19 was used for the interpretation of the data. A descriptive analysis and χ^2-analysis were used.

4. Results

- **Age structure of the mothers:** The age range of mothers carrying fetuses with FHLO was 21–43 years. Under 26 years of age were 24 mothers (22%), 27–35 were 64 (58%) and 36–50 years of age were 21 mothers (19.3%). The average age of the mothers was 29.5 ± 0.72.

- **Number of previous pregnancies of the mothers:** Most of the mothers carrying FHLO had one previous pregnancy (38.1%), followed by mothers with two previous pregnancies (19.5%). The average number of previous pregnancies is 2.50 ± 1.808, with a range of 1 to 5 pregnancies. There were no data for previous pregnancies for only 2.7% of the mothers.

- **Number of previous births of the mothers:** In the studied group, most of the mothers had one previous birth (36.6%), followed by mothers without previous births (31.3%). The average number of births is 1.24 ± 1.23, with a range of 0–5.

- **Blood group of the mothers:** Data were collected for the mothers' blood groups, but unfortunately there is no information for about 21% of the mothers carrying a fetus with FHLO of the studied group. It is noteworthy that most of the mothers were of blood group O(+) – 36 (32.0%), followed by A(+) – 23 (over 20.0%).

- **Consanguinity:** In our study, 27.4% of the marriages were consanguineous, with those of first degree being 15.4%, those of second degree 8.3%, and of third 3.7%.

5. Risk factors

In the present study, 80 of the pregnancies (70.7%) were without risk factors, and only 33 (29.3%) were under the influence of such. The risk factors were grouped into three categories: obstetric risk factors from past events, risk factors due to diseases of the mother, and exogenous risk factors.

1. **Obstetric risk factors.** This group includes spontaneous abortions—13 (11.5%), voluntary abortions—1 (0.9%), birth of a child with malformations—11 (9.8%), stillbirths—2 (1.8%), multifetal pregnancy—2 (1.8%), and multi-year sterility—4 (3.5%).
2. **Endogenous risk factors.** The risk factors from the mother include maternal age, hypertension—1 (0.9%), diabetes mellitus—2 (1.8%), bronchial asthma—2 (1.8%), thalassemia—2 (1.8%), and epilepsy—3 (2.7%).
3. **Exogenous risk factors.** Exogenous risk factors for the pregnancy include pregnancies carried in geographical areas near mines and underground mineral water deposits and consanguineous marriages. In our study, the pregnancies from geographic regions with mining and underwater mineral water deposits were 5 (4.4%). Supplementation with folic acid is mandatory in Tunisia and Bulgaria. There were no women without folic acid supplementation.

The term of pregnancy termination is presented in **Figure 1**. Most interrupted pregnancies are between the 20th and 24th gestational weeks. Six pregnancies were carried to birth.

Motives for pregnancy termination. Interruption of pregnancy due to medical reasons was performed in 87 cases (77%); spontaneous abortions were 13 (11.5%), and there was 1 voluntary abortion (0.9%). There were 2 live births (1.8%) and 2 stillbirths (1.8%). In eight of the cases (7%), there is no information on the motive for pregnancy interruption (**Figure 2**).

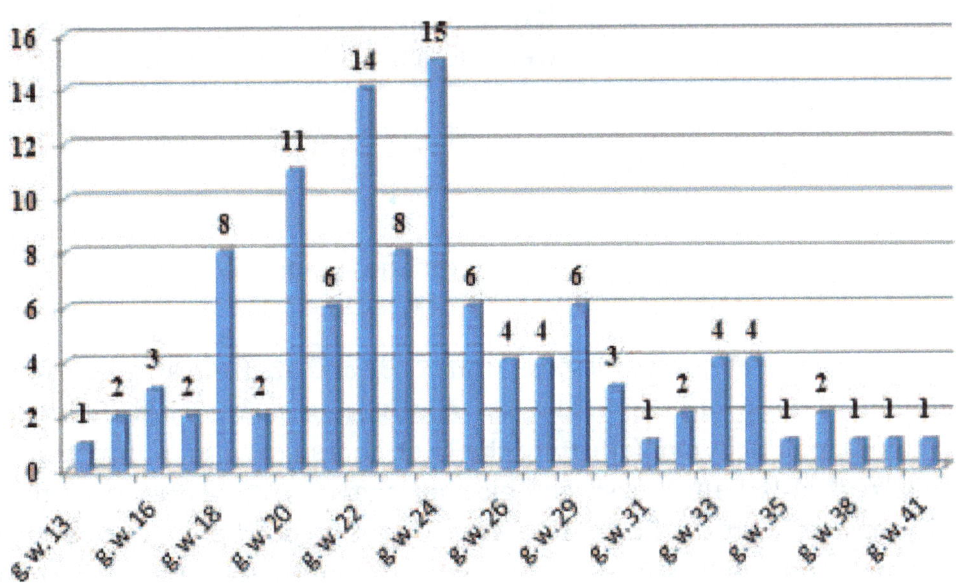

Figure 1. Term of pregnancy termination.

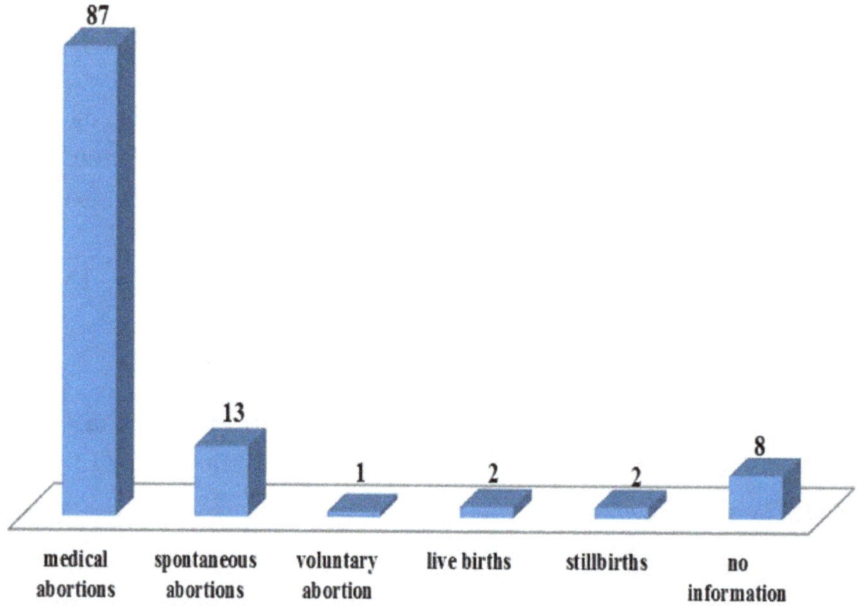

Figure 2. Motives for pregnancy termination.

6. Anthropometric characteristics of the fetuses

Distribution of lethal hydrocephalus by gender (sex ratio). The genders were equally affected, but the mean weight of male fetuses (842.17 ± 115.2) was less than that of female fetuses (892.06 ± 101.1), without the difference being statistically significant ($u = 0.51$, $p > 0.05$).

Age of the fetus. The average pregnancy term in the entire study is 24 ± 0.45 gestational weeks. The fetal expulsion in two-thirds of the cases occurred before the 24th gestational week, with the smallest fetus being 13 gestational weeks (**Figure 1**).

Fetus weight. The average weight of the fetuses is 865.99 ± 809.8 g with a range of 23–3800 g. It is worth noting that 50 fetuses (44.2%) weigh less than the corresponding gestational age.

7. System anomalies of the fetus

The head, extremities, and respiratory system anomalies associated with FHLO are presented in **Table 1**.

The cardiovascular system abnormalities are a total of 32 and are from all groups. The digestive system abnormalities are 56 and are broken down into groups: mesenteric (affecting the small intestine and colon), parenchymal (affecting the liver and spleen), anal imperforation (affecting the terminal part of the intestines), gall bladder agenesis, and situs inversus. The parenchymal and mesenteric abnormalities are evenly distributed. The gender abnormalities are present in both male and female fetuses with a ratio of female to male of 8:7. Hermaphroditism was established in four (3.5%) fetuses. The fatal hydrocephalus-associated anomalies of the cardiovascular, digestive, excretory, and genital systems are presented in **Table 2**.

Association of hydrocephalus with other brain abnormalities. In 85 fetuses (76%), hydrocephalus was associated with other brain abnormalities: polygyria—12 (10.7%); lissencephaly—2 (1.8%); agenesis of corpus callosum—18 (16%); agenesis of the cerebellar vermis—19 (16.9%); diastamatomyelia—1 (0.9%); stenosis of the Sylvian aqueduct—5 (4.4%); holoprosencephaly—1 (0.9%) and cyst of the choroid plexus—2 (1.8%) (**Table 3**, **Figure 4**). The relations between the prenatal and postnatal diagnosis of hydrocephalus-associated brain abnormalities are shown in **Figure 3**.

The hydrocephalus-associated syndromes and malformations are presented in **Table 4**.

Systems	Types of anomalies	Anomalies	N/%
Lips, soft and hard palate	Clefts	Cleft lip	6/5.3
		Cleft palate	3/2.7
		Labia palate cleft	4/3.5
		Uvula cleft palate	1/0.9
	Configurations	High palate	25/22.1
	Total		39/34.5
Anomalies of the nose	Configurations	Snub nose	4/3.5
	Agenesia	Arrhinia	1/0.9
	Atresia	Choanal atresia	1/0.9
	Total		6/5.3
Head and limb abnormalities	Head	Macrocrania	70/61.9
	Limb	Curved foot	23/20.4
	Agenesia	Short limbs	13/11.5
	Clinodactyly	Agenesia of finger	6/5.3
	Polydactyly	Finger clinodactyly	28/24.7
	Syndactyly		6/5.3
	Total		9/7.9
			182/161
Anomalies of the respiratory system	Hypoplasia		21/18.6
	Incorrect lobulation		16/14.2
	Hypoplasia and Incorrect lobulation		6/5.3
	Situs inversus		2/1.8
	Liver agenesis		1/0.9
	Total		46/40.7

Table 1. Hydrocephalus-related abnormalities of the head, extremities, and respiratory system.

Most are neural tube defects followed by trisomies and skeletal dysplasias. The VACTERL association has been established in six fetuses (5.3%), four of which were male and two female, and the Dandy-Walker malformation in four fetuses (3.5%) (**Figure 4**).

The Meckel-Gruber syndrome, which is a ciliopathy, was established six times (5.4%). A karyotype study was performed on 23 fetuses (20.5%)—one by fluorescent in situ hybridization (FISH) and the rest by chromosome study. A magnetic resonance tomography (MRI) was performed in three cases.

Systems	Types of anomalies	Anomalies	N/%
Anomalies of the cardiovascular system	Position	Dextroradia	1/0.9
	Organomegaly	Cardiomegaly	2/1.8
	Defects	Atrial septal defect (ASD)	3/2.7
		Ventricular septal defect (VSD)	11/9.7
		Both together	2/1.8
		Tetralogy of Fallot	2/1.8
		Minor form of AV channel of the heart	2/18
		AV channel of the heart	2/1.8
	Stenoses	Aortic valve stenosis	1/0.9
		Pulmonary valve stenosis	1/0.9
	Transposition	Transposition of the great vessels (TGV)	1/0.9
	Isomerism	Isomerism of incoming vessels of the heart	3/2.7
	Hypoplasia	Hypoplastic right heart syndrome (HRHS)	1/0.9
	Total		32/28.3
Digestive system abnormalities	Mesenterial	Common mesentery	1/0.9
		Hemi-mesenter	22/19.5
	Parenchymal	Hepatomegaly	8/7.1
		Splenomegaly	3/2.7
		Hepato-splenomegaly	5/4.4
		Polysplenia	6/5.3
		Accessory spleen	1/0.9
	Imperforations	Imperforate anus	8/7.1
	Agenesis	Gallbladder Agenesis	1/0.9
	Situs inversus		1/0.9
	Total		56/49.5

Systems	Types of anomalies	Anomalies	N/%
Anomalies of kidney and urinary tract	Kidneys	Ptosis of the kidney	10/8.8
		Horseshoe kidney	4/3.4
		Agenesis (uni- and bilateral)	8/7.1
		Hydrophoresis	5/4.4
		Tubular necrosis	1/0.9
		Dysplasia	2/1.9
		Cystic dysplasia	6/5.3
	Urinary tract	Pelvicalyceal dilatation	4/3.4
		Megaureter	2/1.8
		Mega-bladder	2/1.8
		Hypoplasia of bladder	3/2.7
		Colovesical fistula	1/0.9
		Agenesis of ureter	5/4.4
	Total		53/46.9
Anomalies of the genitals	Female	Bicornuate uterus	5/4.4
		Ovarian hypoplasia Vaginal Atresia	1/0.9
		Hydrocolpos	1/0.9
			2/1.8
	Male	Hypospadias	4/3.4
		Posterior urethral valve	1/0.9
		Cryptorchism	2/1.8
	Hermaphroditism		4/3.4
	Total		19/16.8

Table 2. Hydrocephalus-related abnormalities of cardiovascular, digestive, excretory, and genital systems.

The degree of hydrocephalus according to the fetopathological study is major hydrocephalus (hydrancephaly; >15 mm)—15 cases (13.3%) and ventriculomegaly (>10 mm)—77 cases (69%). Obstructive hydrocephalus as a result of intraventricular hemorrhage was found in 20 fetuses (17.7%) (**Table 5**, **Figure 4**).

The assessment of the significance of spontaneous abortions, abortions due to medical reasons, stillbirth, and a previous child with malformations as risk factors for the occurrence of hydrocephalus was accomplished by means of a χ^2-analysis (**Table 6**).

The proportion of spontaneous abortion is almost four times higher, and the abortion due to medical reasons is more than four times higher, when compared to other risk factors for FHLO. Hydrocephalus is almost three times more likely to develop in cases of previous stillbirths in the obstetric history and more than two times more likely to occur in the presence

Brain associations	Number of cases	%
Polygyria	12	10.6
Lissencephaly	2	1.8
Agenesis of corpus callosum	18	15.9
Agenesis of cerebellar vermis	19	16.8
Cerebellar hypoplasia	25	22.1
Diastematomyelia	1	0.9
Aqueductal stenosis (stenosis of the aqueduct of Sylvius)	5	4.4
Holoprosencephaly	1	0.9
Choroid plexus cysts	2	1.8
Total	85	75.2

Table 3. Distribution of associated brain abnormalities with lethal hydrocephalus.

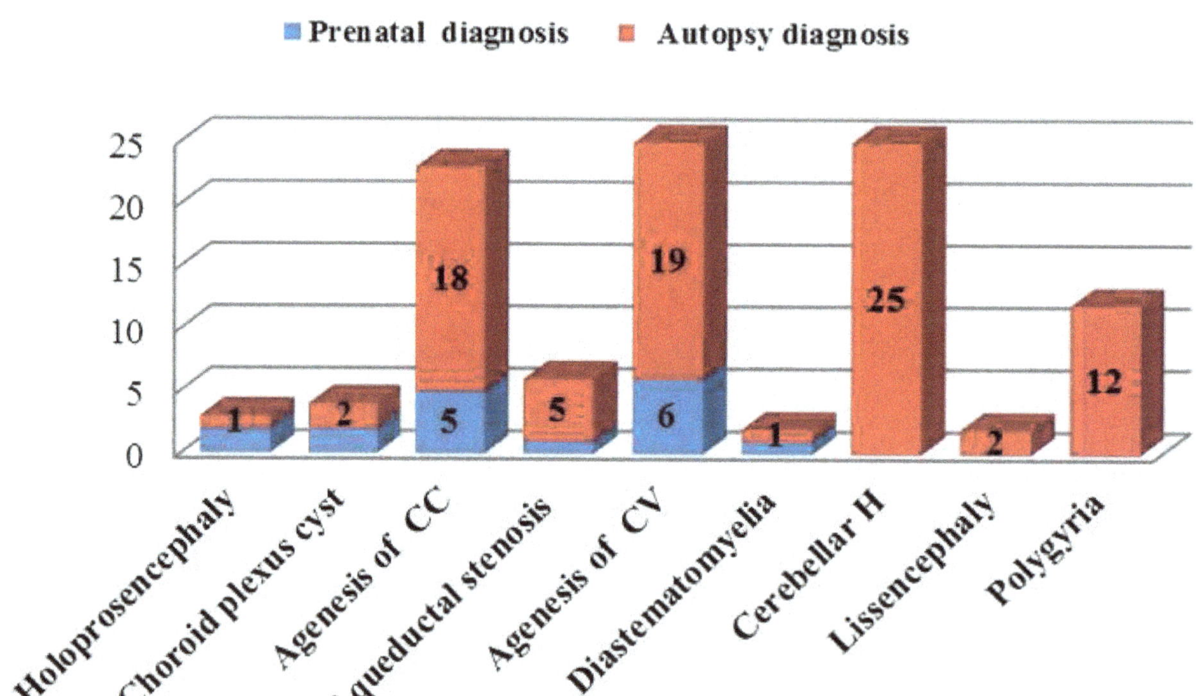

Figure 3. Relations between the prenatal and postnatal diagnosis of hydrocephalus-associated brain abnormalities. Abbreviations: CC, corpus callosum; CV, cerebeller vermis; H, hypoplasia.

of a pre-term birth of a child with a malformation, compared to the studied risk factors. The assessment of the significance of the different degrees of consanguinity in the presence of a child with malformations, epileptic mother, as well as the mother's age is shown in **Table 7**.

The incidence of FHLO is nearly six times higher when it is the result of a consanguineous marriage with a history of a previous pregnancy with a malformation, relative to the presence of hydrocephalus of a non-consanguineous marriage with no such a history. Almost 13 times higher is the incidence of FHLO in cases of maternal epilepsy with a consanguineous marriage of first degree (first cousins), when compared to the proportion of FHLO in a fetus

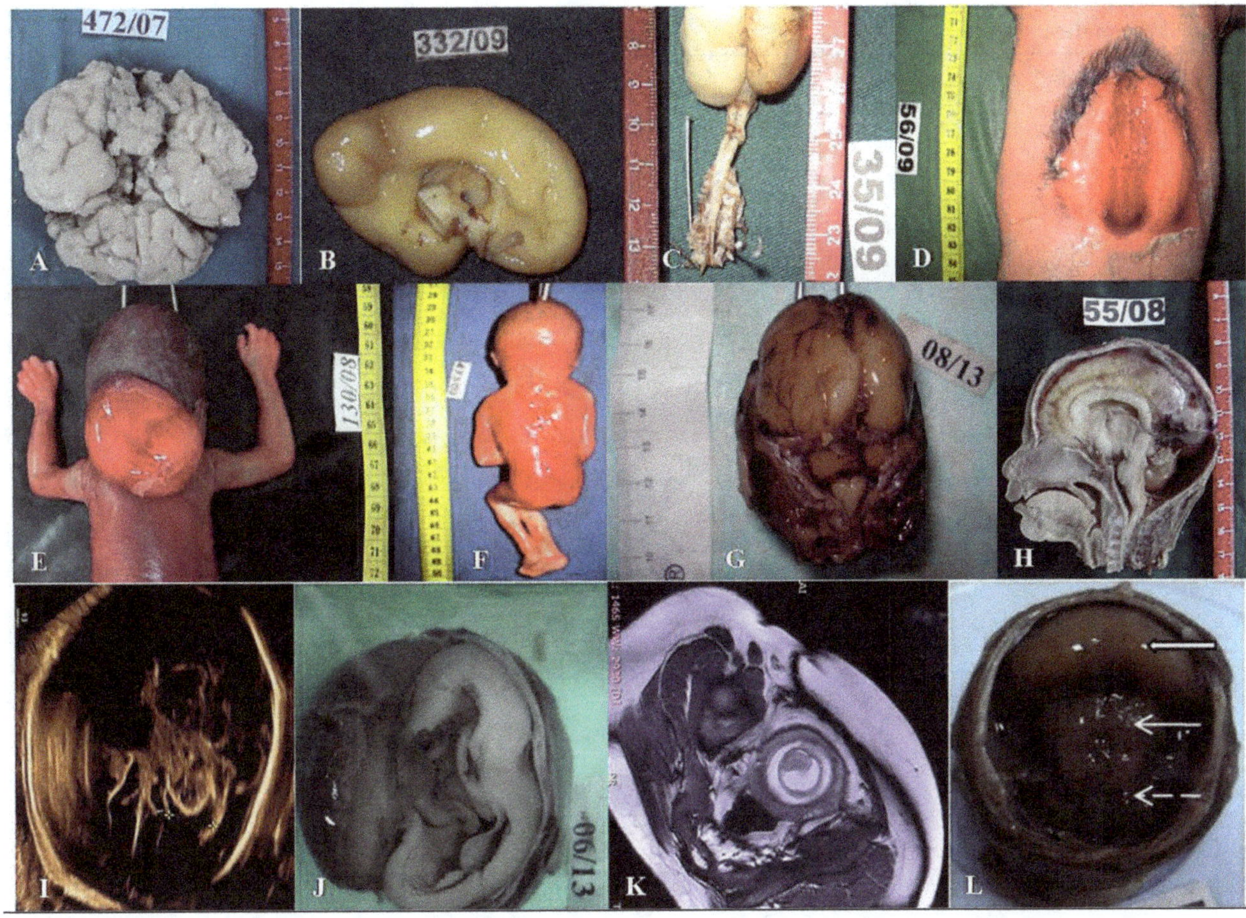

Figure 4. (A) Polygria (inferior view of the brain); (B) Agenesis of corpus callosum (medical view of hemisphere); (C) Extracted brain and spinal cord from the skull and vertebral canal. Split of the cord. Diastematomyelia; (D) Thorac-lumbar spina bifidia; (E) Occipital meningo-encephalocele; (F) Rachischisis; (G) Wedging of the cerebellar tonsils through the foramen magnum. Arnold-Chiari malformation; (H) Cystic dilatation of IVth ventricle, elevating of the tentorium, cerebellar hypoplasia. Dandy-Walker malformation; (I) Ventriculomegaly-ultrasound examination; (J) Ventriculomegaly (horizontal section of the right hemisphere); (K) Holoprosencephaly. Fetal MRI; (L) Holoprosencephaly. Fetal autopsy (White-black arrow—hemisphere, white arrow—brain stem, dotted arrow—cerebellum).

carried by an epileptic mother but not from such a marriage. Over four times higher is the proportion of FHLO in cases of consanguinity of second degree, when compared to hydrocephalus influenced by the other studied maternal risk factors. Almost four times higher is the proportion of FHLO with a maternal age between 27 and 35 years compared to other ages, with maternal risk factors present. The rate of hydrocephalus when the maternal age is over 40 years and with consanguinity of third degree is 13 times greater than women over 40 years of age without the risk factor consanguinity. The assessment of the degree of risk of consanguinity, the presence of spontaneous abortion, and the mother's blood group is presented in **Table 8**.

When the mother is from the A(+) blood group and has a consanguineous marriage (giving second-degree consanguinity in the fetus), FHLO has a two times higher incidence than in cases without consanguinity. Around two times higher is the incidence of FHLO, carried by mothers with O(+) blood group and a history of a previous spontaneous abortion,

Types of anomalies	Anomalies	N/%
Neural tube defects	Spina bifida	10/8.8
	Myelomeningocele	6/5.3
	Encephalocele	6/5.3
	Meningocele	6/5.3
	Rachischisis	5/4.4
	Total	33/29.2
Chromosomal abnormalities	Trisomy 21	4/3.4
	Trisomy 18	18/15.9
	Trisomy 13	2/1.8
	Trisomy 15	1/0.9
	Trisomy 7 + 2	1/0.9
	Triplodia	1/0.9
	Total	27/23.9
Skeletal dysplasias	Ellis-van Creveld syndrome	1/0.9
	Thanatophoric dysplasia	3/2.7
	Osteochondrodysplasia	1/0.9
	Osteogenesis imperfecta	2/1.8
	Arthrogryposis	3/2.7
	Total	10/9.8
VACTERL association		6/5.3
Dandy-Walker malformation		4/3.4
Other syndromes and malformation	DiGeorge syndrome	1/0.9
	Isomerism	3/2.7
	Meckel-Gruber syndrome	6/5.3
	Fraser syndrome	1/0.9
	Fryns syndrome	1/0.9
	Arnold-Chiari malformation	4/3.4
	Total	16/14.2

Table 4. Distribution of syndromes and malformations associated with lethal hydrocephalus.

compared to the occurrence when there is no such history. The degree of significance of the mother's age for the incidence of polygyria and abortions, obstetric and other risk factors, as well as the blood group for the occurrence of agenesis of the cerebellar vermis are shown in **Table 9**.

According to the degree of hydrocephalus	Number of cases	%
Major hydrocephalus (hydranencephaly)	15	13.3%
Ventriculomegaly	78	69.0%
Hydrocephaly due to intraventricular hemorrhage	20	17.7%
Total	113	100.0%

Table 5. Distribution of data on the extent and origin of hydrocephalus.

Indicators	Groups	Without risk factors		Risk factors		Total		χ^2	Fisher	OR
		N	%	N	%	N	%		P	(CI)
Miscarriage	No	78	78	22	22	100	100.0	21.816	0.000	19.500
	There are	2	15.4	11	84.6	13	100.0			(4.020–94.594)
	Total	80	70.8	33	29.2	11	100.0			
Abortion	No	78	81.3	18	18.8	96	100.0	33.727	0.000	32.500
	There are	2	11.8	15	88.2	17	100.0			(6.817–154.954)
	Total	80	70.8	33	29.2	113	100.0			
Stillbirth	No	79	73.1	29	29.6	108	100.0	6.529	0.011	10.897
	There are	1	20	4	80	5	100.0			(1.169–10.564)
	total	80	70.8	33	29.2	113	100.0			
Baby with malformation	No	76	75.4	26	25.5	102	100.0	6.988	0.008	5.385
	There are	4	36.4	7	63.6	11	100.0			(1.385–18.896)
	Total	80	70.8	33	29.2	113	100.0			

Abbreviations: No, number; CI, confidence intervals; OR, odds ratio; χ^2, chi-square; P, sig.

Table 6. Risk factors and lethal hydrocephalus.

The association of FHLO and polygyria is more than three times higher in cases where the mother is over 35 years of age, when compared to cases with a mother's age less than 35 years. More than 2.5 times higher is the incidence of FHLO associated with agenesis of the cerebellar vermis in cases of a mother with a previous abortion, when compared to cases without a previous abortion. In the present study, the incidence of the association FHLO and agenesis of the cerebellar vermis is more than two times higher when exposed to the obstetric risk factors. Almost three times higher is the incidence of the association of FHLO and agenesis of the cerebellum in cases in which the mother's blood group is A(+), when compared to other maternal blood groups. The assessment of the importance of the

Indicators	Groups	No malformation		Baby with malformation		Total		χ^2	Fisher P	OR (CI)
		N	%	N	%	N	%			
Consanguinity	No	74	96.1	3	3.9	77	100.0	9.768	0.002	7.309
	There are	27	77.1	8	22.9	35	100.0			(1.806–29.584)
	Total	101	90.2	11	9.8	112	100.0			
Indicators	**Groups**	**Without epilepsy**		**Epilepsy**		**Total**		χ^2	P	**OR (CI)**
		N	%	N	%	N	%			
Consanguinity first degree	No	77	96.1	3	3.9	77	100.0	25.742	0.000	24.667
	There are	7	50.0	7	50.0	14	100.0			(5.189–117.247)
	Total	84	89.0	10	11.0	94	100.0			
Indicators	**Groups**	**Without risk factors**		**Risk factors**		**Total**		χ^2	P	**OR (CI)**
		N	%	N	%	N	%			
Consanguinity second degree	No	71	93.4	5	6.6	76	100.0	4.014	0.045	75.680 (0.872–36.997)
	There are	5	71.4	2	28.6	7	100.0			
	Total	76	91.6	7	8.4	83	100.0			
Maternal age	Others	81	95.3	4	4.7	85	100.0	4.247	0.039	4.203 (0.977–18.601)
	27–35 years	19	82.6	4	17.4	23	100.0			
	Total	100	92.6	8	7.4	108	100.0			
Indicators	**Groups**	**Under 40 years of age**		**Over 40 years**		**Total**		χ^2	P	**OR (CI)**
		N	%	N	%	N	%			
Consanguinity third degree	No	74	97.4	2	2.6	76	100.0	7.447	0.006	18.500
	There are	2	66.7	1	33.3	3	100.0			(1.146–298.547)
	Total	76	96.2	3	3.8	79	100.0			

Abbreviations: No, number; CI, confidence intervals; OR, odds ratio; χ^2, chi-square; P, sig.

Table 7. Consanguinity, risk factors, and lethal hydrocephalus.

maternal age for the association of hydrocephalus with trisomies, as well as the mother's blood group for the association of hydrocephalus and agenesis of corpus callosum is presented in **Table 10**.

The rate of FTLO associated with trisomy is more than six times higher when the mother's age is over 38 years of age, than in younger than 38-year-old mothers. Almost three times higher is the share of the association of FHLO with agenesis of corpus callosum in the fetus in cases of O(+) maternal blood group.

Indicators.	Groups	Another group		A+		Total		χ^2	P	OR
		N	%	N	%	N	%			(CI)
Consanguinity first degree	No	63	81.8	14	18.2	77	100.0	4.206	0.04	3.375
	First	8	57.1	6	42.9	14	100.0			(1.010–11.279)
	Total	71	78.0	20	22.0	91	100.0			
Indicators	**Groups**	**Another group**		**O+**		**Total**		χ^2	P	**OR**
		N	%	N	%	N	%			(CI)
Miscarriage	No	74	74.0	26	26.0	100		4.315	0.038	3.321
	There are	6	46.2	7	53.8	13				(1.022–10.789)
	Total	80	70.8	33	29.2	113				

Abbreviations: No, number; CI, confidence intervals; OR, odds ratio; χ^2, chi-square; P, sig.

Table 8. Blood groups, risk factors, and lethal hydrocephalus.

Indicators	Groups	Without polygyria		Polygyria		Total		χ^2	P	OR
		N	%	N	%	N	%			(CI)
Maternal age	≤35	82	92.1	7	7.9	89	100.0	4.894	0.027	4.894 (1.094–13.94)
	≥35	15	75.0	5	25.0	20	100.0			
	Total	97	89.1	12	11.0	109	100.0			
Indicators	**Groups**	**Without agenesis of cerebellar vermis**		**Agenesis of cerebellar vermis**		**Total**		χ^2	P	**OR** (CI)
		N	%	N	%	N	%			
Abortion	No	83	86.5	13	13.5	96	100.0	4.886	0.027	3.483
	There are	11	64.7	6	35.3	17	100.0			(1.099–1.040)
	Total	94	83.2	19	16.8	113	100.0			
Obstetric risk factors	No	71	87.7	10	12.3	81	100.0	4.432	0.035	2.905
	There are	22	71.0	9	29.0	31	100.0			(1.048–8.052)
	Total	93	83.0	19	17.0	112	100.0			
Risk factors	No	47	90.4	5	9.6	52	100.0	3.898	0.046	3.463
	There are	19	73.1	7	26.9	26	100.0			(0.977–12.274)
	total	66	84.6	12	15.4	78	100.0			
A+ blood group	No	78	86.7	12	13.3	90	100.0	3.830	0.050	2.844
	There are	16	69.6	7	30.4	23	100.0			(0.969–8.342)
	Total	94	83.2	19	16.8	113	100.0			

Abbreviations: No, number; CI, confidence intervals; OR, odds ratio; χ^2, chi-square; P, sig.

Table 9. Brain abnormalities, risk factors, and lethal hydrocephalus.

Indicators	Groups	Without trisomy		Trisomy		Total		χ^2	P	OR
		N	%	N	%	N	%			(CI)
Maternal age	≤38	88	90.7	9	9.3	97	100.0	20.518	0.000	13.689
	≥38	5	41.7	7	58.3	12	100.0			(3.952–52.122)
	total	93	85.3	16	14.7	109	100.0			

Indicators	Groups	Without agenesis of corpus callosum		Agenesis of corpus callosum		Total		χ^2	P	OR
		N	%	N	%	N	%			(CI)
O+ blood group	No	53	86.9	8	13.1	61	100.0	4.441	0.035	3.614
	There are	11	64.7	6	35.3	17	100.0			(1.044–12.510)
	Total	64	82.1	14	17.9	78	100.0			

Abbreviations: No, number; CI, confidence intervals; OR, odds ratio; χ^2, chi-square; *P*, sig.

Table 10. Risk factors, trisomy, agenesis of corpus callosum, and lethal hydrocephalus.

8. Discussion

Currently, prenatal ultrasound is able to visualize ventriculomegaly. Knowledge of the risk factors associated with CH may increase the success of the prenatal ultrasound study. It has been established that a wide range of factors can cause hydrocephalus in animal experiments including alcohol consumption [7], X-ray [8], infections, food disorders, exposure to chemicals [9] and medications taken during pregnancy [10].

Our study is similar to those of Fernell et al., Stoll et al., and Porto et al. which showed that CH was significantly associated with previous abortions, stillbirth, and birth of a child with a malformation [11–13]. Our findings show that the risk of FHLO is increased in cases of previous spontaneous abortions (odds ratio (OR) = 19.500, confidence interval (CI): 4.020–94.594), stillbirth (OR = 10.897; CI: 1.169–10.564), and births of a child with a malformation (OR = 5.385; CI: 1.385–18.896). Pregnancy complications, such as an increase in the amniotic fluid over 1500 ml (polyhydramnios) or a reduction below 500 ml (oligohydramnios), are also considered as potential risk factors for CH [12, 13].

The role of consanguinity is also known for the occurrence of congenital malformations such as hydrocephalus, postaxial polydactyly of the hands, and defects of the lips and palate [13, 14]. In our study, FHLO is significantly associated with a maternal age over 40 years and third-degree consanguinity of the fetus (OR = 18.500; CI: 1.146–298.547). FHLO, previous pregnancies with malformations, and consanguinity are also significantly associated (OR = 7.309; CI: 1.806–29.584). FHLO with agenesis of the cerebellar vermis is significantly associated with the effect of obstetric risk factors (OR = 2.905; CI: 1.048–8.052).

Almost all studies have documented a slightly higher percentage of male fetuses in cases of CH in live births and stillbirths as well as in fetopathologic autopsies [15–18]. Van Landingham et al. did not find a difference in the genders of the children with hydrocephalus compared to the general population [4].

According to the study of Van Landingham et al. in 2009, the mother's age is not associated with CH, unlike the study by Sipek et al. for the period 1961–2000 in the Czech Republic which found that a mother's age over 37 years was significantly associated with CH [4, 6]. Hydrocephalus is significantly associated with a mother's age above 40 years and third-degree consanguinity, and it is 18 times higher compared to women above 40 years of age without consanguinity (OR = 18.500; CI: 1.146–298.547).

In regard to maternal disease, it is known that mothers suffering from diabetes mellitus have a significantly higher risk for giving birth to a child with congenital malformations, especially cardiovascular and neural tube defects [4, 19, 20].

Hydrocephalus is often divided by genetic specialists into a syndromic and non-syndromic form, depending on the presence of associated malformations [21, 22]. Some authors prefer to differentiate hydrocephalus in which the phenotype is characterized mainly with brain malformations and hydrocephalus which is associated with significant physical anomalies and clinical symptoms [23]. In cases with a specific clinical syndrome or genetic changes, hydrocephalus is best to be defined as hydrocephalus associated with the corresponding syndrome.

Some enzyme mutations result in defective neuron connections with the extracellular matrix, abnormal formation of the limiting glial membrane, and disturbances in the neuronal migration [24, 25]. As a result, characteristic brain malformation develops—loss of cerebral gyrification, abnormal white matter of the hemispheres as well as brainstem anomalies (flat pons, enlarged tectum, and curved medulla oblongata), often associated with an aqueductal stenosis and cerebellar cysts. These findings often cannot be found by the prenatal examination, especially in cases of significant ventriculomegaly, making the MRI study essential [26]. In our study, the risk increases almost five times for the association of FHLO and polygyria when the mother's age is above 35 years (OR = 4.894; CI: 1.094–13.94). The association of FHLO and agenesis of the cerebellar vermis is significantly associated with previous abortions (OR = 3.483; CI: 1.099–1.040) and the effect of risk factors (OR = 3.463; CI: 0.977–12.274). Ventriculomegaly is significantly associated with agenesis of corpus callosum, as well as O(+) blood group of the mother, when compared to other blood groups (OR = 3.614; CI: 1.044–12.510). Hydrocephalus may be associated with other brain malformations such as holoprosencephaly, rhombencephalosynapsis, Aicardi syndrome, agenesis of corpus callosum, and periventricular heterotopia [27–31].

Some cytogenetic malformations are associated with hydrocephalus, including trisomy 13, 18, 21, and triploidy [32]. The trisomies in our study were 27 (24.1%) and their occurrence is significantly associated with a mother's age above 38 years (OR = 13.689; CI: 3.952–52.122).

NTD-associated hydrocephalus has a multifactor genesis. Experiments with animals have found that the intrauterine leak age of cerebrospinal fluid causes the Arnold-Chiari type II malformation, which causes an obstruction of the cerebrospinal fluid flow [33, 34]. Genetic mutations responsible for planar cell polarity such as Fuzzy (FUZ), VANGL1, and CELSR1 add to the development of NTDs [35–37]. Other mutations of genes with a relation to planar cell polarity (CELSR2 and MPDZ) may cause hydrocephalus regardless of the presence of NTDs [38, 39]. The specific pathogenetic mechanism is not completely clear, but it is accepted that a disjunction of the ependymal cilia is present [40]. The neural tube defects in our study were 33 (29.4%), with the most common being spina bifida, followed by myelomeningocele, encephalocele, and meningocele.

9. Conclusion

Congenital hydrocephalus with a lethal outcome is the result of a significant number of risk factors and is often associated with other malformations. Therefore, it is important to perform a prenatal ultrasound study in pregnancies with risk factors to diagnose possible CH or other malformations. Currently, the prenatal ultrasound is able to visualize ventriculomegaly and should be directed toward the search of other associated malformations, and when they are suspected, an MRI study and genetic testing must follow. In cases of medical abortion, stillbirth, or neonatal death, a fetopathological study must be carried out which enriches our knowledge of malformations, complements and completes the ultrasound examination, modifies genetic counseling, and determines the behavior to be followed when taking responsibility for a subsequent pregnancy. It is also important to further study the associated risk factors and the fetopathological changes in CH in order to increase the success of the ultrasound prenatal diagnosis.

Author details

Tanya Kitova[1]*, Borislav Kitov[2], Denis Milkov[4] and Aida Masmoudi[3]

*Address all correspondence to: tanyakitova@yahoo.com

1 Department of Anatomy, Histology and Embryology, Medical University of Plovdiv, Plovdiv, Bulgaria

2 Department of Neurosurgery, Medical University of Plovdiv, Plovdiv, Bulgaria

3 University of Tunis—El Manar, Faculty of Medicine of Tunis, Center of Maternity and Neonatology of Tunis, Tunis, Tunisia

4 Medical Faculty, Medical University of Plovdiv, Plovdiv, Bulgaria

References

[1] Schechtman KB, Gray DL, Baty JD, Rothman SM. Decision-making for termination of pregnancies with fetal anomalies: Analysis of 53 000 pregnancies. Obstetrics and Gynecology. 2002;**99**:216-222. https://doi.org/10.1016/S0029-7844(01)01673-8

[2] Benute GRG, Nomura RMY, Liao AW, et al. Feelings of women regarding end-of-life decision making after ultrasound diagnosis of a lethal fetal malformation. Midwifery. 2012;**28**:472-475. DOI: 10.1016/j.midw.2011.06.011

[3] Jeng S, Gupta N, Wrensch M, et al. Prevalence of congenital hydrocephalus in California, 1991-2000. Pediatric Neurology. 2011;**45**;67-71. DOI: 10.1016/j.pediatrneurol.2011.03.009

[4] Van Landingham M, Nguyen TV, Roberts A, et al. Risk factors of congenital hydrocephalus: A 10 year retrospective study. Journal of Neurology, Neurosurgery, and Psychiatry. 2009; **80**:213-217. DOI: 10.1136/jnnp.2008.148932

[5] Weller S, Gartner J. Genetic and clinical aspects of X-linked hydrocephalus (L1disease): Mutations in the L1CAM gene. Human Mutation. 2001;**18**:1-12. DOI: 10.1002/humu.1144

[6] Sípek A, Gregor V, Horácek J, Masátová D. Congenital hydrocephalus 1961-2000. Incidence, prenatal diagnosis and prevalence based on maternal age. Ceská Gynekologie. 2002;**67**:360-364

[7] Bearer CF. L1 cell adhesion molecule signal cascades: Targets for ethanol developmental neurotoxicity. Neurotoxicology. 2001;**22**:625-633. https://doi.org/10.1016/S0161-813X(01)00034-1

[8] Aolad HM, Inouye M, Hayasaka S, et al. Congenital hydrocephalus caused by exposure to low level X-radiation at early gestational stage in mice. Biological Sciences in Space. 1998;**12**:256-257

[9] Adeloye A, Warkany J. Experimental congenital hydrocephalus. A review withspecial consideration of hydrocephalus produced by zinc deficiency. Child's Brain. 1976;**2**:325-360. DOI: 10.1159/000119630

[10] Kazy Z, Puho E, Czeizel AE. Teratogenic potential of vaginal metronidazole treatment during pregnancy. European Journal of Obstetrics & Gynecology and Reproductive Biology. 2005;**123**:174-178. DOI: 10.1016/j.ejogrb.2005.03.016

[11] Fernell E, Hagberg C, von Wendt L.Epidemiology of infantile hydrocephalus in Sweden II. Origin in infants born at term.Acta paediatrica Scandinavica 1987;**76**:411-417. DOI: 10.11 11/j.1651-2227.1987.tb10491.x

[12] Stoll C, Alembik Y, Dott B, Roth MP. Epidemiologic study of environmental and genetic factors in congenital hydrocephalus. European Journal of Epidemiology. 1992;**8**(6): 797-803. Available from: http://www.jstor.org/stable/3520830

[13] Porto R, Reis FP, Oliveira C, et al. Prevalence and factors associated at presence of central nervous system congenital malformations. British Journal of Medicine & Medical Research. 2015;**6**(10):956-964. DOI: 10.9734/BJMMR/2015/14642

[14] Rittler M, Liascovich R, López Camalo J, Castilla J. Parental consanguinity in specifics types of congenital anomalies. American Journal of Medical Genetics. 2001;**102**:36-43. DOI: 10.1002/1096-8628(20010722)102:1<36::AID-AJMG1394>3.0.CO;2-M

[15] Fernell E, Hagberg B, Hagberg G, von Wendt L. Epidemiology of infantile hydrocephalus in Sweden. III. Origin in preterm infants. Acta Paediatrica Scandinavica. 1987;**76**:418-423. DOI: 10.1111/j.1651-2227.1987.tb10492.x

[16] Kitova T, Kitov B, Milkov D, Cheih N, Gaigi S. Fetal hydrocephalus. Pteridines. 2014;**25**(3-4): 65-68. DOI: 10.1515/pterid-2014-0007

[17] Munch TN, Rostgaard K, Rasmussen M-L H, et al. Familial aggregation of congenital hydrocephalusin a nation wide cohort. Brain. 2012:**135**;2409-2415. DOI: 10.1093/brain/aws158. Epub 2012 Jul 4

[18] Garne E, Loane M, Addor MC, et al. Congenital hydrocephalus – Prevalence, prenatal diagnosis and outcome of pregnancy in four European regions. European Journal of Paediatric Neurology. 2010;**14**:150-155. DOI: 10.1016/j.ejpn.2009.03.005 Epub May 2, 2009

[19] Yang J, Cummings EA, O'Connell C, et al. Fetal and neonatal outcomes of diabetic pregnancies. Obstetrics and Gynecology. 2006;**108**:644-650. DOI: 10.1097/01.AOG.0000231688.08263.47

[20] Macintosh MC, Fleming KM, Bailey JA, et al. Perinatal mortality and congenital anomalies in babies of women with type 1 or type 2 diabetes in England, Wales, and Northern Ireland: Population based study. British Medical Journal. 2006;**333**(177):1-6. DOI: 10.1136/bmj.38856.692986.AE

[21] Verhagen JM, Schrander-Stumpel CT, Krapels IP, et al. Congenital hydrocephalus in clinical practice: A genetic diagnostic approach. European Journal of Medical Genetics. 2011;**54**:e542-e547. DOI: 10.1016/j.ejmg.2011.06.005 Epub 2011 Jul 30

[22] Snijders RJM, Nicolaides KH. Fetal biometry at 14-40 weeks'gestation. Ultrasound in Obstetrics & Gynecology. 1994;**4**:34-48. DOI: 10.1046/j.1469-0705.1994.04010034.x

[23] Tully HM, DobynsWB. Infantile hydrocephalus: A review of epidemiology, classification and causes. European Journal of Medical Genetics. August 2014;**57**(8):359-368. DOI: 10.1016/j.ejmg.2014.06.002. Epub Jun 13, 2014

[24] Dobyns WB, Pagon RA, Armstrong D, et al. Diagnostic criteria for Walker-Warburg syndrome. American Journal of Medical Genetics. 1989;**32**(2):195-210. DOI: 10.1002/ajmg.1320320213

[25] Miller G, Ladda RL, Towfighi J. Cerebro-ocular dysplasia-muscular dystrophy (Walker Warburg) syndrome. Findings in 20-week-old fetus. Acta Neuropathologica. 1991;**82**(3): 234-238. DOI: 10.1007/BF00294451

[26] Longman C, Mercuri E, Cowan F, et al. Antenatal and postnatal brain magnetic resonance imaging in muscle-eye- brain disease. Archives of Neurology. 2004;**61**(8):1301-1306. DOI: 10.1001/archneur.61.8.1301

[27] Plawner LL, Delgado MR,Miller VS, et al. Neuroanatomy of holoprosencephaly as predictor of function Beyond the face predicting the brain.Neurology 2002; **59**(7):1058-1066. DOI: http://dx.doi.org/10.1212/WNL.59.7.1058

[28] Ishak GE, Dempsey JC, Shaw DWW, et al. Rhombencephalosynapsis: A hindbrain malformation associated with incomplete separation of midbrain and forebrain, hydrocephalus and a broad spectrum of severity. Brain. 2012;**135**(Pt 5):1370-1386. DOI: 10.1093/brain/aws065 Epub Mar 26, 2012

[29] Spennato P, La Porta A, Varone A, et al. Aicardi and Turner syndrome in a 45,X0/46,XX female. Clinical Neurology and Neurosurgery 2013;**115**(6):820-822. DOI: 10.1016/j.clineuro.2012.07.030. Epub 2012 Aug 13.

[30] Paul LK, Brown WS, Adolphs R, et al. Agenesis of the corpus callosum: Genetic, developmental and functional aspects of connectivity. Nature Reviews. Neuroscience. 2007;**8**(4):287-299. DOI: 10.1038/NRN2107

[31] Kato M, Das S, Petras K, et al. Mutations of ARX are associated with striking pleiotropy and consistent genotype-phenotype correlation. Human Mutation 2004; **23**(2):147-159. DOI:10.1002/humu.10310

[32] Schrander Stumpel C, Fryns JP. Congenital hydrocephalus: Nosology and guidelines for clinical approach and genetic counselling. European Journal of Pediatrics. 1998;**157**(5):355-362. https://DOI.org/10.1007/s00431005083

[33] McLone DG, Knepper PA. The cause of Chiari II malformation: A unified theory: A unified theory. Pediatric Neuroscience. 1989;**15**(1):1-12. DOI: 10.1159/000120432

[34] Sweeney KJ et al. Spinal level of myelomeningocele lesion as a contributing factor in posterior fossa volume, intracranial cerebellar volume, and cerebellar ectopia. Journal of Neurosurgery. Pediatrics. 2013;**11**(2):154-159. http://thejns.org/doi/abs/10.3171/2012.10.PEDS12177

[35] Seo JH, ZilberY, Babayeva S, et al. Mutations in the planar cell polarity gene, fuzzy, are associated with neural tube defects in humans. Human Molecular Genetics 2011; **20**(22):4324-4333. DOI: 10.1093/hmg/ddr359. Epub Aug 12, 2011.

[36] Bartsch O, Kirmes I, Thiede A, et al. Novel VANGL1 gene mutations in 144 Slovakian, Romanian and German patients with neural tube defects. Molecular Syndromology. 2012;**3**(2):76-81. DOI: 10.1159/000339668 Epub Jul 5, 2012

[37] Allacher R, De Marco P, Merello E, et al. Role of the planar cell polarity gene CELSR1 in neural tube defects and caudal agenesis. Birth Defects Research. Part A, Clinical and Molecular Teratology. 2012;**94**(3):176-181. DOI: 10.1002/bdra.23002 Epub Feb 28, 2012

[38] Tissir F, Qu Y, Montcouquiol M, et al. Lack of cadherins Celsr2 and Celsr3 impairs ependymal ciliogenesis, leading to fatal hydrocephalus. Nature Neuroscience. 2010;**13**(6):700-707. DOI: 10.1038/nn.2555 Epub May 16, 2010

[39] Al-Dosari MS, Mohammed Al-Owain M, Tulbah M, et al. Mutation in MPDZ causes severe congenital hydrocephalus. Journal of Medical Genetics. 2013;**50**(1):54-58. DOI: 10.1136/jmedgenet-2012-101294

[40] Sotak BN, Gleeson JG. Can't get there from here: Cilia and hydrocephalus. Nature Medicine. 2012;**18**(12):1742-1743. DOI: 10.1038/nm.3011

Permissions

All chapters in this book were first published in CAFTETN, by InTech Open; hereby published with permission under the Creative Commons Attribution License or equivalent. Every chapter published in this book has been scrutinized by our experts. Their significance has been extensively debated. The topics covered herein carry significant findings which will fuel the growth of the discipline. They may even be implemented as practical applications or may be referred to as a beginning point for another development.

The contributors of this book come from diverse backgrounds, making this book a truly international effort. This book will bring forth new frontiers with its revolutionizing research information and detailed analysis of the nascent developments around the world.

We would like to thank all the contributing authors for lending their expertise to make the book truly unique. They have played a crucial role in the development of this book. Without their invaluable contributions this book wouldn't have been possible. They have made vital efforts to compile up to date information on the varied aspects of this subject to make this book a valuable addition to the collection of many professionals and students.

This book was conceptualized with the vision of imparting up-to-date information and advanced data in this field. To ensure the same, a matchless editorial board was set up. Every individual on the board went through rigorous rounds of assessment to prove their worth. After which they invested a large part of their time researching and compiling the most relevant data for our readers.

The editorial board has been involved in producing this book since its inception. They have spent rigorous hours researching and exploring the diverse topics which have resulted in the successful publishing of this book. They have passed on their knowledge of decades through this book. To expedite this challenging task, the publisher supported the team at every step. A small team of assistant editors was also appointed to further simplify the editing procedure and attain best results for the readers.

Apart from the editorial board, the designing team has also invested a significant amount of their time in understanding the subject and creating the most relevant covers. They scrutinized every image to scout for the most suitable representation of the subject and create an appropriate cover for the book.

The publishing team has been an ardent support to the editorial, designing and production team. Their endless efforts to recruit the best for this project, has resulted in the accomplishment of this book. They are a veteran in the field of academics and their pool of knowledge is as vast as their experience in printing. Their expertise and guidance has proved useful at every step. Their uncompromising quality standards have made this book an exceptional effort. Their encouragement from time to time has been an inspiration for everyone.

The publisher and the editorial board hope that this book will prove to be a valuable piece of knowledge for researchers, students, practitioners and scholars across the globe.

List of Contributors

Amal Zubani, Irfan Asra and Amjad Kouatli
King Faisal Specialist Hospital and Research Center 'Gen.-Org.', Jeddah, Saudi Arabia

Ples Liana
UMF Carol Davila, Bucharest, Romania

Anca Lesnic
Bucur Maternity, Bucharest, Romania

Sidonia Maria Sandulescu
University of Medicine and Pharmacy, Craiova, Romania

Vaduva Cristian
University of Medicine and Pharmacy, Craiova, Romania
County Clinical Emergency Hospital of Craiova, Craiova, Romania

Ramona Mircea Vicol and Adela Serban
University of Medicine and Pharmacy, Bucharest, Romania
INSMC Alessandrescu-Rusescu, Bucharest, Romania

Andreea Veliscu Carp
University of Medicine and Pharmacy, Bucharest, Romania
Clinical Hospital of Obstetrics and Gynecology Panait Sarbu, Bucharest, Romania

Adrian Claudiu Ratiu
University of Medicine and Pharmacy "Victor Babes", Timisoara, Romania

Mihaela Amelia Dobrescu, Florin Burada, Mihai Gabriel Cucu, Anca Lelia Riza, Gratiela Chelu, Razvan Mihail Plesea, Adela Cucu, Alina Liliana Cimpoeru and Mihai Ioana
Medical Genetics Regional Center (CRGM), Dolj, Human Genomics Laboratory, University of Medicine and Pharmacy of Craiova, Craiova, Romania

Dominic Gabriel Iliescu, Ştefania Tudorache, Ciprian Laurentiu Patru, Roxana Cristina Drăguşin and Maria Sorop-Florea
Department of Obstetrics and Gynaecology, University of Medicine and Pharmacy, Craiova, Romania

Dragos Nemescu
Department of Obstetrics and Gynaecology, University of Medicine and Pharmacy, "Gr.T.Popa", Iasi, Romania

Monica Mihaela Cirstoiu, Iuliana Ceausu and Mona Elena Zvanca
Department of Obstetrics-Gynecology, University of Medicine and Pharmacy, Bucharest, Romania

Simona Vlădăreanu
Department of Neonatology, University of Medicine and Pharmacy, "Carol Davila", Bucharest, Romania

Claudiu Marginean
Department of Obstetrics and Gynaecology, University of Medicine and Pharmacy, Targu-Mures, Romania

Daniel Muresan
Department of Obstetrics and Gynaecology, University of Medicine and Pharmacy, "Iuliu Hatieganu", Cluj-Napoca, Romania

Marius Calomfirescu Vicea
Secretary, Romanian Society of Ultrasound in Obstetrics and Gynecology, Bucharest, Romania

Cezara Muresan
Department of Obstetrics and Gynaecology, University of Medicine and Pharmacy, "Victor Babes", Timisoara, Romania

Laura Monica Cara
Department of Public Health, University of Medicine and Pharmacy, Craiova, Romania

Andreea Ceausescu, Andreea Docea and Marina Dinu
Department of Obstetrics and Gynecology, Emergency University Hospital, Craiova, Romania

Stefan Degeratu
Department of Obstetrics and Gynecology, University Hospital, Craiova, Romania

Dominic Iliescu
Prenatal Diagnostic Unit, University of Medicine and Pharmacy of Craiova, Craiova, Romania

Monica Cara
Department of Public Health, University of Medicine and Pharmacy, Craiova, Romania

Shiori Nakano, Haruyuki Makishima and Shigehito Yamada
Congenital Anomaly Research Center, Kyoto University Graduate School of Medicine, Japan

Tanya Kitova
Department of Anatomy, Histology and Embryology, Medical University of Plovdiv, Plovdiv, Bulgaria

Borislav Kitov
Department of Neurosurgery, Medical University of Plovdiv, Plovdiv, Bulgaria

Aida Masmoudi
University of Tunis—El Manar, Faculty of Medicine of Tunis, Center of Maternity and Neonatology of Tunis, Tunis, Tunisia

Denis Milkov
Medical Faculty, Medical University of Plovdiv, Plovdiv, Bulgaria

Index

www.ingramcontent.com/pod-product-compliance
Lightning Source LLC
LaVergne TN
LVHW060601210926
848485LV00005B/1353